W9-DFQ-893

Instructor's Manual and Resource Guide for

PHARMACOLOGY FOR NURSES

A Pathophysiologic Approach

Third Edition

MICHAEL PATRICK ADAMS, PhD

LELAND NORMAN HOLLAND, JR., PhD

Contributors

Barbara Maxwell, MSN, MS, BSN, RN, LNC
Associate Professor of Nursing SUNY Ulster
Stone Ridge, NY

Rosemary Bakasa, PhD, RN
Nursing Faculty
B&S College Eastlake Campus
Eastlake, OH

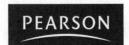

PEARSON

Boston   Columbus   Indianapolis   New York   San Francisco   Upper Saddle River
Amsterdam   Cape Town   Dubai   London   Madrid   Milan   Munich   Paris   Montreal   Toronto
Delhi   Mexico City   Sao Paulo   Sydney   Hong Kong   Seoul   Singapore   Taipei   Tokyo

Notice: Care has been taken to confirm the accuracy of information presented in this book. The authors, editors, and the publisher, however, cannot accept any responsibility for errors or omissions or for consequences from application of the information in this book and make no warranty, express or implied, with respect to its contents.

The authors and publisher have exerted every effort to ensure that drug selections and dosages set forth in this text are in accord with current recommendations and practice at time of publication. However, in view of ongoing research, changes in government regulations, and the constant flow of information relating to drug therapy and reactions, the reader is urged to check the package inserts of all drugs for any change in indications or dosage and for added warning and precautions. This is particularly important when the recommended agent is a new and/or infrequently employed drug.

Publisher: Julie Levin Alexander
Assistant to Publisher: Regina Bruno
Editor-in-Chief: Maura Connor
Assistant to the Editor-in-Chief: Deirdre MacKnight
Executive Acquisitions Editor: Kelly Trakalo
Assistant to the Executive Acquisitions Editor: Lauren Sweeney
Director of Marketing: David Gesell
Marketing Coordinator: Michael Sirinides
Managing Editor, Production: Patrick Walsh
Production Editor: Kim Schmidt, S4Carlisle Publishing Services
Production Liaison: Anne Garcia
Media Project Manager: Rachel Collett
Manufacturing Manager: Ilene Sanford
Senior Design Coordinator: Christopher Weigand
Cover Design: Christine Cantera
Composition: S4Carlisle Publishing Services
Printer/Binder: OPM
Cover Printer: OPM

This work is protected by United States copyright laws and is provided solely for the use of instructors in teaching their courses and assessing student learning. Dissemination or sale of any part of this work (including on the World Wide Web) will destroy the integrity of the work and is not permitted. The work and materials from it should never be made available to students except by instructors using the accompanying text in their classes. All recipients of this work are expected to abide by these restrictions and to honor the intended pedagogical purposes and the needs of other instructors who rely on these materials. Anywhere. All rights reserved.

Copyright © 2011, 2008, 2005 by Pearson Education, Inc., Upper Saddle River, New Jersey 07458. All rights reserved. Printed in the United States of America. This publication is protected by Copyright and permission should be obtained from the publisher prior to any prohibited reproduction, storage in a retrieval system, or transmission in any form or by any means, electronic, mechanical, photocopying, recording, or likewise. For information regarding permission(s), write to: Rights and Permissions Department.

Pearson® is a registered trademark of Pearson plc

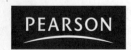

www.pearsonhighered.com

10 9 8 7 6 5 4 3 2 1
ISBN-13: 978-0-13-509130-2
ISBN-10:   0-13-509130-6

CONTENTS

PREFACE

Nurses today must be able to grow and evolve to meet the demands of a dramatically changing health care system. *Pharmacology for Nurses, 3E* addresses the many concepts of contemporary professional nursing that students will need to learn and embrace to be effective members of the collaborative health care team. This Instructor's Manual and Resource Guide is designed to support your teaching in this stepped-up environment and to reduce your preparation for class. It will help you provide an optimal learning experience for your students and their many learning needs.

Each chapter in the Instructor's Manual and Resource Guide is thoroughly integrated with the corresponding chapter in *Pharmacology for Nurses, 3E*. Chapters are organized by learning outcomes, and the teaching unit flows from these outcomes. You will find the following features to support the outcomes.

- **Concepts for Lecture.** This outline of the key concepts presented in each chapter may be used in its entirety or in conjunction with the classroom activities for a mixture of teaching styles that will meet the needs of students with various learning styles.

- **PowerPoint Slides.** The PowerPoint slides contain lecture outlines, integrated images, videos and animations, Connection Checkpoint questions, and classroom response system questions.

- **Suggestions for Classroom and Clinical Activities.** Ideas from educators to address learning styles and make the learning process more interesting.

- **Guide to Resources.** In the margin you will also find a listing of additional resources that pertain to each learning outcome. These include figures, tables, and boxes from the textbook, additional references and websites, animations and videos available from the image library, and more!

- **General Chapter Considerations.** At the end of each chapter is a list of additional resources for you and your students. These include the student workbook, MyNursingKit, Pearson eText, MyNursingLab, and other separate resources. Have your students take advantage of all these resources to help them succeed in the classroom!

This Instructor's Manual and Resource Guide also contains a Strategies for Success module that includes discussion on learning theories, planning for instruction, how to use effective pedagogies, assessing learning, and more.

There is also a guide on *Teaching Students Who Speak English as a Non-native Language*. This tool is intended to guide you in reaching across cultural barriers to train nurses.

The following additional resources are also available to accompany this textbook. For more information or sample copies, please contact your Pearson sales representative or visit *www.mypearsonstore.com*:

- **MyNursingKit (*www.mynursingkit.com*)** This student and instructor resource gives you everything you need in one place! Students can use this site as an online study guide and source for additional resources. Instructors can find chapter-specific PowerPoint lecture notes, test item questions, and instructor manual materials.

- **Student Workbook and Resource Guide.** This workbook incorporates strategies for students to focus their study and increase comprehension of concepts of nursing care. It contains a variety of activities such as multiple-choice, fill-in-the-blank, case studies, and more.

- **Instructor's Resource Kit.** This cross-platform CD-ROM provides lecture note PowerPoint slides; image library PowerPoint Slides; classroom response questions in PowerPoint; test item questions in TestGen, word, and PAR test; and a video and animation library. This supplement is available to faculty upon adoption of the textbook.

- **Online Course Management Systems.** Instructor and student resources are available within our Course Compass platform. For more information on Course Compass and other course management systems such as Blackboard or WebCT, please contact your Pearson sales representative or visit *www.mypearsonstore.com*.

- **MyNursingLab.** A valuable tool for formative assessment and customized student remediation. This online tool gives students the opportunity to test themselves on key concepts and skills in pharmacology. By using MyNursingLab, students can track their own progress through the course and use customized, media-rich study plan activities to help achieve success in the classroom, in clinical, and ultimately on the NCLEX-RN®. MyNursingLab allows instructors to monitor class progress as student's move through the curriculum.

TEACHING NURSING TO STUDENTS WHO SPEAK ENGLISH AS A NON-NATIVE LANGUAGE

We are fortunate to have so many multinational and multilingual nursing students in the United States in the 21st century. As our classrooms become more diverse, there are additional challenges to communication, but we in the nursing education community are ready. Our goal is to educate competent and caring nurses to serve the health needs of our diverse communities.

We know that ENNL students experience higher attrition rates than their native English-speaking counterparts. This is a complex problem. However, there are teaching strategies that have helped many students be successful.

The first step toward developing success strategies is understanding language proficiency. Language proficiency has four interdependent components. Each component is pertinent to nursing education. **Reading** is the first aspect of language. Any nursing student will tell you that there are volumes to read in nursing education. Even native speakers of English find the reading load heavy. People tend to read more slowly in their non-native language. They also tend to recall less. Non-native speakers often spend inordinate amounts of time on reading assignments. These students also tend to take longer to process exam questions.

Listening is the second component of language. Learning from lectures can be challenging. Some students are more proficient at reading English than at listening to it. It is not uncommon for ENNL students to understand medical terminology, but to become confused by social references, slang, or idiomatic expressions used in class. The spoken language of the teacher may be different in accent or even vocabulary from that experienced by immigrant students in their language education. ENNL students may not even hear certain sounds that are not present in their native languages. *Amoxicillin* and *Ampicillin*, for example, may sound the same. Asian languages do not have gender-specific personal pronouns (he, she, him, her, etc.). Asian students may become confused when the teacher is describing a case study involving people of different genders.

Speaking is the third component of language proficiency. People who speak with an accent are often self-conscious about it. They may hesitate to voice their questions or to engage in discussion. Vicious cycles of self-defeating behavior can occur in which a student hesitates to speak, resulting in decreased speaking skills, which results in more hesitation to speak. Students may develop sufficient anxiety about speaking that their academic outcomes are affected. Students tend to form study groups with others who have common first languages. Opportunities to practice English are therefore reduced, and communication errors are perpetuated. When the teacher divides students into small groups for projects, ENNL students often do not participate as much as others. If these students are anxious about speaking, they may withdraw from classroom participation. ENNL students may feel rejected by other students in a small group situation when their input is not sought or understood.

The fourth aspect of language is **writing**. Spelling and syntax errors are common when writing a non-native language. Teachers often respond to student writing assignments with feedback that is too vague to provide a basis for correction or improvement by ENNL students. When it comes to writing lecture notes, these students are at risk of missing important details because they may not pick up the teacher's cues about what is important. They might miss information when they spend extra time translating a word or concept to understand it, or they might just take more time to write what is being said.

Another major issue faced by ENNL nursing students is the culture of the learning environment. International students were often educated in settings where students took a passive role in the classroom. They may have learned that faculty are to be respected, not questioned. Memorization of facts may have been emphasized. It may be a shock to them when the nursing faculty expect assertive students who ask questions and think critically. These expectations cannot be achieved unless students understand them.

Finally, the European American culture, which forms the context for nursing practice, creates challenges. Because they are immersed in Euro-American culture and the culture of nursing, faculty may not see the potential sources of misunderstanding. For example, if a teacher writes a test question about what foods are allowed on a soft diet, a student who understands therapeutic diets may miss the question if he or she does not recognize the names of the food choices. Nursing issues with especially high culture connection are: food, behavior, law, ethics, parenting, games, or choosing the right thing to say. These topics are well represented in psychiatric nursing, which makes it a difficult subject for ENNL students.

MINIMIZING CULTURE BIAS ON NURSING EXAMS

Our goal is not really to eliminate culture from nursing or from nursing education. Nursing exists in a culture-dependent context. Our goal is to practice transcultural nursing and to teach nursing without undue culture bias.

Sometimes our nursing exam questions will relate to culture-based expectations for nursing action. The way to make these questions fair is to teach transcultural nursing and to clarify the cultural expectations of a nursing student in the Euro-American-dominated health care system. Students must learn the cultural aspects of the profession before they can practice appropriately within it. Like other cultures, the professional culture of nursing has its own language (medical terminology and nursing diagnoses, of course). We have our own accepted way of dress, our own implements, skills, taboos, celebrations, and behavior. The values accepted by our culture are delineated in the ANA Code of Ethics, and are passed down to our young during nursing education.

It is usually clear to nursing educators that students are not initially aware of all the aspects of the professional culture, and that these must be taught. The social context of nursing seems more obvious to educators, and is often overlooked in nursing education. Some aspects of the social context of nursing were mentioned previously (food, games, social activities, relationships, behavior, what to say in certain situations). Students must also learn these social behaviors and attitudes if they are to function fully in nursing. If they do not already know about American hospital foods, what to say when someone dies, how to communicate with an authority figure, or what game to play with a 5-year-old child, they must learn these things in nursing school.

Try for yourself the following test. It was written without teaching you the cultural expectations first.

CULTURE BIASED TEST

1. Following radiation therapy, an African American client has been told to avoid using her usual hair-care product due to its petroleum content. Which product should the nurse recommend that she use instead?
   a. Royal Crown hair treatment
   b. Dax Wave and Curl
   c. Long Aid Curl Activator Gel
   d. Wave Pomade

2. A Jewish client is hospitalized for pregnancy-induced hypertension during Yom Kippur. How should the nurse help this client meet her religious needs based on the tradition of this holy day?
   a. Order meals without meat/milk combinations.
   b. Ask a family member to bring a serving of *Marror* for the client.
   c. Encourage her to fast from sunrise to sunset.
   d. Remind her that she is exempt from fasting.

3. Based on the Puerto Rican concept of *compadrazco*, who is considered part of the immediate family and responsible for care of children?
   a. Parents, grandparents, aunts, uncles, cousins, and godparents
   b. Mother and father, older siblings
   c. Mother, father, any blood relative
   d. Parents and chosen friends (*compadres*) who are given the honor of childcare responsibility

4. A 60-year-old Vietnamese immigrant client on a general diet is awake at 11 p.m. on a summer night. What is the best choice of food for the nurse to offer to this client?
   a. warm milk
   b. hot tea
   c. ice cream
   d. iced tea

5. Which of the following positions is contraindicated for a client recovering from a total hip replacement?
   a. side-lying using an abductor pillow
   b. standing
   c. walking to the restroom using a walker
   d. sitting in a low recliner

When you took this test, did it seem unfair? It was intended to test nursing behaviors that were based on culture-specific situations. Your immigrant and ENNL students are likely to face questions like these on every exam.

Item 1 is about hair-care products for black hair. Option C is the only one that does not contain petroleum products. Students could know this, if they were given the information before the exam. Otherwise the item is culture-biased.

Item 2 is about the Jewish holiday Yom Kippur. To celebrate this holiday, it is customary to fast from sunrise to sunset, but people who are sick, such as the client in the question, are exempted from fasting. This question is only unfair if students did not have access to the information.

Item 3 expects you to know about *compadrazco*, in which parents, grandparents, aunts, uncles, cousins, and godparents are all considered immediate family. This can be an important point if you are responsible for visiting policies in a pediatrics unit.

Item 4 tests knowledge about the preferred drink for an immigrant Vietnamese client. Many people in Asia feel comforted by hot drinks and find cold drinks to be unsettling.

Item 5 does not seem so biased. If you understand total hip precautions, it is a pretty simple question, unless you have never heard of a "low recliner." An ENNL student who missed this question said, "I saw the chairs in clinical called 'geri chairs' and I know that the client cannot bend more than 90 degrees, but 'low recliner' was confusing to me. I imagined someone lying down (reclining) and I think this would not dislocate the prosthesis."

The best way to avoid culture bias on exams is to know what you are testing. It is acceptable to test about hip precautions, but not really fair to test about the names of furniture. The same is true of foods. Test about therapeutic diets, but not about the recipes (an African immigrant student advised us to say "egg-based food" instead of custard).

Behavior in social and professional situations is especially culture-bound. Behavior-based questions are common on nursing exams. Make behavior expectations explicit. Especially when a student is expected to act in a way that would be inappropriate in his or her social culture, these are very difficult questions. For example, we expect nurses to act assertively with physicians and clients. It is inappropriate for many Asian students to question their elders. When a client is their elder, these students will choose the option that preserves respect for the client over one that provides teaching. We must make our expectations very clear.

Finally, talk with your ENNL and immigrant students after your exams. They can provide a wealth of information about what confused them or what was ambiguous. Discuss your findings with your colleagues and improve your exams. Ultimately your exams will be clearer and more valid.

SUCCESS STRATEGIES

The following strategies were developed originally to help ENNL students. An interesting revelation is that they also help native English speakers who have learning styles that are not conducive to learning by lecture, or who read slowly, or have learning disabilities or other academic challenges.

STRATEGIES FOR PROMOTING ENNL STUDENT SUCCESS

1. You cannot decrease the reading assignments because some students read slowly, but you can help students prioritize the most important areas.
2. Allow adequate time for testing. The NCLEX® is not a 1-minute-per-question test anymore. Usually 1.5 hours is adequate for a 50-item multiple-choice exam.
3. Allow students to tape lectures if they want to. You might have lectures audiotaped and put in the library for student access.
4. Speak clearly. Mumbling and rapid, anxious speech are difficult to understand. If you have a problem with clarity, provide handouts containing the critical points. Provide the handouts anyway. You want to teach and test nursing knowledge, not note-taking skills.
5. Avoid slang and idiomatic expressions. This is harder than heck to do, but you can do it with practice. When you do use slang, explain it. This is especially important on exams. When in doubt about whether a word is confusing, think about what the dictionary definition would be; if there are two meanings, use another word.
6. Allow the use of translation dictionaries on exams. You can say that students must tell you what they are looking up, so they cannot find medical terminology that is part of the test.
7. Be aware of cultural issues when you are writing exams. Of course you will test on culture-specific issues, but be sure you are testing what you want to test (e.g., the student's knowledge of diets, not of recipes).
8. Feel free to use medical terminology, after all this is nursing school. However, when you use an important new term, write it on the board so students can spell it correctly in their notes.
9. In clinical, make the implied explicit. It seems obvious that safety is the priority, but if a student thinks the priority is respecting her elders, when a client with a new hip replacement demands to get out of bed there could be a disaster.
10. Hire a student who takes clear and accurate lecture notes to post his or her notes for use by ENNL and other students. The students will still attend class and take their own notes, but will have this resource to fill in the details that they miss.
11. SOA (spell out abbreviations).
12. Many international students learned to speak English in the British style. If something would be confusing to a British person, they will find it confusing.
13. Provide opportunities for students to discuss what they are learning with other students and faculty. A faculty member might hold a weekly discussion group where students bring questions. It can be interesting to find a student having no trouble tracing the path of a red cell from the heart to the portal vein, but having difficulty understanding what cream of wheat is ("I thought it was a stalk of grain in a bowl with cream poured on it").
14. Make it clear that questions are encouraged. When a student is not asking questions, and you think he or she may not understand, ask the student after class if he or she has questions. Make it easier for students to approach you by being approachable. Learn their names, and learn to pronounce them correctly. Hearing you try to pronounce their name might be humorous for them, and it will validate how difficult it is to speak other languages.
15. Take another look at basing grades on class participation. You may be putting inordinate demands on the ENNL students. Of course nurses must learn to work with others, but the nurse who talks most is not necessarily the best.
16. Be a role model for communication skills. You might even say in class when you talk about communication that if you respect a person who is trying to communicate with you, you will persist until you understand the message. Say, "Please repeat that," or "I think you said to put a chicken on my head, is that correct?" or "You want me to do what with the textbook?" It may be considered socially rude to ask people to repeat themselves repeatedly. Make it clear that this is not a social situation. In the professional role, we are responsible for effective communication. We cannot get away with smiling and nodding our heads.
17. In clinical, if a student has an accent that is difficult for the staff to understand, discuss clarification techniques (see 16 above) with the student and staff members. Make it explicit that it is acceptable for the student to ask questions and for the staff to ask for clarification.
18. If your college has a writing center where students can receive feedback on grammar and style before submitting papers, have students use it. If you are not so fortunate, view papers as a rough draft instead of a final product. Give specific feedback about what to correct and allow students to resubmit.
19. Make any services available to ENNL students available to all students (such as group discussions and notes). These services may meet the learning needs of many students while preventing the attitude that "they are different and they get something I don't."
20. Faculty attitudes are the most important determinant of a successful program to promote the success of ENNL nursing students. Talk with other faculty about the controversial issues. Create an organized program with a consistent approach among the faculty. The rewards will be well worth the work.

STRATEGIES FOR SUCCESS

Sandra DeYoung, Ed.D., R.N.

IMPROVING OUR TEACHING

Every faculty member wants to be a good teacher, and every teacher wants her or his students to learn. In particular, we want to achieve the student learning outcomes that our educational institutions say that we must achieve. How can we best meet both goals? We cannot just teach as we were taught. We have to learn a variety of teaching methods and investigate best practices in pedagogy. We also have to learn how to measure student learning outcomes in practical and efficient ways. The next few pages will introduce you to principles of good teaching and ways to evaluate learning. Keep in mind that this is only an introduction. For a more extensive study of these principles and pedagogies, you might consult the resources listed at the end of this introduction.

LEARNING THEORY

In order to improve our teaching, we must have some familiarity with learning theory. Nurses who come into educational roles without psychology of learning courses in their background should read at least an introductory-level book on learning theories. You should, for example, know something about stages and types of learning, how information is stored in memory and how it is retrieved, and how knowledge is transferred from one situation to another.

BEHAVIORIST THEORIES

Behaviorist theories are not in as much favor today as they were 25 years ago, but they still help to explain simple learning. Conditioning and reinforcement are concepts with which most educators are familiar. Conditioning explains how we learn some simple movements and behaviors that result in desired outcomes, such as a nurse responding when an alarm sounds on a ventilator. Reinforcement refers to the fact that behavior that is rewarded or reinforced tends to reoccur. Therefore, reinforcement is a powerful tool in the hands of an educator.

COGNITIVE LEARNING THEORIES

Cognitive learning theories are much more sophisticated and deal with how we process information by perceiving, remembering, and storing information. All of these processes are a part of learning. One of the most useful concepts in cognitive theory is that of mental schemata.

Schemata (plural) are units of knowledge that are stored in memory. For example, nurses must develop a schema related to aseptic technique. Once a schema is stored in memory, related information can be built on it. For instance, changing a dressing is easier to learn if the learner already has a schema for asepsis.

Metacognition is another concept identified in cognitive theories. This concept refers to thinking about one's thinking. To help learners who are having difficulty mastering certain material, you might ask them to think about how they learn best and to help them evaluate whether they really understand the material.

Transfer of learning occurs when a learner takes information from the situation in which it is learned and applies it to a new situation. Transfer is most likely to occur if the information was learned well in the first place, if it can be retrieved from memory, and if the new situation is similar to the original learning situation. Educators can teach for transfer by pointing out to students how a concept is applied in several situations so that learners know that the concept is not an isolated one, and the students begin to look for similar patterns in new situations.

ADULT LEARNING THEORIES

Adult learning theories help to explain how learning takes place differently for adults than for children. Adults usually need to know the practical applications for the information they are given. They also want to see how it fits with their life experiences. When teaching young adults and adults, nurse educators need to keep in mind adult motivation for learning.

LEARNING STYLE THEORIES

Learning style theories abound. Research has shown that some learners are visually oriented; some are more auditory or tactile learners; some are individualistic and learn best alone whereas others learn best by collaboration; some deal well with abstract concepts while others learn better with concrete information. Measurement instruments that can determine preferred learning styles are readily available. Although not many educators actually measure their students' learning styles, they should at least keep learning styles in mind when they plan their instruction.

PLANNING FOR INSTRUCTION

With some background knowledge of how students learn, the nurse educator can begin to plan the learning experiences. Planning includes developing objectives, selecting content, choosing pedagogies, selecting assignments, and planning for assessment of learning. All nurse educators come to the teaching process already knowing how to write objectives. Objectives can be written in the cognitive, psychomotor, and affective domains of learning. In the cognitive domain, they can be written at the knowledge, comprehension, application, analysis, and synthesis levels of complexity. The critical aspect of objectives is that you need to keep referring to them as you plan your lesson or course. They will help you focus on the "need to know" versus the "nice to know" material. They will help you decide on which assignments will be most suitable, and they will guide your development of evaluation tools.

SELECTING ASSIGNMENTS

Selecting and developing out-of-class assignments calls for creativity. You may use instructor manuals, such as this one, for ideas for assignments or you may also develop your own. To encourage learning through writing, you can assign short analysis papers, position papers, or clinical journals, all of which promote critical thinking. Nursing care plans of various lengths and complexity may be assigned. You may create reading guides with questions to help students read their textbooks analytically. You might also ask students to interview people or observe people to achieve various objectives.

USING EFFECTIVE PEDAGOGIES

Selecting teaching methods or pedagogies takes considerable time. You must consider what you are trying to achieve. To teach facts, you may choose to lecture or assign a computer tutorial. To change attitudes or motivate learners, you may use discussion, role-playing, or gaming. Developing critical thinking may be done effectively using critical thinking exercises, concept maps, group projects, or problem-based learning. There are what I will call *traditional* pedagogies, *activity-based* pedagogies, and *technology-based* pedagogies.

TRADITIONAL PEDAGOGIES

Traditional pedagogies include lecture, discussion, and questioning. Lecturing is an efficient way to convey a great deal of information to large groups of people. However, the lecture creates passive learning. Learners just sit and listen (or not) and do not interact with the information or the lecturer. Research has shown that students learn more from active learning techniques—that is, from being able to talk about, manipulate, reduce, or synthesize information. So, if you are going to lecture, it would be wise to intersperse lecture with discussion and questioning.

Discussion gives students an opportunity to analyze and think critically about information that they have read or were given in a lecture. By discussing key concepts and issues, they can learn the applicability of the concepts and see how they can transfer to varied situations. Discussions can be formal or informal, but they generally work best if they are planned. For a formal discussion, students must be held accountable for preparing for it. The teacher becomes a facilitator by giving an opening statement or question, guiding the discussion to keep it focused, giving everyone a chance to participate, and summarizing at the end.

Questioning is a skill that develops over time. The first principle to learn is that you have to give students time to answer. Most teachers wait only one second before either repeating the question or answering it themselves. You should wait at least three to five seconds before doing anything, to allow students time to think and prepare a thoughtful answer. Research has revealed that most instructor-posed questions are at a very low level (lower-order), eliciting recall of facts. But questioning can be used to develop critical thinking if it is planned. Higher-order questions are those that require students to interpret information, to apply it to different situations, to think about relationships between concepts, or to assess a situation. If you ask higher-order questions during your classes or clinical experiences, students will rise to the occasion and will be challenged to provide thoughtful answers.

ACTIVITY-BASED PEDAGOGIES

Activity-based teaching strategies include cooperative learning, simulations, games, problem-based learning, and self-learning modules, among others. Cooperative learning is an old pedagogy that has received more research support than any other method. This approach involves learners working together and being responsible for the learning of group members as well as their own learning. Cooperative learning groups can be informal, such as out-of-class study groups, or can be formally structured in-class groups. The groups may serve to solve problems, develop projects, or discuss previously taught content.

Simulations are exercises that can help students to learn in an environment that is low risk or risk free. Students can learn decision making, for example, in a setting where no one is hurt if the decision is the wrong one. Simulations in skills laboratories are frequently used to teach psychomotor skills. Simulations can be written (case studies), acted out (role-playing), computer-based (clinical decision-making scenarios), or complex, technology-based (active simulation mannequins).

Games can help motivate people to learn. Factual content that can be rather boring to learn, such as medical terminology, can be turned into word games such as crossword puzzles or word searches. More complex games can teach problem solving or can apply previously learned information; board games or simulation games can be used for these purposes.

Problem-based learning (PBL) provides students with real-life problems that they must research and analyze and then develop possible solutions for. PBL is a group activity. The instructor presents the students with a brief problem statement. The student groups make lists of what they know and don't know about the problem. They decide what information they must collect in order to further understand the problem. As they collect the information and analyze it, they further refine the problem and begin to investigate possible solutions. The educator serves as a facilitator and resource during the learning process and helps keep the group focused.

Self-learning modules are a means of self-paced learning. They can be used to teach segments of a course or an entire course or curriculum. Modules should be built around a single concept. For example, you might design a module for a skills lab based on aseptic technique; or you could develop a module for a classroom course around

© 2011 Pearson Education, Inc.

the concept of airway impairment. Each module contains components such as an introduction, instructions on how to use the module, objectives, a pretest, learning activities, and a posttest. Learning activities within a module should address various learning styles. You should try to include activities that appeal to visual learners and tactile learners, conceptual learners and abstract learners, and individual and collaborative learners, for example. Those activities could be readings, audiovisuals, computer programs, group discussion, or skills practice. The educator develops and tests the module and then acts as facilitator and evaluator as learners work through the module.

TECHNOLOGY-BASED PEDAGOGIES

Technology-based pedagogies include computer simulations and tutorials, internet use, and distance-learning applications. Computer simulations were discussed briefly in the previous section. They include decision-making software in which a clinical situation is enacted and students are asked to work through the nursing process to solve problems and achieve positive outcomes. They also include simulation games such as SimCity, which can be a useful tool in teaching community health principles. Computer tutorials are useful for individual remedial work such as medication calculations or practice in answering multiple-choice test questions.

The internet is a rich resource for classroom use and for out-of-class assignments. The World Wide Web contains hundreds of websites that can be accessed for health-related information. Students need to be taught how to evaluate the worth of these websites. The criteria they should apply to this evaluation include identifying the intended audience, the currency of the information, the author's credentials or the affiliated organization, and content accuracy. Students may not know how to identify online journal sources compared to other websites. It is worth spending time, therefore, teaching students how to use the Web before giving them assignments that include Web use. If your classroom is internet-access enabled, you can visually demonstrate how to identify and use appropriate websites. For example, if you want students to find relevant information for diabetic teaching, you can show them the differing value of information from official diabetes associations versus pharmaceutical sites versus chat rooms or public forums.

You may be using this instructor manual in a distance-learning course. Distance learning takes the forms of interactive television classes, Webcasting, or online courses. In any form of distance learning, students are learning via the technology, but they are also learning about technology and becoming familiar with several computer applications. Those applications may include synchronous and asynchronous applications, streaming video, and multimedia functions.

ASSESSING LEARNING

You can assess or evaluate learning in a number of ways. Your first decision is whether you are just trying to get informal, ungraded feedback on how well students are learning in your class, or whether you are evaluating the students for the purpose of assigning a grade. Following are a number of techniques that can be used for one or both purposes.

CLASSROOM ASSESSMENT TECHNIQUES

Classroom assessment techniques (CATs) are short, quick, ungraded, in-class assessments used to gauge students' learning during or at the end of class. Getting frequent feedback on students' understanding helps educators to know if they are on the right track and if students are benefiting from the planned instruction. If you wait until you give a formal quiz or examination, you may have waited too long to help some students who are struggling with the material. The most popular CAT is probably the *minute paper*. This technique involves asking students to write down, in one or two minutes, usually at the end of class, the most important thing they learned that day or points that remain unclear. A related technique is the *muddiest point*, in which you ask the class to write down what the "muddiest" part of the class was for them. In nursing, *application cards* can be especially useful. After teaching about a particular concept or body of knowledge, and before you talk about the applications of the information, ask the students to fill out an index card with one possible clinical application of the information. This technique fosters application and critical thinking. Always leave class time during the following session to give feedback on the CAT results.

TESTS AND EXAMINATIONS

Tests and examinations are also used to assess or evaluate learning. Tests should be planned carefully to measure whether learning objectives have been met. You should form a test plan in which you decide the number of test items to include for each objective as well as the complexity of the items. Just as objectives can be written at the knowledge through synthesis levels of knowing, test items can be written at each level, too. Some types of items lend themselves to the lower levels of knowing, such as true-false and matching items, while multiple-choice and essay questions can be used to test higher levels.

TRUE-FALSE QUESTIONS

True-false questions are used simply to assess whether the student can determine the correctness of a fact or principle. This type of question should be used sparingly, because the student has a 50% chance of guessing the correct answer. Well-written true-false questions are clear and unambiguous. The entire statement should be totally true or totally false. An example of a question that is ambiguous is:

(T F) A routine urinanalyis specimen must be collected with clean technique and contain at least 100 mL.

The answer to this question is false because the specimen does not require 100 mL of volume. However, the clean technique part of the question is true. Because part of the statement is true and part is false, the question is misleading. A better question is:

(T F) A routine urinalysis specimen must be collected with clean technique.

True-false questions can be made more difficult by requiring the student to explain why the statement is true or false.

MATCHING QUESTIONS

Matching questions also test a low level of learning—that of knowledge. They are most useful for determining if students have learned definitions or equivalents of some type. They should be formatted in two columns, with the premise words or statements on the left and the definitions or responses on the right. You should have more responses than premises so that matching cannot be done simply by process of elimination. Instructions should be given that indicate whether responses can be used more than once or even not used at all. An example of a matching question is:

Match the definition on the right with the suffix on the left. Definitions can be used only once or not at all.

_____1.	_____-itis	a. presence of
_____2.	_____-stalsis	b. abnormal flow
_____3.	_____-rrhage	c. inflammation
_____4.	_____-iasis	d. discharge or flow
_____5.	_____-ectomy	e. contraction
		f. surgical removal of

MULTIPLE-CHOICE QUESTIONS

Multiple-choice questions can be written at the higher levels of knowing, from application through evaluation. At these higher levels they can test critical thinking. A multiple-choice question has two parts. The first part, the question, is also called the *stem*. The possible answers are called *options*. Among the options, the correct one is called the *answer*, while the incorrect options are termed *distracters*. You can word stems as questions or as incomplete statements that are completed by the options. For example, an item written as a question is:

WHAT IS A QUICK WAY TO ASSESS THE APPROXIMATE LITERACY LEVEL OF A PATIENT?

a. Pay attention to her vocabulary as she speaks.

b. Give her an instruction sheet to read.

c. Administer a literacy test.

d. Ask her whether she graduated from high school.

The same knowledge can be tested by a stem written as an incomplete statement:

A QUICK WAY TO ASSESS THE APPROXIMATE LITERACY LEVEL OF A PATIENT IS TO

a. pay attention to her vocabulary as she speaks.

b. give her an instruction sheet to read.

c. administer a literacy test.

d. ask her whether she graduated from high school.

Notice the differing formats used here. When the stem is a question, each option is capitalized. When the stem is an incomplete statement, it does not end with a period, so the options do not begin with a capital letter. This style may vary. In this manual's test bank, all options begin with a capital letter, regardless of whether the stem is a complete or incomplete sentence. Stems should be kept as brief as possible to minimize reading time. Avoid negatively stated stems. For example, a poor stem would be, "Which of the following is not a good way to assess a patient's literacy level?" It is too easy for readers to miss the word "not" and therefore answer incorrectly. If you feel compelled to write negative stems occasionally, be sure to capitalize or underline the word "not," or use the word "except," as in the following example: "All of the following are good ways to assess a patient's literacy level, EXCEPT." In this case, the reader is less likely to miss the negative word because of the sentence structure and also because the word "except" is capitalized.

Options usually vary from three to five in number. The more options you have, the more difficult the item. However, it is often difficult to write good distracters. Be sure that your options are grammatically consistent with the stem. Next is a test item in which all of the options do not fit grammatically with the stem:

THE LECTURE METHOD OF TEACHING IS BEST SUITED TO

a. when the audience already knows a lot about the topic.

b. large audiences.

c. times when you are in a hurry to cover your material and don't want to be interrupted.

d. young children.

Not only are the options grammatically inconsistent, they are also of varied lengths. Attempt to keep the options about the same length. The following restatement of the item corrects the problems with grammar and with length:

THE LECTURE METHOD OF TEACHING IS BEST SUITED TO

a. an audience that already knows the topic.

b. an audience that is very large.

c. times when you must cover your material quickly.

d. an audience of young children.

Distracters that make no sense should never be used. Instead, try to develop distracters that reflect incorrect ideas that some students might hold about a topic.

© 2011 Pearson Education, Inc.

ESSAY QUESTIONS

Essay-type questions include short answer (restricted-response questions) and full essays (extended-response questions). These types of items can be used to test higher-order thinking. Extended-response essays are especially suited to testing analysis, synthesis, and evaluation levels of thinking. An example of an essay question that might test these higher-order levels of thinking is: "Explain how exogenous cortisone products mimic a person's normal cortisol functions and why long-term cortisone administration leads to complications. Also explain how nursing assessment and intervention can help to reduce those complications."

The educator must plan how the essay is going to be graded before the test is given. An outline of required facts and concepts can be developed and points given to each. Then a decision must be made as to whether it is appropriate to give points for writing style, grammar, spelling, and so on.

TEST ITEM ANALYSIS

After a test is given, an analysis of objective items can be conducted. Two common analyses are *item difficulty* and *item discrimination*. Most instructors want to develop questions that are of moderate difficulty, with around half of the students selecting the correct answer. A mixture of fairly easy, moderate, and difficult questions can be used.

The difficulty index can be easily calculated by dividing the number of students who answered the question correctly by the total number of students answering the question. The resulting fraction, converted to a percentage, gives an estimate of the difficulty, with lower percentages reflecting more difficult questions.

Item discrimination is an estimate of how well a particular item differentiates between students who generally know the material and those who don't. Another way of saying this is that a discriminating item is one that most of the students who got high scores on the rest of the examination got right and most of the students who got low scores got wrong. The discrimination index can be calculated by computer software or by hand using a formula that can be found in tests and measurement textbooks.

These few pages are but an introduction to teaching techniques. For more information, you might consult the following resources:

Book: DeYoung, S. (2003). *Teaching Strategies for Nurse Educators*. Upper Saddle River, NJ: Prentice Hall.

Websites:

www.crlt.umich.edu/tstrategies/teachings.html

www.gmu.edu/facstaff/part-time/strategy.html

www.ic.arizona.edu/ic/edtech/strategy.html

© 2011 Pearson Education, Inc.

CHAPTER 1
INTRODUCTION TO PHARMACOLOGY: DRUG REGULATION AND APPROVAL

LEARNING OUTCOME 1

Identify key events in the history of pharmacology.

Concepts for Lecture

1. The history of pharmacology begins with records describing the use of plants (herbs) to relieve symptoms of disease in every culture dating to antiquity. During the Dark Ages, herbal medicine continued to be practiced, but there are few records.
2. The first recorded reference to pharmacology is found in the text *Pharmacologia sen Manuducto and Materiam Medicum* by Samuel Dale in 1693.
3. Modern pharmacology is thought to have begun in the early 1800s, when chemists were beginning to isolate the pharmacological agents from their natural products and pharmacologists could study their effects in animals or use themselves as test subjects.
4. Pharmacology was officially recognized as a distinct discipline when the first department of pharmacology was established in Estonia in 1847. In 1890 John Jacob Abel, known as the father of American pharmacology, founded the first pharmacology department in the United States at the University of Michigan.
5. Beginning in the 20th century and continuing into the 21st, the mechanism of how drugs produce their effects has been understood, and drugs are now synthesized and tested in a relatively short time. The primary purpose of pharmacology is to focus on the improvement of the patient's quality of life.

 POWERPOINT SLIDES

 SUGGESTIONS FOR CLASSROOM ACTIVITIES

- Have students prepare a time line of the history of pharmacology, including important dates and individuals.
- Invite a representative from a pharmaceutical company to speak to the class on the research and development of a new drug.

 REFERENCE

LEARNING OUTCOME 2

Explain the interdisciplinary nature of pharmacology, giving examples of subject areas needed to learn the discipline well.

Concepts for Lecture

1. Pharmacology is the study of drugs, which includes understanding how drugs are administered, where they travel in the body, and the responses they produce.
2. Several subject areas are interrelated to pharmacology, such as anatomy and physiology, chemistry, microbiology, and pathophysiology.
3. Pharmacology is a challenging, ever-changing subject. Of the over ten thousand drugs currently available, each has its own therapeutic application, interactions, side effects, and mechanisms of action. Many drugs are prescribed for more than one disease. Individual factors, such as age, sex, body mass, health status, and genetics, may elicit different responses.

 POWERPOINT SLIDES

 SUGGESTIONS FOR CLASSROOM ACTIVITIES

- Discuss how knowledge of anatomy and physiology, chemistry, microbiology, and pathophysiology are helpful in understanding pharmacology.
- Discuss why pharmacology is challenging and requires continuous learning.

 SUGGESTIONS FOR CLINICAL ACTIVITIES

- Have students list the drugs their assigned patient is receiving. For each drug identify its therapeutic applications, interactions, side effects, and mechanisms of action. During postclinical conference, have students share this information.
- Discuss why patients receiving the same drug may have different responses.
- Assign each student a drug to look up in the PDR; have students note the drug's chemical structure, what body system(s) it affects, and what disease the drug is used to treat.

© 2011 Pearson Education, Inc.

LEARNING OUTCOME 3

Compare and contrast therapeutics and pharmacology.

Concepts for Lecture

Therapeutics and pharmacology are closely connected. Therapeutics is concerned with the prevention of disease and treatment of suffering, while pharmacotherapy is the application of drugs for the purpose of disease prevention and treatment of suffering.

 POWERPOINT SLIDES

 SUGGESTION FOR CLASSROOM ACTIVITIES

- Discuss different examples of therapeutics and pharmacotherapy and how they prevent disease and treat suffering.

 SUGGESTION FOR CLINICAL ACTIVITIES

- On assigned patients have each student identify therapeutics and pharmacotherapy and how these areas prevent disease and/or treat suffering in the assigned patient.

LEARNING OUTCOME 4

Compare and contrast traditional drugs, biologics, and alternative therapies.

Concepts for Lecture

1. Traditional drugs are chemical agents synthesized in a laboratory that produce biological responses in the body. The responses may be desirable (therapeutic) or undesirable (adverse).
2. Biologics, such as hormones, monoclonal antibodies, natural blood products and components, interferon, and vaccines, are naturally produced in animal cells, microorganisms, or the human body itself and are used to treat a variety of illnesses and conditions.
3. Alternative therapies, such as natural plant extracts, herbs, vitamins, minerals, dietary supplements, acupuncture, hypnosis, biofeedback, and massage, show promise in treating some diseases.

 POWERPOINT SLIDES

 REFERENCE

- National Center for Complementary and Alternative Medicine: *nccam.nih.gov/*

 SUGGESTION FOR CLASSROOM ACTIVITIES

- Divide class into four groups. Assign one complementary therapy (acupuncture, hypnosis, biofeedback, or massage) to each group, and have them provide information on that therapy to the class.

 SUGGESTION FOR CLINICAL ACTIVITIES

- Have students identify any complementary or alternative therapies on assigned patients.

LEARNING OUTCOME 5

Identify the advantages and disadvantages of prescription and over-the-counter (OTC) drugs.

Concepts for Lecture

1. Prescription drugs offer the advantage of the patient's being examined by a health care provider, as well as ensuring that the proper amount and frequency of a drug is prescribed. The patient also receives information on how to take the medication and on potential side effects. Disadvantages of prescription drugs include the need to schedule time for an appointment with a health care provider and only being able to obtain the drug with a prescription.
2. Advantages of OTC drugs include the ability to obtain the drug without seeing a health care provider, and OTC drugs are often less expensive than prescription drugs. Disadvantages of OTC drugs include the possibility of choosing the wrong drug, disease progression, and not knowing side effects and interactions of the drug with both prescription and other OTC drugs.

 POWERPOINT SLIDES

 REFERENCE

- Over-the-counter medications: *www.nlm.nih.gov/medlineplus/overthecountermedicines.html*

SUGGESTIONS FOR CLASSROOM ACTIVITIES

- Discuss why some drugs are prescription drugs and other drugs are OTC drugs. Have students give examples of prescription drugs and OTC drugs.
- Discuss why a prescription drug sometimes becomes an OTC drug. Have students give examples.

© 2011 Pearson Education, Inc.

Learning Outcome 6

Identify key U.S. drug regulations that have ensured the safety and efficacy of medications.

Concepts for Lecture

1. There were few standards or guidelines to protect the public from drug misuse before the 19th century. Some contained hazardous levels of dangerous or addictive substances.
2. The *United States Pharmacopoeia* (USP), established in 1820, was the first comprehensive publication of drug standards in the United States. It summarizes standards of drug purity and strength and directions for synthesis.
3. The National Formulary (NF) was established by the American Pharmaceutical Association (APhA) in 1852, with the focus of the NF on pharmaceutical ingredients. The USP and NF merged in 1975 to form the United States Pharmacopoeia–National Formulary (USP-NF). Official monographs and interim-revision announcements are published regularly, and the full, bound version is printed every five years.
4. The United States began developing and enforcing tougher drug legislation in the 1900s. Some of the laws were the Biologics Control Act (1902), which helped to standardize the quality of serums and other blood products; the Pure Food and Drug Act (1906), which gave the government power to control the labeling of medicines; the Sherley Amendment (1912), which prohibited the sale of drugs labeled with fake therapeutic claims that were intended to defraud the consumer; the Food, Drug, and Cosmetic Act (1938) and its later amendments, which prevented the sale of drugs that had not been thoroughly tested and proven safe and effective; and the Dietary Supplement Health and Education Act (1994), which prevented misleading claims.

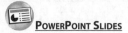
PowerPoint Slides

Suggestions for Classroom Activities
- Have a USP-NF available, and assign students to look for different drugs.
- Design a matching quiz for the different drug acts.

Learning Outcome 7

Discuss the role of the U.S. Food and Drug Administration (FDA) in the drug approval process.

Concepts for Lecture

1. The Food and Drug Administration was officially established as an agency of the U.S. Department of Health and Human Services in 1988.
2. Any pharmaceutical laboratory must solicit approval from the FDA before marketing a drug. The Center for Drug Evaluation and Research (CDER), a branch of the FDA, determines the safety and efficacy of a drug before it is placed on the market.
3. The Center for Biologics Evaluation and Research (CBER) is another branch of the FDA; it regulates the use of biologics, such as serums, vaccines, and blood products. A result of the work of the CBER was the 1986 Childhood Vaccine Act, which authorizes the FDA to oversee all aspects of vaccines.
4. The Center for Food Safety and Applied Nutrition (CFSAN) is the branch of the FDA that oversees herbal and dietary products. In 1994 the Dietary and Supplemental Health and Education Act was established, but this act does not regulate dietary and herbal supplements as closely as the Food, Drug, and Cosmetic Act regulates drugs.

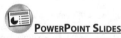
PowerPoint Slides

Reference
- Food and Drug Administration: *www.fda.gov/*

LEARNING OUTCOME 8

Explain the four stages of approval for therapeutic and biologic drugs.

Concepts for Lecture

1. The FDA reviews therapeutic and biologic drugs for approval in four phases. These phases include the preclinical investigation, clinical investigation, review of the new drug application (NDA), and postmarketing surveillance. The amount of time that this process takes depends on several checkpoints.
2. The preclinical investigation involves extensive laboratory research on human and microbial cells cultured in the laboratory and several species of animals, in order to examine the drug's effectiveness at various doses and to examine the side effects. Since this testing is not performed on humans, preclinical tests are always considered inconclusive.
3. The clinical investigation, which is the longest part of the drug approval process, takes place in three different stages, termed "clinical phase trials," and evaluates the drug's effectiveness and safety in humans.
4. The new drug application (NDA) is reviewed by the FDA and either is approved and continues to the final stage or is rejected and the process is suspended until concerns are addressed by the pharmaceutical company. The average NDA review time is 17 to 24 months.
5. Postmarketing surveillance, the last stage of the approval process, begins after the clinical trials and NDA review are completed; this stage surveys for harmful drug effects on a larger population.

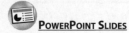

REFERENCE
- Food and Drug Administration: *www.fda.gov/*

SUGGESTIONS FOR CLASSROOM ACTIVITIES
- Discuss why it takes so long for drugs to be approved by the FDA.
- Discuss why newly approved drugs are so expensive to the consumer.
- Have students research drugs that have been removed from the market because of harmful effects and present their findings to the class.

SUGGESTION FOR CLINICAL ACTIVITIES
- Discuss the MedWatch program and its purpose.

LEARNING OUTCOME 9

Discuss how the FDA has increased the speed with which new drugs reach consumers.

Concepts for Lecture

1. Reasons identified for the delays in the FDA drug approval process were outdated guidelines, poor communications, and insufficient staff to handle the workload.
2. The Prescription Drug User Fee Act, established on a five-year trial basis in 1992, required drug and biologic manufacturers to pay yearly product-user fees to the FDA. The fee allowed the FDA to hire more employees and to restructure its organization to handle more drug applications.
3. The results were a success. From 1992 to 1996, the FDA approved double the number of drugs and cut some review times by half.
4. The FDA Modernization Act in 1997 reauthorized the Prescription Drug User Fee Act.

POWERPOINT SLIDES

REFERENCE
- Food and Drug Administration: *www.fda.gov/*

SUGGESTION FOR CLASSROOM ACTIVITIES
- Discuss how the user fee increases the cost of prescription drugs.

© 2011 Pearson Education, Inc.

LEARNING OUTCOME 10

Identify the nurse's role in the drug approval process.

Concepts for Lecture

1. Discuss the role of the nurse during the postmarketing surveillance period of phase IV.
2. Discuss the role of the nurse in reporting adverse effects of trial drugs.

GENERAL CHAPTER CONSIDERATIONS

1. Have students study and learn key terms listed at the beginning of the chapter.
2. Have students complete end-of-chapter exercises either in their book or on the MyNursingKit website.
3. Use the Classroom Response Questions provided in PowerPoint to assess students prior to lecture.

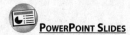 **POWERPOINT SLIDES**

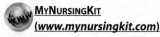 **SUGGESTION FOR CLASSROOM ACTIVITIES**

- Have students identify the role of the nurse in drug research and postmarketing surveillance.

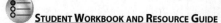 **MYNURSINGKIT (www.mynursingkit.com)**

- Websites
- NCLEX® questions
- Critical Thinking Questions
- Case Studies
- Animations and Videos
- Drug Prototype Questions

 MYNURSINGLAB (www.mynursinglab.com)

- Knowledge Quick Check
- Pre/Posttests
- Customized study plans
- *Separate purchase*

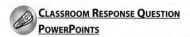 **STUDENT WORKBOOK AND RESOURCE GUIDE**

- Chapter 1 activities
- *Separate purchase*

PEARSON NURSE'S DRUG GUIDE

- *Separate purchase*

 PEARSON eTEXT

- Students can search, highlight, take notes, and more all in electronic format.
- *Separate purchase*

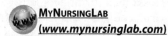 **CLASSROOM RESPONSE QUESTION POWERPOINTS**

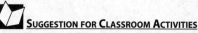 **TESTBANK**

CHAPTER 2
DRUG CLASSES AND SCHEDULES

LEARNING OUTCOME 1

Explain the basis for placing drugs into therapeutic and pharmacologic classes.

Concepts for Lecture

1. Drugs can be organized by therapeutic classification and pharmacologic classification.
2. The therapeutic classification is based on what a particular drug does clinically. Examples of therapeutic classifications are anticoagulants, antidepressants, and antineoplastics.
3. The pharmacologic classification of a drug refers to how a drug produces its effect in the body, such as at the molecular, tissue, or body-system level. This classification is more specific than a therapeutic classification and requires an understanding of biochemistry and physiology.
4. Examples of pharmacologic classifications are calcium channel blockers, angiotensin-converting enzyme inhibitors, and proton-pump inhibitors.

LEARNING OUTCOME 2

Discuss the prototype approach to drug classification.

Concepts for Lecture

1. A "prototype" drug is one drug from a class of drugs that is well understood and serves as a model for other drugs in that pharmacologic class to be compared to. By knowing the prototype drug, the actions and adverse effects of other drugs in that class can be predicted.
2. Newer drugs in the same class may replace prototype drugs because they are more effective, have a more favorable safety profile, or have a longer duration of action.

LEARNING OUTCOME 3

Describe what is meant by a drug's mechanism of action.

Concepts for Lecture

A drug's mechanism of action is how the drug produces its effect in the body.

 POWERPOINT SLIDES

Table 2.1 Organizing Drug Information by Therapeutic Classification
Table 2.2 Organizing Drug Information by Pharmacologic Classification

 SUGGESTIONS FOR CLASSROOM ACTIVITIES

- Have students provide examples of therapeutic classifications of central nervous system (CNS) drugs, gastrointestinal (GI), etc.
- Have students provide examples of pharmacologic classifications for antidepressant agents, diuretics, antihypertensive agents, etc.

 SUGGESTION FOR CLINICAL ACTIVITIES

- Ask students to classify the drugs their assigned patient has ordered.

 POWERPOINT SLIDES

 SUGGESTION FOR CLASSROOM ACTIVITIES

- Discuss the prototype drug for different pharmacologic classes. Is the original prototype drug still being used or has it been replaced by a newer drug in that pharmacologic class? If the prototype drug has been replaced, why?

 POWERPOINT SLIDES

 SUGGESTION FOR CLASSROOM ACTIVITIES

- Briefly describe two or three mechanisms of action.

© 2011 Pearson Education, Inc.

LEARNING OUTCOME 4

Distinguish between a drug's chemical name, generic name, and trade name.

Concepts for Lecture

1. Most drugs have a chemical name, a generic name, and a trade name.
2. A drug has one chemical name, which is assigned using standard nomenclature established by the International Union of Pure and Applied Chemistry (IUPAC). The chemical name describes the physical and chemical properties of the drug but is often complicated and difficult to remember and pronounce. For example, the chemical name for diazepam is 7-chloro-1,3-dihydro-1-methyl-5-phenyl-2H-1,4-benzodiazepin-2-one.
3. Drugs are sometimes classified by their chemical group name, which is a portion of their chemical structure. Some common examples are phenothiazines, cephalosporins, and benzodiazepines.
4. A drug has one generic name, which is assigned by the U.S. Adopted Name Council and used by many organizations, including the U.S. Food and Drug Administration, the U.S. Pharmacopoeia, and the World Health Organization. The generic name is less complicated and easier to remember. It describes the active ingredient of the drug and is written in lowercase. An example of this is the drug name diazepam.
5. The company marketing the drug assigns the trade name of a drug, which is usually short and easy to remember. The trade name is sometimes called the proprietary or product or brand name. In the United States a drug developer has exclusive rights to name and market a drug for 17 years after a new drug application is submitted to the FDA. After 17 years, competing drug companies may sell a generic equivalent drug using a different trade name approved by the FDA. The trade name is capitalized. For example, the trade name for diazepam is Valium.

LEARNING OUTCOME 5

Explain why generic drug names are preferred to trade-name drugs.

Concepts for Lecture

1. Drugs have several trade names but only one generic name that is assigned by the U.S. Adopted Name Council. These names are generally less complicated than chemical names, making them easier to remember.
2. Communication is enhanced between health care providers and other health organizations by utilizing the generic drug names. Generic names are always written in lowercase letters.

LEARNING OUTCOME 6

Discuss why drugs are sometimes placed on a restrictive list and the controversy surrounding this issue.

Concepts for Lecture

1. Some states have compiled a negative formulary list, which is a list of trade-name drugs that pharmacists may not dispense as generic drugs. The bioavailability (physiologic ability of a drug to reach its target cells and produce the desired effect) of a drug is the reason for the negative formulary list.

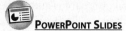
POWERPOINT SLIDES

Table 2.3 Examples of Brand-Name Products Containing Popular Generic Substances

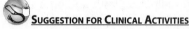
SUGGESTIONS FOR CLASSROOM ACTIVITIES

- Assign each student a selected drug to present to the class, identifying its chemical name, generic name, and trade name, plus its pharmacologic and therapeutic classifications.
- Discuss why drug companies may have selected the trade names of several drugs.
- Discuss what combination drugs are and why it is difficult to match one generic name with one product name. Give examples of combination drugs.

SUGGESTION FOR CLINICAL ACTIVITIES

- Have students prepare drug cards for assigned patients, including the chemical, generic, brand, and trade names.

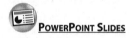
POWERPOINT SLIDES

SUGGESTION FOR CLASSROOM ACTIVITIES

- Have students compare five common drugs, looking at their generic names versus all trade names.

SUGGESTION FOR CLINICAL ACTIVITIES

- Have students present in post-conference the medication list for their assigned patient, listing both the generic and trade names of each drug.

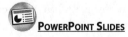
POWERPOINT SLIDES

SUGGESTIONS FOR CLASSROOM ACTIVITIES

- Display a negative formulary list. Discuss why the selected trade-name drugs are on the list.
- Discuss bioavailability and bioequivalence as they relate to trade-name drugs and generic-name drugs.

2. Pharmaceutical companies and some health care practitioners support a negative formulary list because they claim that generic drugs could adversely affect patient outcomes in those with critical conditions or illnesses due to possible differences in the bioequivalency between generic and trade-name drugs.

LEARNING OUTCOME 7

Explain the meaning of a controlled substance.

Concepts for Lecture

1. Controlled substances refer to drugs that are frequently abused or have a high potential for addiction or dependence. Dependence is a physical or psychological need for a substance. These drugs are restricted for use in situations of medical necessity, if allowed at all, and are placed into five schedules (categories) by law.
2. Not all drugs with an abuse potential, such as tobacco, alcohol, and caffeine, are regulated or placed into schedules.

 POWERPOINT SLIDES

 SUGGESTIONS FOR CLASSROOM ACTIVITIES

- Ask students to give examples of controlled substances.
- Discuss why tobacco, alcohol, and caffeine, which have abuse potential, are not regulated. Should they be regulated? Why or why not?
- Divide students into five groups. Assign each group a controlled substance schedule, and have them present information on each, including drug examples.

 SUGGESTION FOR CLINICAL ACTIVITIES

- Have students observe nursing personnel procedure for obtaining a controlled substance for patient administration.

LEARNING OUTCOME 8

Explain the U.S. Controlled Substance Act of 1970 and the role of the U.S. Drug Enforcement Agency in controlling drug abuse and misuse.

Concepts for Lecture

1. The Controlled Substance Act of 1970, also known as the Comprehensive Drug Abuse Prevention and Control Act, restricts the use of drugs with a significant potential for abuse. These drugs are placed into five schedules. Under this law, hospitals and pharmacies must maintain complete records of all controlled substances purchased and sold. Schedule II drugs require a special order form to obtain, orders must be written and signed by the health care provider, telephone orders to pharmacies are not permitted, refills are not permitted, and patients must visit their health care provider first.
2. Anyone convicted of unlawful manufacturing, distributing, and dispensing of controlled substances faces severe penalties.
3. The Drug Enforcement Administration (DEA) regulates the Controlled Substance Act. Hospitals and pharmacies must register with the DEA and use assigned registration numbers to purchase scheduled drugs.

 POWERPOINT SLIDES

 SUGGESTIONS FOR CLASSROOM ACTIVITES

- Discuss the need for the Controlled Substance Act.
- Display forms that hospitals and pharmacies must maintain for controlled substances.

 SUGGESTION FOR CLINICAL ACTIVITIES

- Assign students to observe how controlled substances are monitored in the hospital and/or at a pharmacy.

LEARNING OUTCOME 9

Identify the five drug schedules and give examples of drugs at each level.

Concepts for Lecture

1. Schedule I drugs have the highest potential for abuse and physical and psychological dependency. This schedule of drugs has limited or

 POWERPOINT SLIDES

Table 2.4 U.S. Drug Schedules and Examples

© 2011 Pearson Education, Inc.

no therapeutic use. Examples of schedule I drugs are heroin, LSD, and methaqualone.

2. Schedule II drugs have a high potential for abuse and physical and psychological dependency. Schedule II drugs may be used therapeutically with a prescription, but some are no longer used. Examples of Schedule II drugs are morphine, PCP, cocaine, methadone, and methamphetamine.

3. Schedule III drugs have moderate potential for abuse, moderate physical dependency, and high psychological dependency. This schedule of drugs is used therapeutically with a prescription. Examples of Schedule III drugs are anabolic steroids, codeine and hydrocodone with aspirin or Tylenol, and some barbiturates.

4. Schedule IV drugs have a lower potential for abuse and physical and psychological dependency. This schedule of drugs is used therapeutically with a prescription. Examples of Schedule IV drugs are dextropropoxyphene, pentazocine, meprobamate, diazepam, and alprazolam.

5. Schedule V drugs have the lowest potential for abuse, physical, and psychological dependency. This schedule of drugs is used therapeutically without a prescription. Examples of Schedule V are OTC cough medicines with codeine.

GENERAL CHAPTER CONSIDERATIONS

1. Have students study and learn key terms listed at the beginning of the chapter.
2. Have students complete end-of-chapter exercises either in their book or on the MyNursingKit website.
3. Use the Classroom Response Questions provided in PowerPoint to assess students prior to lecture.

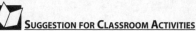

SUGGESTION FOR CLASSROOM ACTIVITIES

- Discuss the importance of knowing what drugs are controlled substances.

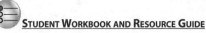

MYNURSINGKIT
(*www.mynursingkit.com*)

- Websites
- NCLEX® questions
- Critical Thinking Questions
- Case Studies
- Animations and Videos
- Drug Prototype Questions

MYNURSINGLAB
(*www.mynursinglab.com*)

- Knowledge Quick Check
- Pre/Posttests
- Customized study plans
- *Separate purchase*

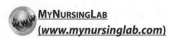

STUDENT WORKBOOK AND RESOURCE GUIDE

- Chapter 2 activities
- *Separate purchase*

PEARSON NURSE'S DRUG GUIDE

- *Separate purchase*

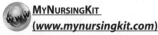

PEARSON eTEXT

- Students can search, highlight, take notes, and more all in electronic format.
- *Separate purchase*

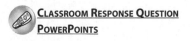

CLASSROOM RESPONSE QUESTION POWERPOINTS

TESTBANK

CHAPTER 3
PRINCIPLES OF DRUG ADMINISTRATION

LEARNING OUTCOME 1

Discuss drug administration as a component of safe, effective nursing care, utilizing the nursing process.

Concepts for Lecture

1. In order to provide safe and effective nursing care, the nurse utilizes the nursing process when administering drugs. Before drug administration, the nurse should assess the patient, plan the drug administration, then administer the drug, and finally evaluate the effects of the drug.
2. It is the nurse's responsibility to have an understanding of the pharmacotherapeutic principles of the medications being administered.

 POWERPOINT SLIDES

 SUGGESTION FOR CLASSROOM ACTIVITIES

- Divide the students into four groups. Assign one of the steps of the nursing process to each group. Have each group describe its step of the nursing process and how it relates to drug administration to the rest of the class.

LEARNING OUTCOME 2

Describe the roles and responsibilities of the nurse regarding drug administration.

Concepts for Lecture

1. The nurse is responsible for knowing the drug classification, actions, side effects, drug preparation, and safe administration and evaluate the patient's response to the medication.
2. Discuss the difference between an allergic reaction and anaphylaxis.
3. Discuss the nursing interventions needed to treat anaphylaxis.

 POWERPOINT SLIDES

 SUGGESTIONS FOR CLASSROOM ACTIVITIES

- Ask students what a nurse should know before administering a drug.
- Discuss the signs and symptoms of an allergic reaction and an anaphylactic reaction.
- Ask students what steps they would take if a patient developed side effects related to a medication.

 SUGGESTION FOR CLINICAL ACTIVITIES

- Have students research a selected drug for their assigned patient and have the student identify what patient teaching they would do.

LEARNING OUTCOME 3

Explain how the five rights of drug administration affect patient safety.

Concepts for Lecture

The five rights of drug administration offer guidance for nurses for safe drug preparation, delivery, and administration. The five rights are right patient, right medication, right dose, right route of administration, and right time of delivery.

 POWERPOINT SLIDES

 SUGGESTIONS FOR CLASSROOM ACTIVITIES

- Demonstrate the three checks of drug administration. Then allow time for students to practice the three checks of drug administration.
- Discuss the additional rights—the right to refuse medication, the right to receive drug education, the right preparation, and the right documentation—that may be included.

 SUGGESTION FOR CLINICAL ACTIVITIES

- Have students demonstrate the five rights and three checks of drug administration and the right documentation on selected patients.

© 2011 Pearson Education, Inc.

LEARNING OUTCOME 4

Give specific examples of how the nurse can increase patient compliance in taking medications.

Concepts for Lecture

1. Specific examples of how the nurse can increase patient compliance in taking medications are telling the patient the name of the drug; why it has been ordered; expected drug actions; associated side effects; and potential interactions with other medications, foods, herbal supplements, or alcohol.
2. Patients need to be reminded that they have an active role in ensuring their own medication effectiveness and safety.

LEARNING OUTCOME 5

Interpret drug orders that contain abbreviations.

Concepts for Lecture

1. Review common abbreviations that relate to universally scheduled times in Table 3.1 and the abbreviations that should not be used.
2. Interpret the meaning of STAT, ASAP, and PRN.

LEARNING OUTCOME 6

Compare and contrast the three systems of measurement used in pharmacology.

Concepts for Lecture

1. Three systems of measurement are used in pharmacology: metric, apothecary, and household. The metric system is the most common system of drug measurement; the apothecary and household are older systems of measurement.
2. The nurse must recognize dosages based on all three systems of measurement until the metric system replaces the other two systems.

 POWERPOINT SLIDES

 SUGGESTION FOR CLASSROOM ACTIVITIES

- Ask students to give examples of instances in which they or a family member or friend have not complied with pharmacotherapy.

 SUGGESTION FOR CLINICAL ACTIVITIES

- Have students prepare and present a medication-teaching plan for an assigned patient.

 POWERPOINT SLIDES

Table 3.1 Drug Administration Abbreviations

 SUGGESTIONS FOR CLASSROOM ACTIVITIES

- Design a matching quiz for drug administration abbreviations.
- Review the Joint Commission Do Not Use List.

 SUGGESTIONS FOR CLINICAL ACTIVITIES

- Have students interpret drug administration abbreviations of medications for assigned patients.
- Have students review the institution's policy on medical abbreviations.

 REFERENCE

- The Joint Commission: *www.jointcommission.org/patientsafety/donotuselist/*

 POWERPOINT SLIDES

Table 3.2 Metric, Apothecary, and Household Approximate Measurement Equivalents

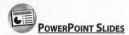 **SUGGESTIONS FOR CLASSROOM ACTIVITIES**

- Display the different devices (droppers, minim cup, and so on) to measure metric, apothecary, and household units.
- Have students convert between the three systems of measurements.

Approximate equivalents between metric, apothecary, and household units of volume and weight are listed in Table 3.2.

LEARNING OUTCOME 7

Explain the proper methods of administering enteral, topical, and parenteral drugs.

Concepts for Learning

1. All routes of drug administration have common protocols and techniques to be followed. Students should review drug administration guidelines prior to administering any type of medication. General guidelines include but are not limited to reviewing the medication order and drug allergies; washing hands and using gloves when appropriate; and identifying the patient appropriately. In addition, the patient should be informed of the medication she is receiving, the patient should be positioned properly for administration, and the nurse should document the administration of the medication and any pertinent patient response.

2. The enteral route includes drugs given orally and through nasogastric or gastrostomy tubes. Enteral drug administration includes tablets or capsules, sublingual and buccal, and nasogastric and gastronomy drug administration. To ensure safe administration for drugs that are given orally, the nurse should assess the patient's level of consciousness and ability to follow instructions, remain with the patient until medications are taken, and offer the patient a glass of water, if desired. Some key guidelines for administration of drugs via the nasogastric or gastronomy routes include administering liquid forms when possible, assessing and verifying tube placement, keeping the head of the bed (HOB) elevated for 1 hour after administration, and fusing the tubing after medication administration. In regard to topical medication administration, key guidelines include rotating sites to prevent skin irritation for transdermal medications, placing the patient in a supine position with the head tilted back for ophthalmic (eye) medications, and avoiding placing drops on the tympanic membrane when administering otic (ear) medications. Additional guidelines include instructing the patient to open and breathe through the mouth with nasal and respiratory medications, placing the patient in a supine position with knees bent and separated for vaginal medications, and placing the patient on the left side for rectal medications. Guidelines for administering drugs via the enteral route can be found in Table 3.3.

3. Topical drugs are applied to the skin or the membranous linings of the eye, ear, nose, respiratory tract, urinary tract, vagina, and rectum. Applications include dermatologic preparations, instillations and irrigations, and inhalations. Vaginal and rectal drug administration are also considered to be in the category of topical drug administration. Information on administration of drugs via the topical route can be found in Table 3.4.

4. Parenteral drugs are administered via a needle into the skin layers (intradermally), subcutaneous tissue, muscles, or veins. Because parenteral drug administration is more invasive than topical or enteral administration, aseptic techniques must be applied. In addition, the nurse must know anatomical locations, the correct equipment, and the procedure for disposing of hazardous equipment. Intradermal injections are administered into the dermal layer of the skin, subcutaneous injections are administered into the deepest layers of the skin, and intramuscular injections are administered into specific muscles. Intravenous medications are administered directly into the bloodstream.

SUGGESTION FOR CLINICAL ACTIVITIES

- Have students convert metric liquid measure to household liquid measures.

POWERPOINT SLIDES

Table 3.3 Enteral Drug Administration
Table 3.4 Topical Drug Administration
Table 3.5 Parenteral Drug Administration
Figure 3.2 Transdermal Patch Administration
Figure 3.3 Instilling Eye Ointment
Figure 3.4 Instilling Ear Drops
Figure 3.5 Nasal Drug Administration
Figure 3.6 Vaginal Drug Administration
Figure 3.7 Intradermal Drug Administration
Figure 3.8 Subcutaneous Drug Administration
Figure 3.9 Intramuscular Drug Administration
Figure 3.10 Secondary Intravenous Lines
Figure 3.11 Baxter Infusion Pump
Figure 3.12 IV Bolus Administration

SUGGESTIONS FOR CLASSROOM ACTIVITIES

- Display equipment and supplies used for each of the routes of drug administration.
- Demonstrate for students each of the routes of drug administration.
- Using models, allow students to practice the parenteral routes of drug administration.

SUGGESTIONS FOR CLINICAL ACTIVITIES

- Assign students to observe the different routes of drug administration.
- With supervision, have students administer drugs to assigned patients.

© 2011 Pearson Education, Inc.

Information on administration of drugs via the parenteral route can be found in Table 3.5.

LEARNING OBJECTIVE 8

Compare and contrast the advantages and disadvantages of each route of drug administration.

Concepts for Lecture

1. Advantages of the enteral route of drug administration: It is the most convenient route; it is usually the least costly of all routes and the safest route because the skin barrier is not compromised; the oral mucosa, stomach, and small intestines have vast absorptive surfaces, so drugs enter the body quickly; in the case of an overdose, medication remaining in the stomach can be retrieved by inducing vomiting. Advantages of the sublingual and buccal routes are that the surfaces provide excellent absorption for certain drugs and medications are not destroyed by digestive enzymes or the liver. The sublingual route provides a rapid onset of action.

2. Disadvantages of the enteral route of drug administration: Some patients have difficulty swallowing tablets or capsules; some drugs are inactivated when tablets are crushed or capsules are opened; some drugs severely irritate the stomach mucosa and cause nausea and vomiting, irritate the oral mucosa, are extremely bitter, or contain dyes that stain the teeth; some drugs are inactivated by digestive enzymes in the stomach and small intestines or are inactivated by the liver before reaching the target organs; there are differences in bioavailability because of patient variations in gastrointestinal motility and ability to absorb medications. Additionally, these drugs cannot be given to a patient who is unconscious or is unable to swallow. Few drugs can be administered by the sublingual or buccal routes.

3. The advantage of topical drug administration is that there are fewer side effects compared with oral or parenteral administration of the same drug because the drug is absorbed very slowly and a minimal amount reaches the general circulation. Rectal administration of drugs is a safe and effective way to deliver drugs to patients who are comatose or who are experiencing nausea and vomiting.

4. The disadvantage of topical drug administration is that drugs should not be applied to abraded or denuded skin unless directions are given to the contrary. The disadvantages of rectal administration are that sometimes a patient may not be able to retain a rectal medication, and drug absorption is slower.

5. Advantages of parenteral administration are that drugs are rapidly absorbed, so there is a rapid onset of action, and drugs are not inactivated by digestive enzymes or metabolized by the liver.

6. Disadvantages of parenteral drug administration are that pathogenic microbes may be introduced directly into the blood or body tissues and that once medication is injected, it cannot be retrieved.

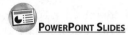

POWERPOINT SLIDES

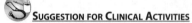

SUGGESTIONS FOR CLASSROOM ACTIVITIES

- Divide the class into three groups. Assign one group each to research the advantages and disadvantages of enteral drug administration, topical drug administration, and parenteral drug administration. Allow each group to share this information with the rest of the class.
- Design a quiz regarding the advantages and disadvantages of each route of drug administration.

SUGGESTION FOR CLINICAL ACTIVITIES

- Have students note the advantages and disadvantages of the drug routes of administration on assigned patients.

GENERAL CHAPTER CONSIDERATIONS

1. Have students study and learn key terms listed at the beginning of the chapter.
2. Have students complete end-of-chapter exercises either in their book or on the MyNursingKit website.
3. Use the Classroom Response Questions provided in PowerPoint to assess students prior to lecture.

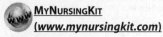

MyNursingKit (www.mynursingkit.com)

- Websites
- NCLEX® questions
- Critical Thinking Questions
- Case Studies
- Animations and Videos
- Drug Prototype Questions

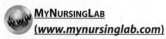

MyNursingLab (www.mynursinglab.com)

- Knowledge Quick Check
- Pre/Posttests
- Customized study plans
- *Separate purchase*

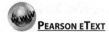

STUDENT WORKBOOK AND RESOURCE GUIDE

- Chapter 3 activities
- *Separate purchase*

PEARSON NURSE'S DRUG GUIDE

- *Separate purchase*

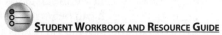

PEARSON eTEXT

- Students can search, highlight, take notes, and more all in electronic format.
- *Separate purchase*

CLASSROOM RESPONSE QUESTION POWERPOINTS

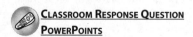

TESTBANK

© 2011 Pearson Education, Inc.

CHAPTER 4
PHARMACOKINETICS

LEARNING OUTCOME 1

Explain the applications of pharmacokinetics to clinical practice.

Concepts for Lecture

Pharmacokinetics is the movement of drugs through the body and how the body handles medication. Knowing pharmacokinetics allows the nurse to better understand the actions and side effects of medications in patients and the many obstacles, such as membranes, barriers, fluids, and physiological processes, a drug faces to reach its target cells.

POWERPOINT SLIDES

SUGGESTION FOR CLASSROOM ACTIVITIES

- Have students describe the obstacles drugs face that are administered orally, topically, and intravenously to reach target cells.

SUGGESTIONS FOR CLINICAL ACTIVITIES

- Have students identify potential or actual obstacles of assigned patients that may interfere with the pharmacokinetics of prescribed medications.
- Using the PDR, have students select a drug that an assigned patient is receiving and describe the pharmacokinetics of that drug.

LEARNING OUTCOME 2

Identify the four components of pharmacokinetics.

Concepts for Lecture

Identify the four components of pharmacokinetics.

POWERPOINT SLIDES

Figure 4.1 Four Processes of Pharmacokinetics

SUGGESTIONS FOR CLASSROOM ACTIVITIES

- Select different drugs and ask students to compare and contrast the absorption, distribution, metabolism, and excretion of each drug.
- Divide the class into four groups. Assign one of the processes of pharmacokinetics to each group to research and report their findings to the rest of the class.

SUGGESTION FOR CLINICAL ACTIVITIES

- On assigned patients have students describe the absorption, distribution, metabolism, and excretion of the drugs that the patient is receiving.

LEARNING OUTCOME 3

Explain how substances travel across plasma membranes.

Concepts for Lecture

1. Most drugs must cross plasma membranes to produce their effects. Drugs use one of two processes to cross body membranes: diffusion, or passive transport, and active transport.

POWERPOINT SLIDES

SUGGESTION FOR CLASSROOM ACTIVITIES

- Display or demonstrate examples of passive and active transport.

2. Diffusion is movement of chemicals from an area of higher concentration to an area of lower concentration. Drug molecules that are small, nonionized, and lipid soluble will usually pass through plasma membranes by diffusion.
3. Active transport is the movement of a chemical against a concentration or electrochemical gradient. Drug molecules that are large, ionized, or water-soluble pass through the plasma membrane by active transport or carrier proteins.

LEARNING OUTCOME 4

Discuss factors affecting drug absorption.

Concepts for Lecture

Most drugs need to be absorbed to produce an effect. Absorption of medications occurs by the movement of a substance from its site of administration, across body membranes, to circulating fluids. Absorption is the primary pharmacokinetic factor determining the length of time it takes a drug to produce its effect. The following factors can affect drug absorption: route of administration; drug formulation; drug dosage; digestive motility; exposure to enzymes in the digestive tract; blood flow to the site of drug administration; degree of ionization of a drug; pH of local environment; and drug–drug, food–drug, or dietary supplement/herbal product–drug interactions.

LEARNING OUTCOME 5

Explain the metabolism of drugs and its application to pharmacotherapy.

Concepts for Lecture

1. Metabolism, also called biotransformation, is the process of chemically converting a drug to a form that is more easily removed from the body. The liver is the primary site of drug metabolism. Biochemical reactions such as hydrolysis, oxidation, and reduction occur to medications as they pass through the liver.
2. Most metabolism in the liver is accomplished by the hepatic microsomal enzyme system, which is sometimes called the P-450 system. This system inactivates drugs and accelerates their excretion.
3. Oral drugs enter the hepatic-portal circulation before being distributed to other body tissues. This first-pass effect can metabolize many oral drugs to an inactive form, so other routes of delivery (i.e., sublingual, rectal, or parenteral routes) need to be considered. This process occurs by the drug's being absorbed and entering the hepatic-portal circulation to go directly to the liver. Here the hepatic microsomal enzymes metabolize drugs to inactive forms and the drug then conjugates and leaves the liver. The final step distributes the drug to the general circulation. See Figure 4.4.
4. Other factors that may affect the pharmacotherapy of drugs metabolized by the liver are chemical alterations that make some drugs more active than the original form; some drugs increase metabolic activity in the liver. Infants and elderly patients have decreased hepatic metabolic activity, patients with severe liver damage have decreased metabolic activity, and

SUGGESTION FOR CLINICAL ACTIVITIES
• Have students select a drug their assigned patient is receiving and determine how the drug crosses the plasma membrane.

POWERPOINT SLIDES

Figure 4.2 Effects of pH on Drug Absorption

SUGGESTION FOR CLASSROOM ACTIVITIES
• Divide class into groups of two or three. Assign each group a factor affecting drug absorption, and ask them to explain and give examples to the rest of the class.

SUGGESTION FOR CLINICAL ACTIVITIES
• Have students identify any factors that may affect drug absorption on their assigned patients, and have them advise their patients of the factor if appropriate.

POWERPOINT SLIDES

SUGGESTION FOR CLASSROOM ACTIVITIES
• Discuss the reason for decreased metabolic activity in infants, the elderly, and patients with severe liver damage and why drug dosages may need to be lowered.

SUGGESTION FOR CLINICAL ACTIVITIES
• Have students develop a nursing care plan for an infant or elderly patient receiving oral drugs or a patient with severe liver damage receiving oral drugs.

© 2011 Pearson Education, Inc.

patients with certain genetic disorders lack specific metabolic enzymes. In all of these cases, the drug dosage may need to be adjusted.

LEARNING OUTCOME 6

Discuss how drugs are distributed throughout the body.

Concepts for Lecture

1. Medications are distributed or transported throughout the body by the blood. The greater the blood flow to an area, the higher concentration of a drug is delivered to that area.
2. Lipid-soluble drugs are more completely distributed to body tissues and are not limited by the barriers that stop water-soluble drugs.

LEARNING OUTCOME 7

Describe how plasma proteins affect drug distribution.

Concepts for Lecture

1. Many drugs bind with plasma proteins to form drug–protein complexes. These complexes are too large to cross capillary membranes, so the drug is not distributed to body tissues. Drugs bound to proteins circulate in the plasma until they are released or displaced from the drug–protein complex.
2. Drugs and other chemicals compete with each other for plasma–protein binding sites. Some agents have a greater affinity for the binding sites and displace other agents from the plasma proteins. The displaced drug can reach high levels and produce adverse effects.

LEARNING OUTCOME 8

Identify major processes by which drugs are excreted.

Concepts for Lecture

1. The primary site of excretion is the kidney. Ionized and water-soluble drugs are filtered at the glomerulus and remain in the filtrate for excretion. Drug–protein complexes are sometimes secreted into the distal tubule of the nephron. Secretion mechanisms are less active in infants and older adults. Certain drugs may be excreted more quickly if the pH of the filtrate is changed.
2. Renal failure will diminish excretion of medications, and drugs are retained for extended times, so dosages must be reduced.
3. Drugs may be excreted by other organs. Drugs that can be changed into a gaseous form are excreted by the respiratory system. Respiratory

POWERPOINT SLIDES

SUGGESTIONS FOR CLASSROOM ACTIVITIES

- Have students give examples of drugs that are lipid soluble.
- Discuss what drugs are stored in adipose tissues.

SUGGESTION FOR CLINICAL ACTIVITIES

- Have students develop a nursing care plan instructing a pregnant woman about the risk of using any types of drugs, alcohol, tobacco products, or herbal products while pregnant.

POWERPOINT SLIDES

Figure 4.3 Plasma–Protein Binding and Drug Availability
Figure 4.4 First-Pass Effect

SUGGESTION FOR CLASSROOM ACTIVITIES

- Discuss why it is important for the anticoagulant warfarin (Coumadin) to remain bound to plasma proteins.

SUGGESTION FOR CLINICAL ACTIVITIES

- Have students research the percentage of medication bound to plasma proteins in patients receiving multiple drugs that are highly bound and the possible adverse effects.

POWERPOINT SLIDES

SUGGESTION FOR CLASSROOM ACTIVITIES

- Divide the class into four groups. One group will present examples of drugs secreted into the distal tubule, and the second group will present examples of drugs filtered at the glomerulus. The third group will present examples of drugs excreted through the respiratory system, and the fourth group will present examples of drugs excreted through glandular activity.

excretion of drugs depends on diffusion, gas solubility, and pulmonary blood flow. Water-soluble drugs may be eliminated in glandular secretions such as saliva, sweat, or breast milk. Some drugs are eliminated through biliary excretion.

LEARNING OUTCOME 9

Explain how enterohepatic recirculation might affect drug activity.

Concepts for Lecture

Some drugs are secreted in the bile. Most of the bile is circulated back to the liver by enterohepatic recirculation. A percentage of the drug may be recirculated with the bile numerous times and prolong the activity of the drug for several weeks after therapy has been discontinued.

LEARNING OUTCOME 10

Explain the applications of a drug's plasma half-life ($t_{1/2}$) to pharmacotherapy.

Concepts for Lecture

Plasma half-life is the length of time required for a medication to decrease concentration in the plasma by one-half after administration. The plasma half-life describes a drug's duration of action. The greater the half-life, the longer it takes a medication to be excreted. Drugs with short half-lives need to be given more frequently than drugs with long half-lives. The plasma half-life of a drug will increase in a patient with renal or hepatic disease, and to prevent toxic drug levels the drug is given less frequently or the dosage is reduced.

LEARNING OUTCOME 11

Explain how a drug reaches and maintains its therapeutic range in the plasma.

Concepts for Lecture

Repeated doses result in an accumulation of a drug in the bloodstream. A plateau is reached, and the level of the drug in the plasma is maintained continuously within the therapeutic range. At this level equilibrium occurs where the amount of drug administered is equal to the amount of drug eliminated, and there is a continuous therapeutic level of the drug that is being distributed to body tissues.

SUGGESTION FOR CLINICAL ACTIVITIES

- Have students develop a teaching plan for nursing mothers who are taking prescription drugs, OTC drugs, or herbal supplements.

POWERPOINT SLIDES

Figure 4.5 Enterohepatic Recirculation

SUGGESTION FOR CLASSROOM ACTIVITIES

- Discuss examples of drugs that have a prolonged activity because of enterohepatic recirculation.

SUGGESTION FOR CLINICAL ACTIVITIES

- Have students identify drugs of assigned patients who may undergo enterohepatic recirculation and the potential effects that may occur.

POWERPOINT SLIDES

Figure 4.6 Single-Dose Drug Administration

SUGGESTION FOR CLASSROOM ACTIVITIES

- Assign students selected drugs to research the plasma half-life of the drug. Have the students share the information in class and compare and contrast the frequency of the drugs.

SUGGESTION FOR CLINICAL ACTIVITIES

- Have students research the plasma half-life of the drugs on their assigned patients and the frequency of the drugs.

POWERPOINT SLIDES

SUGGESTION FOR CLASSROOM ACTIVITIES

- Present several situations with selected drugs, such as antibiotics, antihypertensive agents, antiasthma agents, and so on, when the therapeutic range was not maintained. Ask students what the resulting consequences to the patient could be.

© 2011 Pearson Education, Inc.

LEARNING OUTCOME 12

Differentiate between loading and maintenance doses.

Concepts for Lecture

1. A loading dose is a higher amount of drug given once or twice so the plateau is reached faster and the drug quickly produces a therapeutic response.
2. Maintenance doses are given to keep the plasma–drug concentration in the therapeutic range.

GENERAL CHAPTER CONSIDERATIONS

1. Have students study and learn key terms listed at the beginning of the chapter.
2. Have students complete end-of-chapter exercises either in their book or on the MyNursingKit website.
3. Use the Classroom Response Questions provided in PowerPoint to assess students prior to lecture.

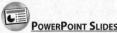

POWERPOINT SLIDES

Figure 4.7 Multiple-Dose Drug Administration

SUGGESTIONS FOR CLASSROOM ACTIVITIES

- Ask students for situations when a loading dose and when a maintenance dose of a drug are used.
- Invite a health care provider to speak to the class on the process and importance of loading and maintenance dosing of medications.

SUGGESTION FOR CLINICAL ACTIVITIES

- Have students research orders for specific cases of drugs ordered with a loading and a maintenance dose.

MYNURSINGKIT
(*www.mynursingkit.com*)

- Websites
- NCLEX® questions
- Critical Thinking Questions
- Case Studies
- Animations and Videos
- Drug Prototype Questions

MYNURSINGLAB
(*www.mynursinglab.com*)

- Knowledge Quick Check
- Pre/Posttests
- Customized study plans
- *Separate purchase*

STUDENT WORKBOOK AND RESOURCE GUIDE

- Chapter 4 activities
- *Separate purchase*

PEARSON NURSE'S DRUG GUIDE

- *Separate purchase*

PEARSON ETEXT

- Students can search, highlight, take notes, and more all in electronic format
- *Separate purchase*

CLASSROOM RESPONSE QUESTION POWERPOINTS

TESTBANK

Chapter 5
Pharmacodynamics

Learning Outcome 1

Apply principles of pharmacodynamics to clinical practice.

Concepts for Lecture

Knowing the principles of pharmacodynamics helps to predict whether a drug will produce a significant change in patients and provide safe and effective treatment for patients.

Learning Outcome 2

Discuss how frequency response curves may be used to explain how patients respond differently to medications.

Concepts for Lecture

A frequency distribution curve is a graphical representation of the number of patients responding to a drug action at different doses. The peak of the curve indicates the largest number of patients responding to the drug. See Figure 5.1.

Learning Outcome 3

Explain the importance of the median effective dose (ED_{50}) to clinical practice.

Concepts for Lecture

1. A drug's median effective dose (ED_{50}) is found in the middle of the frequency distribution curve and represents the dose required to produce a specific therapeutic response in 50 percent of a group of patients. Drug guides sometime report the ED_{50} as the "average" or "standard" dose. Many patients will require more or less than the average dose for optimum pharmacotherapy.
2. The skill of the nurse in observing the patient, taking vital signs, and monitoring laboratory data is critical in determining whether the average dose is effective for the patient.

 POWERPOINT SLIDES

 POWERPOINT SLIDES

Figure 5.1 Frequency Distribution Curve: Interpatient Variability in Drug Response

 SUGGESTION FOR CLASSROOM ACTIVITIES

- Display frequency distribution curves for different drugs, and ask students to explain the curves.

 SUGGESTION FOR CLINICAL ACTIVITIES

- For an assigned patient, have students select a drug, view the frequency distribution curve for that drug, and determine where on the curve the assigned patient is.

 POWERPOINT SLIDES

 SUGGESTION FOR CLASSROOM ACTIVITIES

- Ask students to determine the median effective dose in the frequency distribution curves displayed.

 SUGGESTION FOR CLINICAL ACTIVITIES

- Assign students a select drug, and have them determine its median effective dose. Then have the students check the medication reports of patients receiving that drug and what dosage the patient is receiving.

© 2011 Pearson Education, Inc.

LEARNING OUTCOME 4

Compare and contrast median lethal dose (LD_{50}) and median toxicity dose (TD_{50}).

Concepts for Lecture

1. The nurse can predict whether the dose is safe by looking at the frequency distribution curve of the drug. The median lethal dose (LD_{50}), as determined in preclinical trials, is the dose that will be lethal in 50 percent of a group of animals. It cannot be experimentally determined in humans.
2. The median toxicity dose (TD_{50}) is the dose that will produce a given toxicity in 50 percent of a group of patients. The median toxicity dose is a more practical value in a clinical setting. This value is extrapolated from animal data or based on adverse effects recorded in patient clinical trials.

LEARNING OUTCOME 5

Discuss how a drug's therapeutic index is related to its margin of safety.

Concepts for Lecture

1. The therapeutic index is a measure of a drug's safety margin; the higher the value, the safer the medication.
2. A drug's therapeutic index is the ratio of a drug's LD_{50} to its ED_{50}.
3. For example, if the therapeutic index of a drug were 4, it would take an error in magnitude of approximately four times the average dose to be lethal. See Figure 5.2 for examples of therapeutic indexes.

LEARNING OUTCOME 6

Identify the significance of the graded dose–response relationship to clinical practice.

Concepts for Lecture

There are three distinct phases of a dose–response curve that have relevance to clinical practice. Phase 1 occurs at the lowest doses, when few target cells have been affected by the drug. Phase 2 shows a linear relationship between the amount of drug administered and the degree of response obtained from the patient and is the most desirable range of doses for pharmacotherapeutics. In phase 3 a plateau is reached in which increasing the drug dose produces no additional therapeutic response. This may occur because all the receptors for the drug are occupied or the drug has brought 100 percent relief. In phase 3 increasing the dose does not result in a more therapeutic effect but may produce adverse effects. See Figure 5.3.

 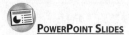
PowerPoint Slides

Suggestion for Classroom Activities

- Ask students to determine the median lethal dose and the median toxicity dose on the frequency distribution curves displayed.

Suggestion for Clinical Activities

- Assign students selected drugs, and ask them to determine the median lethal dose and the median toxicity dose of the selected drugs.

PowerPoint Slides

Figure 5.2 Therapeutic Index

Suggestion for Classroom Activities

- Have students calculate the therapeutic index for drugs in the same classification, such as antihypertensives, diuretics, or analgesics, and determine the drugs' margins of safety.

Suggestion for Clinical Activities

- Have students determine the therapeutic index of the drugs administered to assigned patients.

PowerPoint Slides

Figure 5.3 Dose-Response Relationship

Learning Outcome 7

Compare and contrast the terms *potency* and *efficacy*.

Concepts for Lecture

1. There are two ways to compare medications within therapeutic and pharmacologic classes: potency and efficacy.
2. A drug that is more potent will produce a therapeutic effect at a lower dose, compared to another drug in the same class. See Figure 5.4a.
3. Efficacy is the magnitude of maximal response that can be produced from a particular drug. See Figure 5.4b.
4. From a pharmacotherapeutic perspective, efficacy is almost always more important than potency.

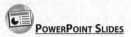

POWERPOINT SLIDES

Figure 5.4 Potency and Efficacy

Learning Outcome 8

Distinguish between an agonist, a partial agonist, and an antagonist.

Concepts for Lecture

1. An agonist is a drug that binds to a receptor and produces the same type of response as the endogenous chemical. Agonists sometimes produce a greater maximal response than the endogenous chemical.
2. A partial agonist is a drug that binds to a receptor and produces a weaker, or less efficacious, response than an agonist.
3. An antagonist is a drug that occupies a receptor and prevents the endogenous chemical from acting. Antagonists often compete with agonists for the receptor. Functional antagonists inhibit the effects of an agonist by changing pharmacokinetic factors.

POWERPOINT SLIDES

SUGGESTIONS FOR CLASSROOM ACTIVITIES

- Provide examples of drugs that act as agonists, antagonists, or partial agonists and the reasons for using these drugs.
- Have students provide examples of drug–drug interactions and drug–food interactions that act like agonists and antagonists.

SUGGESTION FOR CLINICAL ACTIVITIES

- On assigned patients have students determine if the drugs their patients are receiving act as agonists, partial agonists, or antagonists, and have them identify any drug–drug interactions or drug–food interactions that could act as agonists or antagonists.

Learning Outcome 9

Explain the relationship between receptors and drug action.

Concepts for Lecture

1. A receptor is a cellular macromolecule to which a drug binds to cause a change in body chemistry or physiology. The receptors' normal function is to bind endogenous molecules such as hormones, neurotransmitters, and growth factors. Most drug receptors are proteins. Receptors are associated with cellular plasma membranes and intracellular molecules such as DNA or enzymes in the cytoplasm.
2. A drug attaches to its receptor much like a key does to a lock. This triggers a series of second messenger events within the cell, which initiate the drug's action by either stimulating or inhibiting a normal activity of the cell.

POWERPOINT SLIDES

SUGGESTION FOR CLASSROOM ACTIVITIES

- Divide students into two groups. Have one group explain to the other students what happens when a drug attaches to a receptor in the cellular plasma membrane, and the other group explains what happens when a drug attaches to an intracellular molecule.

SUGGESTION FOR CLINICAL ACTIVITIES

- On an assigned patient have students explain the relationship of a drug action and receptor for a selected drug the patient is receiving.

© 2011 Pearson Education, Inc.

LEARNING OUTCOME 10

Explain possible future developments in the field of pharmacogenetics.

Concepts for Lecture

1. Pharmacogenetics is the area of pharmacology that examines the role of heredity in drug response. The greatest advances in pharmacogenetics have been the identification of subtle genetic differences in drug-metabolizing enzymes that are responsible for a significant portion of drug-induced toxicity.
2. Pharmacogenetics may someday allow for customized drug therapy by allowing patients to take a DNA test before receiving a drug, thus preventing idiosyncratic responses.

GENERAL CHAPTER CONSIDERATIONS

1. Have students study and learn key terms listed at the beginning of the chapter.
2. Have students complete end-of-chapter exercises either in their book or on the MyNursingKit website.
3. Use the Classroom Response Questions provided in PowerPoint to assess students prior to lecture.

POWERPOINT SLIDES

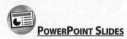
SUGGESTION FOR CLASSROOM ACTIVITIES

- Invite a pharmacist to speak about pharmacogenetics and drug therapy.

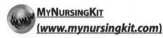
MYNURSINGKIT
(www.mynursingkit.com)

- Websites
- NCLEX® questions
- Critical Thinking Questions
- Case Studies
- Animations and Videos
- Drug Prototype Questions

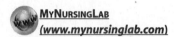
MYNURSINGLAB
(www.mynursinglab.com)

- Knowledge Quick Check
- Pre/Posttests
- Customized study plans
- *Separate purchase*

STUDENT WORKBOOK AND RESOURCE GUIDE

- Chapter 5 activities
- *Separate purchase*

PEARSON NURSE'S DRUG GUIDE

- *Separate purchase*

PEARSON eTEXT

- Students can search, highlight, take notes, and more all in electronic format
- *Separate purchase*

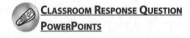
CLASSROOM RESPONSE QUESTION POWERPOINTS

TESTBANK

CHAPTER 6
THE NURSING PROCESS IN PHARMACOLOGY

LEARNING OUTCOME 1

Compare and contrast the different steps of the nursing process.

Concepts for Lecture

Review the steps of the nursing process: Assessment, diagnosis, outcome identification and planning, implementation, and evaluation.

POWERPOINT SLIDES

Figure 6.1 The Nursing Process

SUGGESTIONS FOR CLASSROOM ACTIVITIES

- Divide the class into five groups. Assign a step of the nursing process to each group to present to the entire class.
- Present a case study to the class, and ask the students to apply the steps of the nursing process to the case study.

SUGGESTION FOR CLINICAL ACTIVITIES

- Have students apply the steps of the nursing process to an assigned patient.

LEARNING OUTCOME 2

Identify assessment data that is pertinent to medication administration.

Concepts for Lecture

Assessment data that are pertinent to medication administration are health history information, physical assessment data, lab values and other measurable data, and assessment of medications' therapeutic effects and side effects.

POWERPOINT SLIDES

Table 6.1 Health History Assessment Questions Pertinent to Drug Administration

SUGGESTION FOR CLASSROOM ACTIVITIES

- Provide case studies, and have students identify pertinent data in administration of medication.

SUGGESTION FOR CLINICAL ACTIVITIES

- On an assigned patient, have students identify pertinent data in the administration of medication.

LEARNING OUTCOME 3

Develop appropriate nursing diagnoses for patients receiving medications.

Concepts for Lecture

1. Nursing diagnoses for drug administration are the same as diagnoses written for other patient condition-specific responses. They may address actual problems; focus on potential, or risk, problems; or deal with maintaining the patient's current level of wellness.

POWERPOINT SLIDES

Table 6.2 Common Nursing Diagnoses Applicable to Drug Administration

© 2011 Pearson Education, Inc.

2. Actual problems include the diagnostic statement, related factor or inferred cause, and evidence gathered to support the chosen statement.
3. Risk problems include the diagnostic statement and a related factor, or inferred cause.
4. Most common nursing diagnoses for medication administration are Knowledge Deficient and Noncompliance.
5. Nursing diagnoses applicable to drug administration are often collaborative problems that require communication with other health care providers.
6. Table 6.2 provides a list of some of the North American Nursing Diagnosis Association (NANDA)—approved diagnoses appropriate to drug administration. Examples include *Activity Intolerance, Risk for Falls, Urinary Incontinence,* and *Oral Mucous Membrane Impaired.* Consult books on nursing diagnoses for more information.

LEARNING OUTCOME 4

Plan realistic goals and outcomes for patients receiving medications.

Concepts for Lecture

1. Goals based on the nursing diagnosis established from the assessment data should be realistic and focus on what the patient should be able to achieve and do. These goals should be prioritized and discussed with the patient or caregiver. Goals may be short term or long term depending on the setting and situation. Safe and effective administration of medications is the overall goal. Goals should focus first on the therapeutic outcomes of medications, then on the treatment of side effects.
2. Outcomes provide the specific, measurable criteria that will be used to evaluate the degree to which the goal was met. Outcomes should be realistic and focus on what the patient will achieve or do. These outcomes should be discussed with the patient or caregiver. The written outcomes should include the subject, the actions required by the subject and under what circumstances, the expected performance, and the specific time frame in which the performance will be accomplished.

LEARNING OUTCOME 5

Discuss key intervention strategies to be implemented for patients receiving medications.

Concepts for Lecture

1. Interventions are aimed at returning the patient to an optimal level of wellness through the safe and effective administration of medications.
2. Key intervention strategies include the five rights and the techniques of administering medications discussed in Chapter 3, monitoring drug effects, documenting medications, and patient teaching.
3. Monitoring drug effects is a primary intervention. This includes identifying therapeutic effects, reassessing the patient's physical condition, taking vital signs, determining body weight, checking lab values and/or serum drug levels, taking a statement from the patient, and monitoring side and adverse effects.
4. Documentation is completed during the intervention phase. This includes documenting the when, where, and how of medication administration,

SUGGESTIONS FOR CLASSROOM ACTIVITIES

- Using the same case studies as in Objective 2, have the students develop nursing diagnoses for patients receiving medications.
- Divide students into two groups. Assign one group to develop a nursing diagnosis for a patient who lacks knowledge of a medication he is receiving. Assign the other group to develop a nursing diagnosis for a patient who is noncompliant regarding a medication.

SUGGESTION FOR CLINICAL ACTIVITIES

- Using the assigned patient in Objective 2, have students develop appropriate nursing diagnoses for the patient receiving medications.

POWERPOINT SLIDES

SUGGESTION FOR CLASSROOM ACTIVITIES

- Using the same case studies as in Objective 2, have students develop goals and outcomes for the patient receiving medications.

SUGGESTION FOR CLINICAL ACTIVITIES

- Using the same assigned patient in Objective 2, have students develop goals and outcomes during the planning stage for the patient receiving medications.

POWERPOINT SLIDES

Table 6.3 Important Areas of Teaching for a Patient Receiving Medications

SUGGESTION FOR CLASSROOM ACTIVITIES

- Using the same case studies in Objective 2, have students develop intervention strategies to be implemented for the patient receiving medications.
- Direct students to develop a teaching plan for a patient receiving medications who is noncompliant, for an elderly patient receiving medications, or a pediatric patient receiving medications.

both therapeutic and adverse effects; patient's statements; and objective assessment data, such as vital signs.

5. Patient teaching is a vital component of the interventions for the patient receiving medications. Knowledge deficit and noncompliance are directly related to the type and quality of medication education the patient receives. Elderly and pediatric patients present special challenges to patient teaching. The nurse may need to coteach the patient's caregiver.

LEARNING OUTCOME 6

Evaluate the outcomes of medication administration.

Concepts for Lecture

1. Evaluation is a checkpoint when the nurse considers the overall goal of safe and effective administration of medications, with the best therapeutic outcome possible, and takes the steps necessary to ensure success.

2. Evaluation begins a new cycle as new assessment data are gathered and analyzed, nursing diagnoses are reviewed or rewritten, goals and outcomes are refined, and new interventions are carried out.

GENERAL CHAPTER CONSIDERATIONS

1. Have students study and learn key terms listed at the beginning of the chapter.

2. Have students complete end-of-chapter exercises either in their book or on the MyNursingKit website.

3. Use the Classroom Response Questions provided in PowerPoint to assess students prior to lecture.

 SUGGESTIONS FOR CLINICAL ACTIVITIES

- Using the same assigned patient as in Objective 2, have the students implement intervention strategies for the receiving of medications.
- Have students develop a teaching plan for an assigned patient receiving medications.

 POWERPOINT SLIDES

 SUGGESTION FOR CLASSROOM ACTIVITIES

- Using the same case studies as in Objective 2, ask students what they would evaluate to determine if the goals and outcomes of administration of medications had been met.

 SUGGESTION FOR CLINICAL ACTIVITIES

- Using the same assigned patient in Objective 2, have the student evaluate the goals and outcomes and note any changes.

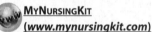 **MYNURSINGKIT (www.mynursingkit.com)**

- Websites
- NCLEX® questions
- Critical Thinking Questions
- Case Studies
- Animations and Videos
- Drug Prototype Questions

 MYNURSINGLAB (www.mynursinglab.com)

- Knowledge Quick Check
- Pre/Posttests
- Customized study plans
- *Separate purchase*

 STUDENT WORKBOOK AND RESOURCE GUIDE

- Chapter 6 activities
- *Separate purchase*

PEARSON NURSE'S DRUG GUIDE

- *Separate purchase*

 PEARSON ETEXT

- Students can search, highlight, take notes, and more all in electronic format
- *Separate purchase*

 CLASSROOM RESPONSE QUESTION POWERPOINTS

 TESTBANK

CHAPTER 7
DRUG ADMINISTRATION THROUGHOUT THE LIFESPAN

LEARNING OUTCOME 1

Describe physiological changes during pregnancy that may affect the absorption, distribution, metabolism, and excretion of drugs.

Concepts for Lecture

1. Absorption of medications takes longer due to the physiological and hormonal changes of pregnancy.
2. Distribution and metabolism of medications are directly related to hemodynamic changes in the pregnant patient.
3. Increased excretion of medications alters drug effectiveness.

POWERPOINT SLIDES

SUGGESTION FOR CLASSROOM ACTIVITIES

- Have students review anatomical changes of pregnancy and impact on specific drug classifications.

LEARNING OUTCOME 2

Describe the placental transfer of drugs from mother to infant.

Concepts for Lecture

1. The semipermeable membrane of the placenta allows substances to readily pass from the mother to the fetus.
2. Water-soluble drugs and those bound to plasma are less likely to cross the placenta.

POWERPOINT SLIDES

SUGGESTION FOR CLASSROOM ACTIVITIES

- Have students review the different types of transport across cell walls and membranes.

LEARNING OUTCOME 3

Match the five FDA pregnancy risk categories with their definitions.

Concepts for Lecture

1. The FDA has developed five pregnancy categories for drugs (A, B, C, D, and X) that classify medications according to their risks during pregnancy (see Table 7.1). Agents that cause fetal malformations are called teratogens.
2. Category A drugs: adequate, well-controlled studies with pregnant women have not shown an increased risk of fetal abnormalities.
3. Category B drugs: animal studies have revealed no harm to the fetus; however, there are no adequate, well-controlled studies with pregnant women—*or* animal studies have shown an adverse effect, but adequate, well-controlled studies with pregnant women have failed to demonstrate a risk to the fetus.
4. Category C drugs: animal studies have shown an adverse effect, and there are no adequate, well-controlled studies with pregnant women—*or* no animal studies have been conducted, and there are no adequate, well-controlled studies with pregnant women.
5. Category D drugs: studies, either adequate, well-controlled or observable, with pregnant women have demonstrated a risk to the fetus; however, the benefits of therapy may outweigh the potential risks.

POWERPOINT SLIDES

Table 7.1 FDA Pregnancy Categories

SUGGESTION FOR CLASSROOM ACTIVITIES

- Divide students into five groups. Assign a pregnancy drug category to each group and have the group give examples of drugs in the assigned category to the class.

SUGGESTION FOR CLINICAL ACTIVITIES

- Have students prepare a teaching plan for an assigned pregnant patient regarding drugs that are safe to take during pregnancy and drugs that are a potential risk or contraindicated during pregnancy.

LEARNING OUTCOME 4

Identify factors that influence the transfer of drugs into breast milk.

Concepts for Lecture

1. Drugs that are water soluble, ionized, and bound to plasma protein are less likely to enter breast milk.
2. Lipid-soluble medications are present in breast milk.
3. Timing of medication directly impacts transfer to breast milk.

LEARNING OUTCOME 5

Identify techniques that the breast-feeding mother can use to reduce drug exposure to the newborn.

Concepts for Lecture

The nurse will complete a thorough history and prenatal assessment to identify potential risks to the mother and unborn child.

LEARNING OUTCOME 6

Explain how differences in pharmacokinetic variables can impact drug response in pediatric patients.

Concepts for Lecture

Physiological changes, immature body systems, and greater fluid distribution in children directly impact the pediatric patient's response to medication.

LEARNING OUTCOME 7

Discuss the nursing and pharmacologic implications associated with each pediatric developmental age group.

Concepts for Lecture

Refer to Chapters 13–48 for care plans specific to medications found in each chapter.

POWERPOINT SLIDES

Table 7.2 Selected Drugs Associated with Adverse Effects During Breast-feeding

SUGGESTION FOR CLASSROOM ACTIVITIES

- Assign students different classifications of drugs. Have students identify the influence these meds have on breast milk and the risk to the infants.

SUGGESTION FOR CLINICAL ACTIVITIES

- Have students prepare a teaching plan for a breast-feeding mother and include substances that may appear in milk and cause adverse effects in the infant.

POWERPOINT SLIDES

SUGGESTION FOR CLASSROOM ACTIVITIES

- Have students identify the components of a thorough prenatal assessment and practice taking a thorough assessment. Discuss how the nurse would ask questions related to substance abuse and recreational drug usage.

SUGGESTION FOR CLINICAL ACTIVITIES

- Have students review records of assigned patients to determine risk factors to the mother and unborn child or infant.

POWERPOINT SLIDES

© 2011 Pearson Education, Inc.

LEARNING OUTCOME 8

Describe the physiological and biochemical changes that occur in the older adult, and how these affect pharmacotherapy.

Concepts for Lecture

1. Absorption of drugs is affected by delayed gastric emptying, changes in gastric pH and reduced blood flow to the GI tract.
2. Changes in body fat, alterations in production of proteins by the liver result in decreased protein-binding ability and increased circulation of free medications.
3. The aging liver has a decreased rate of metabolism of medications that reduces the first-pass metabolism resulting in a more prolonged and intensified drug response.
4. Excretion of medications through the kidneys results from diminished renal blood flow and glomerular filtration rate. The older adult patient is at an increased risk for drug toxicity.

LEARNING OUTCOME 9

Develop nursing interventions that maximize pharmacotherapeutic outcomes in the older adult.

Concepts for Lecture

1. Identify the risk factors associated with polypharmacy in the older adult.
2. Discuss factors that impact the older adult's ability to safely manage self-medication administration.
3. Identify nursing interventions that can enhance patient safety with self-medication administration.

 POWERPOINT SLIDES

 SUGGESTION FOR CLASSROOM ACTIVITIES

- Have students develop a patient teaching plan on medication safety for the older adult.

 SUGGESTION FOR CLINICAL ACTIVITIES

- Have students review the medications ordered for an older adult patient and review laboratory results related to liver and renal function. Have students assess patients for signs of drug toxicity related to the medications ordered.

 REFERENCE

- Drug metabolism and drug interactions in the elderly: *www.ncbi.nlm.nih.gov/pubmed/11866484*

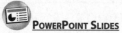 **POWERPOINT SLIDES**

SUGGESTIONS FOR CLASSROOM ACTIVITIES

- Have students divide into groups and assign each group a major body system. The group can identify changes in the system and how they impact effectiveness in the older adult.
- Each group can identify teaching strategies to overcome the changes they have identified.

GENERAL CHAPTER CONSIDERATIONS

1. Have students study and learn key terms listed at the beginning of the chapter.
2. Have students complete end-of-chapter exercises either in their book or on the MyNursingKit website.
3. Use the Classroom Response Questions provided in PowerPoint to assess students prior to lecture.

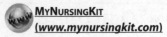

MyNursingKit
(www.mynursingkit.com)

- Websites
- NCLEX® questions
- Critical Thinking Questions
- Case Studies
- Animations and Videos
- Drug Prototype Questions

MyNursingLab
(www.mynursinglab.com)

- Knowledge Quick Check
- Pre/Posttests
- Customized study plans
- *Separate purchase*

STUDENT WORKBOOK AND RESOURCE GUIDE

- Chapter 7 activities
- *Separate purchase*

PEARSON NURSE'S DRUG GUIDE

- *Separate purchase*

PEARSON eTEXT

- Students can search, highlight, take notes, and more all in electronic format
- *Separate purchase*

CLASSROOM RESPONSE QUESTION
POWERPOINTS

TESTBANK

© 2011 Pearson Education, Inc.

CHAPTER 8
PSYCHOSOCIAL, GENDER, AND CULTURAL INFLUENCES ON PHARMACOTHERAPY

LEARNING OUTCOME 1

Describe fundamental concepts underlying a holistic approach to patient care and their importance to pharmacotherapy.

Concepts for Learning

The holistic approach to pharmacology helps us better understand how established risk factors influence pharmacotherapeutic outcomes. These risk factors are age, genetics, biologic characteristics, personal habits, lifestyle, and environment. Each person must be viewed as an integrated biological, psychosocial, cultural, and communicating whole person.

POWERPOINT SLIDES

SUGGESTION FOR CLASSROOM ACTIVITIES

- Divide the class into six groups. Assign a risk factor to each group, and ask the group to give examples of the assigned risk factor and how the examples influence pharmacotherapeutic outcomes. Provide time for groups to share information with the class.

SUGGESTION FOR CLINICAL ACTIVITIES

- On an assigned patient, have the student identify the risk factors and evaluate how the risk factors influence the patient's pharmacotherapeutic outcomes.

LEARNING OUTCOME 2

Describe the components of the human integration pyramid model.

Concepts for Lecture

1. The human integration pyramid model (Figure 10.1) provides a basic framework of the functional environment and interrelationships in which human beings exist. These dimensions can greatly impact the success of pharmacotherapy, but unfortunately, they are often overlooked.
2. The human integration pyramid model includes age, gender, genetic predisposition, community-environment factors, cultural and ethnic perspectives, and psychological-social-spiritual needs.

POWERPOINT SLIDES

Figure 8.1 The Human Integration Pyramid Care Model

SUGGESTION FOR CLASSROOM ACTIVITIES

- Divide the class into six groups. Assign one of the categories of the human integration pyramid to each group, and have the group describe the category, with examples to the class.

SUGGESTION FOR CLINICAL ACTIVITIES

- On an assigned patient, have the student use the human integration pyramid model to describe how these dimensions might affect the outcomes of pharmacotherapy for the patient

LEARNING OUTCOME 3

Identify psychosocial and spiritual factors that can affect pharmacotherapeutics.

Concepts for Lecture

1. Strong spiritual or religious beliefs can affect the outcomes of pharmacotherapy. Issues such as suffering, loneliness, despair, death, and hope can impact pharmacotherapy.

POWERPOINT SLIDES

SUGGESTION FOR CLASSROOM ACTIVITIES

- Ask students to describe psychosocial and spiritual factors that influence their pharmacotherapy outcomes.

© 2011 Pearson Education, Inc.

2. Patients who are convinced that their treatment is important and beneficial to their well-being demonstrate better compliance with drug therapy.
3. Outcomes of pharmacotherapy are influenced by issues such as past experiences with medications or acceptability of taking drugs at school or in the workplace. In addition, certain medications may carry a social stigma for some patients, and they may resist taking these drugs. A patient's attitude toward her personal health and expectations regarding the result of pharmacotherapy may also impact outcomes.

 SUGGESTION FOR CLINICAL ACTIVITIES

- On an assigned patient, have students identify psychosocial and spiritual factors that can influence the outcome of the patient's pharmacotherapy.

LEARNING OUTCOME 4

Explain how ethnicity can affect pharmacotherapeutic outcomes.

Concepts for Lecture

1. Ethnicity refers to biologic and genetic similarities of a community of people and sharing of distinctive social and cultural traditions. The beliefs also include a shared perception of health and illness.
2. Structural variants in metabolic enzymes appear more frequently in certain ethnic groups and have an impact on pharmacotherapeutics.
3. Some variables among a cultural or ethnic group that may impact pharmacotherapy include diet, alternative therapies, beliefs of health and disease, and genetics.

 POWERPOINT SLIDES

 SUGGESTION FOR CLASSROOM ACTIVITIES

- Divide the class into several groups. Assign a specific culture or ethnic group to each group. Have each group identify variables based on the cultural or ethnic beliefs that may impact pharmacotherapy outcomes.

 SUGGESTION FOR CLINICAL ACTIVITIES

- Have students identify cultural or ethnic variables on assigned patients that may impact pharmacotherapy.

LEARNING OUTCOME 5

Identify examples of how cultural values and beliefs can influence pharmacotherapeutic outcomes.

Concepts for Lecture

1. Every culture has a unique set of foods and spices, which may affect pharmacotherapy.
2. Many cultural groups believe in using herbs and other alternative therapies, either along with or in place of modern medicines.
3. Each culture has distinct ways of viewing sickness and health.

 POWERPOINT SLIDES

 SUGGESTION FOR CLASSROOM ACTIVITIES

- Divide the class into three groups. Assign one group to research diets of different cultures and the effect on pharmacotherapeutics, one group to research alternative therapies used by different cultures and the effect on pharmacotherapeutics, and one group to research different cultural views of sickness and health and the effect on pharmacotherapeutics. Provide time for groups to share information with the entire class. Invite people from different cultures to share information regarding diet, alternative therapies, and beliefs of health and disease.

 SUGGESTION FOR CLINICAL ACTIVITIES

- On an assigned patient, have the student identify cultural values and beliefs that can influence pharmacotherapeutic outcomes.

© 2011 Pearson Education, Inc.

LEARNING OUTCOME 6

Explain how community and environmental factors can affect health care outcomes.

Concepts for Lecture

1. Population growth, complex technology advances, and evolving globalization patterns affect health care.
2. Urbanization levels, age distributions, socioeconomic levels, occupational patterns, and industrial growth of communities have the potential to affect health and access to pharmacotherapy.
3. Access to health care is one of the most significant community-related influences on pharmacotherapy. Several obstacles, such as inadequate health insurance, cost of treatment and drugs, and limited medical care in rural areas, may prevent patients from obtaining appropriate health care.
4. Literacy is another community-related influence on pharmacotherapy. As much as 48 percent of the population of English-speaking patients are not functionally literate. This factor may prevent the patient from being able to read drug labels, understand written treatment instructions, read brochures regarding medication or disease, or understand the importance of pharmacotherapy.

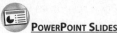
POWERPOINT SLIDES

SUGGESTIONS FOR CLASSROOM ACTIVITIES

- Have students identify community and environmental factors in the surrounding area that have the potential to affect health and access to pharmacotherapy.
- Have a local community-health representative speak to the students regarding community and environmental factors that influence pharmacotherapy in your community.

SUGGESTION FOR CLINICAL ACTIVITIES

- On an assigned patient, ask students to identify community and environmental factors that have the potential to affect health and access to pharmacotherapy.

LEARNING OUTCOME 7

Convey how genetic polymorphisms can influence pharmacotherapy.

Concepts for Lecture

1. Genetic polymorphisms are created when a mutation occurs in the portion of DNA responsible for encoding a certain metabolic enzyme. A single-base mutation in DNA may result in an amino acid change in the enzyme, which changes its function.
2. The change in the enzyme may increase or decrease the metabolism of certain drugs, depending on the exact type of genetic polymorphism.
3. The genetic polymorphisms are most often identified in specific ethnic groups and can be amplified within an ethnic population because people in an ethnic group are located in the same geographical area and marry others within the same ethnic group for hundreds of generations.

POWERPOINT SLIDES

Table 8.1 Enzyme Polymorphisms of Importance to Pharmacotherapy

SUGGESTIONS FOR CLASSROOM ACTIVITIES

- Ask students to identify genetic polymorphisms within ethnic groups that can affect drug metabolism.
- Invite a specialist in pharmacogenetics to speak to the class on genetic polymorphisms within specific ethnic groups and how metabolism of certain drugs can be affected.

SUGGESTION FOR CLINICAL ACTIVITIES

- On an assigned patient, have students identify possible genetic polymorphisms related to the patient's ethnic group and if any of the medications the patient is receiving may be involved.

LEARNING OUTCOME 8

Relate the implications of gender to the actions of certain drugs.

Concepts for Lecture

1. Acceptance or rejection of the use of particular categories of medications may be gender based because of the side effects associated with certain medications.

POWERPOINT SLIDES

SUGGESTION FOR CLASSROOM ACTIVITIES

- Have students research FDA studies that identify gender-specific actions of certain drugs and present this information to the class.

© 2011 Pearson Education, Inc.

2. Local and systemic responses in some medications can differ between genders. These response differences may be based on differences in body composition, cerebral blood-flow variances, or differences in elimination rate of a drug.
3. Since 1993 the FDA has required drug-research studies to include subjects of both genders, do analyses of clinical data by gender and assessment of potential pharmacokinetic and pharmacodynamic differences between genders, and conduct additional studies specific to women's health. Employers' health plans cannot exclude prescription drug coverage because of gender.

GENERAL CHAPTER CONSIDERATIONS

1. Have students study and learn key terms listed at the beginning of the chapter.
2. Have students complete end-of-chapter exercises either in their book or on the MyNursingKit website.
3. Use the Classroom Response Questions provided in PowerPoint to assess students prior to lecture.

SUGGESTION FOR CLINICAL ACTIVITIES

- After the FDA studies presentations listed in Suggestions for Classroom Activities have been presented, have students identify any gender-specific actions of drugs on assigned patients.

MYNURSINGKIT (*www.mynursingkit.com*)

- Websites
- NCLEX® questions
- Critical Thinking Questions
- Case Studies
- Animations and Videos
- Drug Prototype Questions

MYNURSINGLAB (*www.mynursinglab.com*)

- Knowledge Quick Check
- Pre/Posttests
- Customized study plans
- *Separate purchase*

STUDENT WORKBOOK AND RESOURCE GUIDE

- Chapter 8 activities
- *Separate purchase*

PEARSON NURSE'S DRUG GUIDE

- *Separate purchase*

PEARSON eTEXT

- Students can search, highlight, take notes, and more all in electronic format
- *Separate purchase*

CLASSROOM RESPONSE QUESTION POWERPOINTS

TESTBANK

© 2011 Pearson Education, Inc.

CHAPTER 9
MEDICATION ERRORS AND RISK REDUCTION

LEARNING OUTCOME 1

Define medication error.

Concepts for Lecture

1. A medication error is "any preventable event that may cause or lead to inappropriate medication use or patient harm while the medication is in the control of the health care professional, patient, or consumer." This definition comes from the National Coordinating Council for Medication Error Reporting and Prevention and may be applied to misinterpretations, miscalculations, misadministration, handwriting misinterpretation, and misunderstanding of verbal or phone orders.
2. Medication errors impede pharmacotherapeutic outcomes, possibly leading to illness or death. In addition, medication errors may result in legal ramifications for the nurse, physician, and/or health care agency. Medication errors continue to be a significant problem in health care.

LEARNING OUTCOME 2

Identify factors that contribute to medication errors.

Concepts for Lecture

1. Factors that may contribute to medication errors by the health care provider include omitting one of the five rights of drug administration. See Chapter 4 for a review of the five rights. Additional factors are failing to perform an agency system check; failing to take into account patient variables such as age, body size, and renal or hepatic function; giving medications based on verbal orders or phone orders, which may be misinterpreted or go undocumented; giving medication based on an incomplete order or an illegible order; and when the nurse is unsure of the correct drug, dosage, or administration method and is practicing under stressful work conditions.
2. The patient contributes to medication errors by taking drugs prescribed by several practitioners without informing those health care providers about all prescribed medications; getting prescriptions filled at more than one pharmacy; not filling or refilling prescriptions; and taking medications incorrectly or taking medications that may be left over from a previous illness or were prescribed for something else.

POWERPOINT SLIDES

Figure 9.1 Medication Error Index

SUGGESTIONS FOR CLASSROOM ACTIVITIES

- Review the roles of the nurse when administering a medication.
- Invite an attorney to speak to students about the possible legal ramifications of medication errors.

SUGGESTION FOR CLINICAL ACTIVITIES

- Have students observe administration of medication on an assigned patient.

POWERPOINT SLIDES

Table 9.1 Abbreviations to Avoid in Medication Administration

SUGGESTIONS FOR CLASSROOM ACTIVITIES

- Discuss the importance of the five rights in drug administration.
- Have the students practice the five rights of drug administration in the laboratory setting.

SUGGESTION FOR CLINICAL ACTIVITIES

- Supervise the student demonstrating the five rights of drug administration on an assigned patient.

LEARNING OUTCOME 3

Describe specific categories of medication errors.

Concepts for Lecture

Examples of common errors related in medication administration include giving an incorrect dose, not giving an ordered dose, and giving an unordered drug. In order to help prevent medication errors, pharmacists and nurses should collaborate on checking the accuracy and appropriateness of drug orders prior to administration. Nurses not reviewing recent laboratory data and other pertinent data in the patient's chart prior to medication administration make additional medication errors. Verbal and telephone orders that have not been written by the prescriber and lack of clarifying questions regarding correct drugs, dosages, and/or routes of administration may also lead to medication errors. Errors also occur when an incomplete or illegible order is received or when confusing abbreviations are used. Additionally, nurses should not administer medications they are not familiar with until they consult a drug reference. See Table 9.1 for a complete list of recommendations.

LEARNING OUTCOME 4

Explain the impact of medication errors on all aspects of a health care agency.

Concepts for Lecture

Medication errors are the most common cause of morbidity and preventable death within hospitals. The repercussions of an error are emotionally devastating for the nurse and extend beyond the particular nurse and patient involved. The error can increase the patient's length of stay in the hospital, which increases costs and the time a patient is separated from his family. If a high error rate occurs within a particular unit, the nursing unit may develop a poor reputation within the facility. If frequent medication errors are publicized, the reputation of the facility may suffer. Administration personnel may also be penalized because of errors within their department or hospital as a whole.

LEARNING OUTCOME 5

Describe methods of documenting medication errors and occurrences.

Concepts for Lecture

1. It is always the nurse's legal and ethical responsibility to report all occurrences of medication errors. Facility policies and procedures provide information on reporting medication errors. Documentation should occur in a factual manner: The nurse should avoid blaming or making judgments. Documentation in the medical record must include specific nursing interventions that were implemented following the error to protect patient safety, such as monitoring vital signs and assessing the patient for possible complications. Failure to document nursing actions implies negligence or failure to acknowledge that the incident occurred. Document all individuals who were notified of the error. The medication administration record (MAR) is a source that should contain information about what medication was given or omitted.

 POWERPOINT SLIDES

Table 9.1 Abbreviations to Avoid in Medication Administration

 SUGGESTION FOR CLASSROOM ACTIVITIES

- Design a quiz reviewing approved abbreviations for medication orders.

 SUGGESTION FOR CLINICAL ACTIVITIES

- Have each student demonstrate the three checks of drug administration on an assigned patient.

 POWERPOINT SLIDES

 SUGGESTIONS FOR CLASSROOM ACTIVITIES

- Have students divide into teams to represent the patient, nurse, nursing manager, and administration to discuss the impact of various medication errors on each individual.
- Invite a local hospital's risk manager to speak about medication errors and the impact on all persons involved.

 POWERPOINT SLIDES

 SUGGESTION FOR CLASSROOM ACTIVITIES

- Practice proper charting of a medication error.

 SUGGESTION FOR CLINICAL ACTIVITIES

- Review the facility's policy and procedure for reporting a medication error.

© 2011 Pearson Education, Inc.

2. In addition to documentation in the patient's medical record, the nurse making or observing the medication error should complete a written incident report. Again, the details should be recorded in a factual and objective manner. The incident report allows the nurse an opportunity to identify factors that contributed to the medication error. This report is not included in the patient's record.

3. Accurate documentation is essential for legal reasons. The documentation verifies that the patient's safety was protected and serves as a tool to improve medication administration processes. Hospital and agencies monitor medication errors through quality-improvement programs. Specific solutions can be created to reduce the number of medication errors.

4. Sentinel events require an investigation and implementation of interventions to prevent a reoccurrence.

LEARNING OUTCOME 6

Describe strategies that the nurse can implement to reduce medication errors and incidents.

Concepts for Lecture

Avoiding medication errors and promoting safe administration begins with utilizing the nursing process. The four steps involved are assessment, planning, implementation, and evaluation. The assessment step could include asking the patient about allergies to food or medication, current health concerns, and use of over-the-counter medications and herbal supplements. Ensure that the five rights of administration are followed. Review recent physical assessment of the patient, as well as recent laboratory tests, and determine if impairment is noted that could impact pharmacotherapy. Identify patients' need of education concerning their medication regimen. The planning step can minimize factors that contribute to medication errors: Avoid using abbreviations that can be misunderstood, question unclear orders, do not accept verbal orders, and follow specific facility policies and procedures related to medication administration. Ask the patient to participate by restating the right time and dose of medication. The implementation step would include being aware of potential distractions during medication administration and removing the distractions, if possible. Focus on the task of administering medications. Practice the five rights of medication administration. The evaluation step would be to assess the patient for expected outcomes and determine if any adverse effects have occurred.

LEARNING OUTCOME 7

Identify patient teaching information that can be used to reduce medication errors and incidents.

Concepts for Lecture

1. An important strategy for avoiding medication errors is to educate the patient. The nurse needs to provide written, age-appropriate handouts, and/or audiovisual teaching aids about the medications and provide contact information about whom to notify in the event of an adverse reaction.

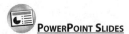 **POWERPOINT SLIDES**

 SUGGESTION FOR CLASSROOM ACTIVITIES

- Have the students break into four teams, with each team being assigned a specific step of the nursing process, and identify ways to reduce medication errors and promote patient safety.

 SUGGESTION FOR CLINICAL ACTIVITIES

- Have students discuss their plan for having a safe medication pass on their assigned patients.

 POWERPOINT SLIDES

 SUGGESTION FOR CLASSROOM ACTIVITIES

- Simulate a patient-teaching situation.

SUGGESTION FOR CLINICAL ACTIVITIES

- Have the student observe or participate in a patient-teaching situation concerning the patient's medications, and report it to the class.

2. Additionally, nurses should teach the patient to:
   a. Know the names of all medications they are taking, their use, when they should be taken, and their doses
   b. Know what side effects need to be reported immediately
   c. Read the label prior to each drug administration, and use the medication device that comes with liquid medications rather than household measuring spoons
   d. Carry a list of all medications, including OTC drugs, as well as herbal and dietary supplements that are being taken; if possible, use one pharmacy for all prescriptions
   e. Ask questions; health care providers want to be partners in maintaining safe medication principles

LEARNING OUTCOME 8

Identify efforts recommended by the FDA to monitor medication errors and incidents and provide information to health care providers.

Concepts for Lecture

The FDA's Med Watch, the Institute of Safe Medication Practices (ISMP), and MedMarx are three agencies that track medication errors and provide a database of error incidents, types, and levels of harm for health care professionals and/or consumers.

LEARNING OUTCOME 9

Explain strategies used by health care organizations to reduce the number of medication errors and incidents.

Concepts for Lecture

Health care organizations are using various methods to reduce the number of medication errors and incidents. The trend is for automated, computerized, locked cabinets for medication storage on patient-care units. Each nurse has a code for accessing the cabinet and removing the medication dose. This system also maintains an inventory of drug supplies. Some large health care agencies have risk-management departments to examine risks and minimize the number of medication errors. The risk-management personnel investigate incidents, track data, identify problems, and provide recommendations for improvement. They collaborate with nursing to modify policies and procedures.

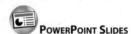

POWERPOINT SLIDES

SUGGESTION FOR CLASSROOM ACTIVITIES

- Separate students into three evenly divided groups. Assign each group one of the agencies that collect and report medication errors, and have them present their information to the class.

SUGGESTION FOR CLINICAL ACTIVITIES

- Have students attend a risk-management team meeting.

© 2011 Pearson Education, Inc.

General Chapter Considerations

1. Have students study and learn key terms listed at the beginning of the chapter.
2. Have students complete end-of-chapter exercises either in their book or on the MyNursingKit website.
3. Use the Classroom Response Questions provided in PowerPoint to assess students prior to lecture.

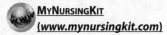 **MyNursingKit (www.mynursingkit.com)**

- Websites
- NCLEX® questions
- Case studies
- Making the Patient Connection

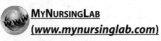 **MyNursingLab (www.mynursinglab.com)**

- Knowledge Quick Check
- Pre/Posttests
- Customized study plans
- *Separate purchase*

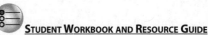 **Student Workbook and Resource Guide**

- Chapter 9 activities
- *Separate purchase*

Pearson Nurse's Drug Guide

- *Separate purchase*

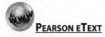 **Pearson eText**

- Students can search, highlight, take notes, and more all in electronic format
- *Separate purchase*

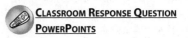 **Classroom Response Question PowerPoints**

 Testbank

CHAPTER 10
HERBAL AND ALTERNATIVE THERAPIES

LEARNING OUTCOME 1

Explain the role of complementary and alternative medicine in promoting patient wellness.

Concepts for Lecture

1. Complementary and alternative medicine (CAM) was considered to be outside mainstream health care, but given its growing popularity with both health care providers and their patients, the dividing line between the two is constantly changing. The major characteristics of CAM include focusing on treating each person as an individual, considering the health of the whole person, and emphasizing the integration of mind and body. Additional characteristics of CAM are promoting disease prevention, self-care, and self-healing and recognizing the role of spirituality in health and healing.
2. There has not been sufficient research on CAM therapies to definitively determine their effectiveness or lack of effectiveness.
3. CAM healing methods include biologically based therapies, such as herbal therapies, nutritional supplements, and special diets; alternate health care systems, including naturotherapy, homeopathy, chiropractic, Native American medicine (sweat lodges and medicine wheels), and Chinese traditional medicine (acupuncture and Chinese herbals); manual healing, such as massage, pressure-point therapies, and hand-medicated biofield therapies; mind-body interventions, including yoga, meditation, hypnotherapy, guided imagery, biofeedback, and movement-oriented therapies (music and dance); spiritual methods, which include shamans, faith, and prayer; and other therapies such as bioelectromagnetics, detoxifying therapies, and animal-assisted therapy.

POWERPOINT SLIDES

Table 10.1 Complementary and Alternative Therapies

SUGGESTION FOR CLASSROOM ACTIVITIES

- Have students discuss their opinions regarding the use of CAM.

SUGGESTION FOR CLINICAL ACTIVITIES

- Have students interview assigned patients regarding their understanding of CAM.

LEARNING OUTCOME 2

Analyze reasons why herbal and dietary supplements have increased in popularity.

Concepts for Lecture

1. One of the main reasons CAM has increased in popularity is the reduced need for medications. This reduction leads to fewer adverse side effects from medications, which lead to better compliance with those medications that are still taken in combination with the CAM.
2. Other factors that have contributed to the rise in the use of herbal and dietary supplements include increased availability of products, aggressive marketing, increased attention to natural alternatives, and renewed interest in preventive medicine.
3. The aging population is looking for therapeutic alternatives for chronic conditions such as pain, arthritis, hormone replacement therapy, and prostate difficulties.
4. The high cost of prescription medicines has also led patients to seek CAM therapies as alternatives that are less costly.

POWERPOINT SLIDES

Table 10.2 Best-selling Herbal Supplements, in Rank Order

SUGGESTION FOR CLASSROOM ACTIVITIES

- Have students list any types of CAM they use and any types of CAM that their family or friends use.

SUGGESTIONS FOR CLINICAL ACTIVITIES

- Have students assess their assigned patient's records and interview their patient regarding the use of any CAM therapies.
- Have students research the cost of selected prescription medications and alternative herbal or dietary supplements.

© 2011 Pearson Education, Inc.

LEARNING OUTCOME 3

Identify the parts of an herb that may contain active ingredients and the types of formulations made from these parts.

Concepts for Lecture

1. An herb, also referred to as a botanical, is a plant product with a useful purpose, for instance, as a food enhancer or as a medicine. Examples of herbal supplements and their applications include garlic, used to reduce blood cholesterol and blood pressure; soy, a source of protein, which is used for relief of menopausal symptoms and prevention of cardiovascular disease; St. John's wort, used to reduce depression and anxiety and as an anti-inflammatory; cranberry, which is used to prevent urinary tract infections; ginseng, believed to relieve stress and fatigue and to enhance the immune system; and bilberry, which is used to terminate diarrhea and improve and protect vision and which is also an antioxidant.

2. The active ingredient(s) in herbs may be present in only one specific part of the plant or in all parts; therefore, it is important for patients who use herbs for home use to know which portion of the plant contains the active ingredient.

3. Solid and liquid are the two basic formulations of herbs. Solid products made from dried herbs include pills, tablets, and capsules. Solids are also used topically and include salves and ointments. Liquids are made by extracting active chemicals from the plant and mixing the chemicals with a solvent (refer to Table 11.4). Examples of liquids include tea, made from fresh or dried herbs and soaked in hot water for five to ten minutes; infusions, made from fresh or dried herbs soaked in hot water for at least 15 minutes; decoctions, made with fresh or dried herbs boiled in water for 30 to 60 minutes; tinctures, which are soaked in alcohol; and extracts, which use organic solvents to extract active ingredients from herbs.

LEARNING OUTCOME 4

Analyze the strengths and weaknesses of the Dietary Supplement Health and Education Act (DSHEA) of 1994.

Concepts for Lecture

1. The DSHEA is a less rigid regulatory act than the Food, Drug, and Cosmetic Act of 1936 (FDA) that approves prescription and over-the-counter (OTC) drugs. According to the DSHEA, dietary supplements are exempted from the FDA. Dietary supplements are defined by the FDA as diet enhancers or supplements and include herbs, vitamins, minerals, and metabolites.

2. Weaknesses of the DSHEA that mean the patient is less protected when using dietary supplements include lack of mandatory testing prior to marketing, as well as the manufacturer's not being mandated to prove efficacy or safety. In addition, the DSHEA does not ensure that the label of the product is accurate with regard to the product listed or amounts listed. Limitations of the DSHEA also allow labels to claim such effects as promoting a healthy immune system, reducing stress, aiding in maintaining cardiovascular function, and reducing pain and inflammation.

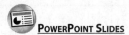

POWERPOINT SLIDES

Table 10.3 Standardization of Selected Herb Extracts

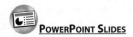

SUGGESTION FOR CLASSROOM ACTIVITIES

- Have students visit a health food store to determine five common herbal supplements and their uses.

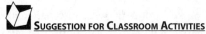

POWERPOINT SLIDES

Table 10.4 Liquid Formulations of Herbal Products

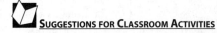

SUGGESTIONS FOR CLASSROOM ACTIVITIES

- Have students visit a health food store and read the label on five dietary supplements for product listings of amounts of active ingredients and components.
- Have students research DSHEA online, utilizing at least three sources.

Learning Outcome 5

Describe adverse effects that may be caused by herbal and dietary supplements.

Concepts for Learning

1. A key concept with alternative therapies is that "natural" does not always mean safer or better because some of the active chemicals are the same strength as those in currently approved prescription and OTC medications.
2. Allergic reactions can occur with the use of natural products. Most herbal products contain several different chemicals from the plants from which they are made. Therefore, it is better if initially the patient takes the smallest dose of an herbal therapy to determine if he has any allergies to the product.
3. "Specialty" supplements, such as chondroitin and glucosamine, are substances that occur naturally in the body. Taking additional amounts may or may not be beneficial and is generally not harmful unless taken in excessive amounts.

Learning Outcome 6

Discuss the role of the nurse in teaching patients about complementary and alternative therapies.

Concepts for Lecture

1. Nurses should not be judgmental of patients who utilize CAM therapies; rather, nurses should try to understand the patient's goal for the therapy.
2. Nurses need to seek the latest medical information on CAM therapies, since many patients are utilizing these therapies.
3. Nurses should educate patients on the strengths and weaknesses of CAM therapies and encourage patients to seek health information from reputable sources before making decisions on therapies.
4. Nurses should ensure that the patient does not have false hope of an easy cure for chronic conditions when using CAM therapy.
5. Nurses should take a complete health history of patients, being sure to ask specifically about the use of any CAM therapy. This action can avoid possible drug interactions as well as help the nurse in identifying any adverse reactions from the supplement alone.

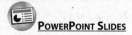
POWERPOINT SLIDES

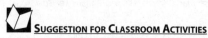
SUGGESTION FOR CLASSROOM ACTIVITIES

- Give students a list of specialty supplements to research to determine their action in the body.

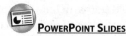
POWERPOINT SLIDES

Table 10.6 Selected Specialty Supplements

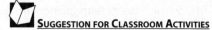
SUGGESTION FOR CLASSROOM ACTIVITIES

- Divide students into groups of three to five individuals, and assign specific CAM therapies to each group for students to present a teaching plan to the class.

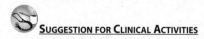
SUGGESTION FOR CLINICAL ACTIVITIES

- Have the students develop a teaching plan for assigned patients who are using CAM therapy.

© 2011 Pearson Education, Inc.

LEARNING OUTCOME 7

Identify common drug–herbal interactions.

Concepts for Learning

When obtaining a patient's health history, be sure to ask about the use of any dietary supplements, since many herbal products interact with prescription drugs. Common herbs that can cause drug-herbal interactions include (refer to Table 11.5 for a more complete list) echinacea, which interacts with amiodarone and anabolic steroids, resulting in possible increased hepatotoxicity; feverfew, ginger, ginkgo, and garlic interact with aspirin, heparin, NSAIDs, and warfarin, resulting in possible increased bleeding potential; garlic and ginseng interact with insulin and oral hypoglycemic agents, resulting in possible increased hypoglycemic effects. Additional herbs that can bring about drug-herbal interactions include ginkgo, which reacts with anticonvulsants, resulting in possible decreased anticonvulsant effectiveness, and with tricyclic antidepressants, possibly resulting in a decreased seizure threshold; ginseng and goldenseal, which react with diuretics, resulting in possible attenuation of diuretic effects; St. John's wort, ginseng, valerian, and kava kava, which react with CNS depressants, resulting in possible potentiation of sedation.

LEARNING OUTCOME 8

Explain how some herbal products are standardized based on specific active ingredients.

Concepts for Lecture

1. Herbs may contain many active chemicals that work together synergistically, but if isolated, do not have the same activity as modern drugs. The strength of herbal preparations may vary, depending on where they were grown and how they were collected and stored.
2. A marker substance has been used on some herbs to assist in standardization. Standardization, however, is difficult in herbal preparations because of the number of active ingredients in an herb, as opposed to a single active ingredient in most medications. One example is the attempted standardization of the ginkgo leaf. In 60 mg of the extract of a 50:1 ginkgo leaf, 24 percent ginkgo flavonglycosides are identified in standardization. Until further research is completed, the entire herb is considered the active ingredient rather than a single chemical.

POWERPOINT SLIDES

Table 10.5 Documented Herb-Drug Interactions

SUGGESTION FOR CLASSROOM ACTIVITIES

- Develop a *Jeopardy*-type game with common drug-herbal interactions.

SUGGESTION FOR CLINICAL ACTIVITIES

- Have students obtain a medication list and dietary supplement list from their assigned patients and determine possible drug-herbal interactions.

POWERPOINT SLIDES

Table 10.6 Selected Specialty Supplements

SUGGESTION FOR CLASSROOM ACTIVITIES

- Have students read the label on five herbal products and list the active ingredients and standardization markers, if present.

REFERENCE

- Herbal Remedies: Drug-Herb Interactions: *ccn.aacnjournals.org/cgi/content/full/22/2/22*

GENERAL CHAPTER CONSIDERATIONS

1. Have students study and learn key terms listed at the beginning of the chapter.
2. Have students complete end-of-chapter exercises either in their book or on the MyNursingKit website.
3. Use the Classroom Response Questions provided in PowerPoint to assess students prior to lecture.

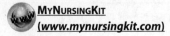

MYNURSINGKIT
(www.mynursingkit.com)

- Websites
- NCLEX® questions
- Critical Thinking Questions
- Case Studies
- Animations and Videos
- Drug Prototype Questions

MYNURSINGLAB
(www.mynursinglab.com)

- Knowledge Quick Check
- Pre/Posttests
- Customized study plans
- *Separate purchase*

STUDENT WORKBOOK AND RESOURCE GUIDE

- Chapter 10 activities
- *Separate purchase*

PEARSON NURSE'S DRUG GUIDE

- *Separate purchase*

PEARSON ETEXT

- Students can search, highlight, take notes, and more all in electronic format
- *Separate purchase*

CLASSROOM RESPONSE QUESTION
POWERPOINTS

TESTBANK

© 2011 Pearson Education, Inc.

CHAPTER 11
SUBSTANCE ABUSE

LEARNING OUTCOME 1

Explain underlying causes of addiction.

Concepts for Lecture

1. Addiction is an overwhelming compulsion that drives someone to repetitive drug-taking behavior, despite serious health and social consequences.
2. Addiction depends on multiple, complex, interacting variables such as agent or drug factors, user factors, and environmental factors.
3. The therapeutic use of scheduled drugs rarely causes addiction when they are used according to accepted medical protocols. Prescription medications having a potential for abuse are prescribed at the lowest effective dose and for the shortest time necessary to treat the medical problem.

LEARNING OUTCOME 2

Compare and contrast psychologic and physical dependence.

Concepts for Lecture

1. Substance dependence occurs when a person has an overwhelming desire to take a drug and cannot stop. It is classified in two categories: physical dependence and psychological dependence.
2. Physical dependence is an altered physical condition caused by the adapting of the nervous system to repeated substance use. Uncomfortable withdrawal symptoms result when the agent is discontinued. Opioids, alcohol, sedatives, some stimulants, and nicotine may easily produce physical dependence with extended use.
3. Psychological dependence produces no obvious signs of physical discomfort after each agent is discontinued. The user has an overwhelming desire to continue substance use despite obvious negative economic, physical, or social consequences. This strong psychological craving may be associated with the patient's home environment or social contacts. This craving may continue for months or even years and is often responsible for relapses during substance abuse therapy and a return to drug-seeking behavior. Psychological dependence usually occurs with high doses of marijuana or antianxiety drugs used for a prolonged time.

LEARNING OUTCOME 3

Compare withdrawal syndromes for the various substance abuse classes.

Concepts for Lecture

1. Withdrawal symptoms of opioids are excessive sweating, restlessness, dilated pupils, agitation, goose bumps, tremor, violent yawning, increased heart rate and blood pressure, nausea/vomiting, abdominal cramps and pain, muscle spasms, and weight loss.

 POWERPOINT SLIDES

 SUGGESTION FOR CLASSROOM ACTIVITIES

- Invite a nurse or counselor from a drug and/or alcohol treatment facility to speak about addiction and its causes.

 SUGGESTION FOR CLINICAL ACTIVITIES

- Assign students to observe and note the causes of addiction of patients at a drug and/or alcohol treatment facility.

 POWERPOINT SLIDES

 SUGGESTION FOR CLASSROOM ACTIVITIES

- Invite a nurse or counselor from a drug and/or alcohol treatment facility to talk about physical dependence and psychological dependence.

 SUGGESTION FOR CLINICAL ACTIVITIES

- Ask students to observe and note physical dependence and psychological dependence in patients at a drug and/or alcohol treatment facility.

 POWERPOINT SLIDES

Table 11.1 Selected Drugs of Abuse, Withdrawal Symptoms and Characteristics

© 2011 Pearson Education, Inc.

2. Withdrawal symptoms of barbiturates and similar sedative-hypnotics are insomnia, anxiety, weakness, abdominal cramps, tremor, anorexia, seizures, skin-hypersensitivity reactions, hallucinations, and delirium.
3. Withdrawal symptoms of benzodiazepines are insomnia, restlessness, abdominal pain, nausea, sensitivity to light and sound, headache, fatigue, and muscle twitches.
4. Withdrawal symptoms of alcohol are tremors, fatigue, anxiety, abdominal cramping, hallucinations, confusion, seizures, and delirium.
5. Withdrawal symptoms of cocaine and amphetamines are mental depression, anxiety, extreme fatigue, and hunger.
6. Withdrawal symptoms of nicotine are irritability, anxiety, restlessness, headache, increased appetite, insomnia, inability to concentrate, and a decrease in heart rate and blood pressure.
7. Withdrawal symptoms of marijuana are irritability, restlessness, insomnia, tremor, chills, and weight loss.
8. Withdrawal symptoms of hallucinogens are rarely observed and are dependent on the specific drug.

LEARNING OUTCOME 4

Discuss how nurses can recognize drug tolerance in patients.

Concepts for Lecture

1. Tolerance is a biological condition that occurs when the body adapts to a substance after repeated administration. Higher doses of the agent are required to produce the same initial effect. Development of tolerance is common for substances that affect the nervous system. Tolerance is not evidence of addiction or substance abuse.
2. Tolerance does not develop at the same rate for all actions of a drug. Tolerances to some drug effects develop quickly, while other tolerances to a drug develop slowly or not at all.
3. Cross-tolerance may develop in closely related drugs, requiring adjustments in dosage to obtain the maximum therapeutic effect.
4. Immunity and resistance should not be used interchangeably with tolerance. These terms apply to the immune system or to infections, whereas tolerance applies to drugs.

LEARNING OUTCOME 5

In the following drug classes, explain the major characteristics of abuse, dependence, and tolerance: alcohol, nicotine, marijuana, hallucinogens, CNS stimulants, sedatives, and opioids.

Concepts for Lecture

1. Alcohol is a CNS depressant. Effects of alcohol are directly proportional to the amount consumed and include relaxation, sedation, memory impairment, loss of motor coordination, reduced judgment, and decreased inhibition. Chronic alcohol consumption produces both psychological and physiological dependence. The alcohol-withdrawal syndrome is severe and may be life-threatening.
2. Nicotine is legal, strongly addictive, and highly carcinogenic. Nicotine affects the nervous, cardiovascular, and endocrine systems. Effects on the nervous system are increased alertness and ability to focus, feelings of relaxation, and light-headedness. Cardiovascular effects are increased heart rate and blood pressure. The effect on the endocrine system is an

SUGGESTION FOR CLASSROOM ACTIVITIES

- Invite a nurse or counselor at a drug and/or alcohol treatment facility to talk about the different withdrawal symptoms for selected drugs of abuse.

SUGGESTION FOR CLINICAL ACTIVITIES

- Assign students to observe at a drug and/or alcohol treatment facility and note withdrawal symptoms among the patients.

POWERPOINT SLIDES

Table 11.1 Selected Drugs of Abuse, Withdrawal Symptoms and Characteristics

SUGGESTIONS FOR CLASSROOM ACTIVITIES

- Ask students to give examples of drugs to which tolerance may develop.
- Ask students to give examples of tolerances to drugs that develop quickly, slowly, or not at all and examples of drugs with cross-tolerance.

SUGGESTION FOR CLINICAL ACTIVITIES

- Ask students to observe for drug tolerance in assigned patients.

POWERPOINT SLIDES

SUGGESTION FOR CLASSROOM ACTIVITIES

- Ask a nurse or counselor at a drug and/or alcohol treatment facility to speak about the major characteristics of abuse, dependence, and tolerance for alcohol, nicotine, marijuana, hallucinogens, CNS stimulants, sedatives, and opioids.

SUGGESTION FOR CLINICAL ACTIVITIES

- Have students observe patients at a drug and/or alcohol treatment facility and note characteristics of abuse, dependence, and tolerance of alcohol, nicotine, marijuana, hallucinogens, CNS stimulants, sedatives, and/or opioids.

© 2011 Pearson Education, Inc.

increase in basal metabolic rate. Both psychological and physical dependence occur quickly.

3. Marijuana is the most commonly used illicit drug in the United States. Use of marijuana slows motor activity; decreases coordination; causes disconnected thoughts, feelings of paranoia, euphoria, thirst and craving for chocolate and other candies, and red or bloodshot eyes. Marijuana produces little physical dependence or tolerance.

4. Hallucinogens are Schedule I drugs. Effects are highly variable and dependent on the mood and expectations of the user and the surrounding environment in which the substance is used. Flashbacks, tolerance, and moderate-to-high psychological dependence may occur but little or no physical dependence.

5. CNS stimulants increase the activity of the central nervous system and produce a sense of exhilaration, improve mental and physical performance, reduce appetite, prolong wakefulness, or simply cause the user to "get high." CNS stimulants have high psychological dependence and less-severe physical signs.

6. Sedatives are prescribed for sleep disorders and certain forms of epilepsy. Physical dependence, psychological dependence, and tolerance develop when these agents are taken for extended periods at high doses. They are commonly combined with other drugs of abuse, such as CNS stimulants or alcohol. There is moderate-to-high psychological dependence and moderate-to-extreme physical signs of withdrawal with sedatives.

7. Opioids are prescribed for severe pain, persistent cough, and diarrhea. A range of CNS effects from extreme pleasure to slowed body activities and profound sedation occur with opioids. Signs include constricted pupils, an increase in the pain threshold, and respiratory depression. Addiction can occur rapidly, and withdrawal can produce intense symptoms. Opioids have a high psychological dependence.

LEARNING OUTCOME 6

Describe the role of the nurse in delivering care to individuals who have substance abuse issues.

Concepts for Lecture

1. The nurse serves a key role in the prevention, diagnosis, and treatment of substance abuse.
2. In the case of IV-drug users, the nurse must consider the possibility of HIV infection, hepatitis, and tuberculosis.
3. The nurse must build a trusting relationship with patients.
4. The nurse serves an important role in educating patients about the consequences of drug abuse and in recommending appropriate treatment.

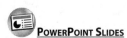
POWERPOINT SLIDES

SUGGESTION FOR CLASSROOM ACTIVITIES
- Present different case studies dealing with substance-abuse issues, and ask students how they would handle the situation.

SUGGESTION FOR CLINICAL ACTIVITIES
- Have students develop a teaching plan dealing with the consequences of substance abuse.

GENERAL CHAPTER CONSIDERATIONS

1. Have students study and learn key terms listed at the beginning of the chapter.
2. Have students complete end-of-chapter exercises either in their book or on the MyNursingKit website.
3. Use the Classroom Response Questions provided in PowerPoint to assess students prior to lecture.

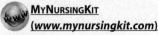

MyNursingKit
(www.mynursingkit.com)

- Websites
- NCLEX® questions
- Critical Thinking Questions
- Case Studies
- Animations and Videos
- Drug Prototype Questions

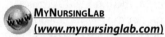

MyNursingLab
(www.mynursinglab.com)

- Knowledge Quick Check
- Pre/Posttests
- Customized study plans
- *Separate purchase*

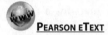

STUDENT WORKBOOK AND RESOURCE GUIDE

- Chapter 11 activities
- *Separate purchase*

PEARSON NURSE'S DRUG GUIDE

- *Separate purchase*

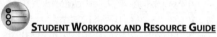

PEARSON eTEXT

- Students can search, highlight, take notes, and more all in electronic format
- *Separate purchase*

CLASSROOM RESPONSE QUESTION POWERPOINTS

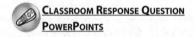

TESTBANK

© 2011 Pearson Education, Inc.

CHAPTER 12
EMERGENCY PREPAREDNESS AND POISONINGS

LEARNING OUTCOME 1

Explain why drugs are important in the context of emergency preparedness.

Concepts for Lecture

1. Drugs are powerful tools in preventing or controlling global disease outbreaks caused by biological, chemical, or nuclear attacks.
2. Medical personnel need to be able to identify, isolate, and treat the cause of global diseases, or a major incident could overwhelm health care resources and produce a catastrophic loss of life.

LEARNING OUTCOME 2

Discuss the role of the nurse in preparing for and responding to a bioterrorist act.

Concepts for Lecture

The key roles of a nurse in preparing for and responding to a bioterrorist act are education, resources, diagnosis and treatment, and planning. Education includes being knowledgeable regarding the emergency management involved in bioterrorist activities. Nurses must maintain a current listing of contacts in their community, both in health and in law enforcement, that would assist in an emergency situation. Nurses must also be knowledgeable about signs, symptoms, and treatment of chemical and biological agents. In addition, nurses should contribute to the development of emergency management plans.

LEARNING OUTCOME 3

Identify the purpose and components of the Strategic National Stockpile (SNS).

Concepts for Lecture

1. The Strategic National Stockpile is a program designed to ensure the immediate deployment of essential medical materials to a community in the event of a large-scale chemical or biological attack. The SNS is managed by the U.S. Centers for Disease Control and Prevention (CDC). The stockpile consists of antibiotics, vaccines, and medical, surgical, and patient-support supplies.
2. The SNS has two components, a push package and a vendor-managed inventory (VMI). The push package consists of a preassembled set of supplies and pharmaceuticals designed to meet the needs of an unknown biological or chemical threat. This component can reach any community in the United States within 12 hours after an attack. The VMI packages are shipped after the chemical or biological threat has

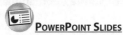
POWERPOINT SLIDES

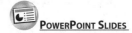
SUGGESTIONS FOR CLASSROOM ACTIVITIES

- Discuss examples and causes of global diseases.
- Discuss bioterrorism and what the goals of a bioterrorist are.

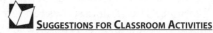
POWERPOINT SLIDES

Table 12.2 Categories of Infectious Agents

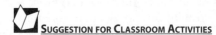
SUGGESTION FOR CLASSROOM ACTIVITIES

- Have the local emergency management officer speak to students regarding the community's emergency management plan.

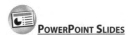
POWERPOINT SLIDES

SUGGESTION FOR CLASSROOM ACTIVITIES

- Discuss why it is not recommended that local hospitals, clinics, and individuals stockpile antibiotics and vaccines.

been more clearly identified. This component consists of supplies and pharmaceuticals more specific to the chemical or biological agent used in the attack. VMI packages can arrive within 24 to 36 hours.

LEARNING OUTCOME 4

Explain the threat of anthrax contamination and how it is transmitted.

Concepts for Lecture

1. Anthrax is caused by the bacterium *Bacillus anthracis*, which is spore forming. The anthrax spores can remain viable in the soil for hundreds or even thousands of years. These spores are responsible for causing anthrax infections.
2. Anthrax can be transmitted to humans by exposure to an open wound, through contaminated food, or by inhalation.

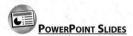 **POWERPOINT SLIDES**

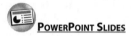 **SUGGESTION FOR CLASSROOM ACTIVITIES**
- Discuss ways anthrax can be transmitted by inhalation.

LEARNING OUTCOME 5

Discuss the clinical manifestations and treatment of anthrax exposure.

Concepts for Lecture

1. Manifestations of every form of anthrax are pain, swelling, and restriction of activity. Clinical manifestations of cutaneous anthrax are small skin lesions that turn into black scabs. Clinical manifestations of gastrointestinal anthrax are sore throat, difficulty swallowing, cramping, diarrhea, and abdominal swelling. Clinical manifestations of inhalation anthrax are initially fever and fatigue, followed by persistent cough and shortness of breath.
2. Ciprofloxacin (Cipro) is used for anthrax prophylaxis and treatment. For prophylaxis, the usual dosage is 500 mg PO, every 12 hours for 60 days. For confirmed cases, the dosage is 400 mg IV, every 12 hours. Other antibiotics that are effective are penicillin, vancomycin, ampicillin, erythromycin, tetracycline, and doxycycline. In inhalation anthrax, the FDA has approved the use of ciprofloxacin and doxycycline in combination for treatment.

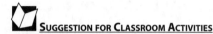 **POWERPOINT SLIDES**

Table 12.3 Clinical Manifestations of Anthrax

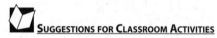 **SUGGESTIONS FOR CLASSROOM ACTIVITIES**
- Discuss the pathophysiology of inhalation anthrax.
- Discuss why the public is discouraged from taking antibiotics prophylactically if exposure to anthrax has not been confirmed.

LEARNING OUTCOME 6

Identify specific viruses that would most likely be used in a bioterrorist act.

Concepts for Lecture

The viruses that cause polio and smallpox would most likely be the viruses used in a bioterrorist act.

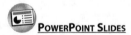 **POWERPOINT SLIDES**

SUGGESTIONS FOR CLASSROOM ACTIVITIES
- Discuss reasons why polio and smallpox viruses would be the most likely viruses used in a bioterrorist act.
- Divide the class into two groups. Assign one group to research how the polio virus is transmitted and the manifestations and treatment for polio. The second group would research the same factors for smallpox. Have both groups report their information to the entire class.

© 2011 Pearson Education, Inc.

LEARNING OUTCOME 7

Explain the advantages and disadvantages of vaccination as a means of preventing illness due to bioterrorist attacks.

Concepts for Lecture

1. The advantage of vaccination as a means of preventing illnesses that are due to bioterrorist attacks is that they stimulate the body's immune system to make antibodies to certain microorganisms before the body is exposed to the microorganism.
2. The disadvantages of vaccination as a means of preventing illness due to bioterrorist attacks are (1) safety concerns with some vaccines, such as those for anthrax and smallpox; (2) lack of information as to whether certain vaccines, such as that for anthrax, are effective; (3) the fact that some vaccines require a series of the vaccine over a certain length of time to stimulate the immune system to produce enough antibodies, plus booster vaccines to maintain the antibody level; and (4) concerns that mutant strains of a microorganism could be developed and the vaccine would not be effective.

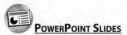

POWERPOINT SLIDES

SUGGESTIONS FOR CLASSROOM ACTIVITIES

- Discuss who should not receive vaccinations.
- Discuss whether vaccinations should be available to everyone or just to health care providers and law enforcement employees who might be exposed to infected patients. Why or why not?

LEARNING OUTCOME 8

Provide examples of chemical agents that might be used in a bioterrorism incident, and their treatments.

Concepts for Lecture

1. Examples of nerve agents are GA (tabun) (liquid), GB (sarin) (gaseous, liquid), GD (soman) (liquid), and VX (gaseous, liquid). The treatment involves an injection of atropine, flushing eyes with water, applying sodium bicarbonate or 5 percent liquid bleach solution to the skin, and no induction of vomiting.
2. Examples of blood agents are hydrogen cyanide (liquid) and cyanogens chloride (gas). Treatment for hydrogen cyanide involves flushing the eyes and washing the skin with water; if inhaled as a mist, oxygen and amyl nitrate may be given; if ingested, 1 percent sodium thiosulfate may be given to induce vomiting. Treatment for cyanogens chloride involves giving oxygen and amyl nitrate; give milk or water but do not induce vomiting.
3. Examples of choking/vomiting agents are phosgene (gas) and adamsite (DM) (crystalline dispensed in aerosol). Treatment for phosgene involves providing fresh air, administering oxygen, flushing eyes with normal saline or water, and keeping the patient warm and calm. Treatment for adamsite (DM) involves rinsing the nose and throat with saline, water, or 10 percent solution of sodium bicarbonate and treating the skin with borated talcum powder.
4. Examples of blister/vesicant agents are phosgene oxime (crystalline or liquid), mustard-Lewisite mixture (HL), nitrogen mustard (HN-1, HN-2, HN-3), and sulfur-mustard agents. Treatment for phosgene oxime involves flushing affected area with large amounts of water; if ingested, do not induce vomiting. Treatment for the other blister/vesicant agents involves flushing the affected area with water, treating the skin with a 5 percent solution of sodium hypochlorite or household bleach or if the agent is Lewisite, use a 10 percent solution of sodium carbonate. Milk should be given for ingestion of Lewisite, but vomiting should not be induced.

POWERPOINT SLIDES

Table 12.4 Chemical Warfare Agents and Treatments

SUGGESTIONS FOR CLASSROOM ACTIVITIES

- Discuss the manifestations of each of the chemical agents that might be used in a bioterrorism incident.
- Ask students to research how these chemical agents are dispensed.

LEARNING OUTCOME 9

Describe the symptoms of acute radiation exposure and the role of potassium iodide (KI) in preventing thyroid cancer.

Concepts for Lecture

1. Immediate symptoms of acute radiation exposure are nausea, vomiting, and diarrhea. These symptoms may occur within hours or days after receiving extreme doses of radiation.
2. Later symptoms of acute radiation exposure are weight loss, anorexia, fatigue, and bone marrow suppression.
3. Those that survive acute radiation exposure are at high risk for developing cancers, particularly leukemia.
4. A single 130-mg dose of potassium iodide (KI), if taken prior to or immediately following a nuclear incident, can prevent radioactive iodine (I-131) from entering the thyroid gland and damaging thyroid cells.

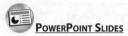 **POWERPOINT SLIDES**

 SUGGESTIONS FOR CLASSROOM ACTIVITIES

- Discuss what radioisotopes are and the therapeutic use of radioisotopes.
- Ask students to research the later effects on those who survived the atomic bombs in Hiroshima and Nagasaki and the effects on those living near the Three Mile Island nuclear accident.

LEARNING OUTCOME 10

List top substances that represent human poison exposures.

Concepts for Lecture

Discuss the different categories of poisonings and their impact on the population.

 POWERPOINT SLIDES

Table 12.5 2006 Data: Top Twenty-five Substances

 SUGGESTIONS FOR CLASSROOM ACTIVITIES

- Have students identify accessibility to the top substances related to poison exposures and how many they have in their own homes.
- Identify safety measures within the home to prevent accidental poisoning from these substances.

LEARNING OUTCOME 11

Explain fundamental elements of toxicity treatment provided by the nurse.

Concepts for Lecture

1. Differentiate the levels of care required to treat acute poisoning.
2. Discuss the different methods used to treat ingested poisons.
3. Identify measures to be used to treat topical exposure to potential poisons.

 POWERPOINT SLIDES

 SUGGESTION FOR CLASSROOM ACTIVITIES

- Invite a representative from Poison Control to discuss the role of the poison control coordinator for your community.

LEARNING OUTCOME 12

Describe specific antidotes used to treat common overdosed substances and toxins.

Concepts for Lecture

Identify specific antidote treatments for selected toxicities.

 POWERPOINT SLIDES

Table 12.6 Examples of Specific Antidotes for Overdosed Substances or Toxins

 SUGGESTION FOR CLASSROOM ACTIVITIES

- Have students identify specific Internet resources to obtain information related to antidotes for specific toxins.

© 2011 Pearson Education, Inc.

General Chapter Considerations

1. Have students study and learn key terms listed at the beginning of the chapter.
2. Have students complete end-of-chapter exercises either in their book or on the MyNursingKit website.
3. Use the Classroom Response Questions provided in PowerPoint to assess students prior to lecture.

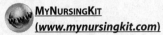 **MyNursingKit**
(www.mynursingkit.com)

- Websites
- NCLEX® questions
- Critical Thinking Questions
- Case Studies
- Animations and Videos
- Drug Prototype Questions

 MyNursingLab
(www.mynursinglab.com)

- Knowledge Quick Check
- Pre/Posttests
- Customized study plans
- *Separate purchase*

 Student Workbook and Resource Guide

- Chapter 12 activities
- *Separate purchase*

Pearson Nurse's Drug Guide

- *Separate purchase*

 Pearson eText

- Students can search, highlight, take notes, and more all in electronic format
- *Separate purchase*

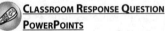 **Classroom Response Question PowerPoints**

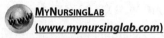 **Testbank**

CHAPTER 13
DRUGS AFFECTING THE AUTONOMIC NERVOUS SYSTEM

LEARNING OUTCOME 1

Identify the basic functions of the nervous system.

Concepts for Lecture

The three basic functions of the nervous system are recognizing changes in the internal and external environments, processing and integrating the environmental changes, and reacting to the environmental changes by producing an action. See Figure 13.1 for the functional divisions of the peripheral nervous system.

 POWERPOINT SLIDES

 SUGGESTION FOR CLASSROOM ACTIVITIES

• Discuss examples of the three basic functions of the nervous system.

LEARNING OUTCOME 2

Identify important divisions of the peripheral nervous system.

Concepts for Lecture

1. The divisions of the peripheral nervous system are the somatic nervous system and the autonomic nervous system.
2. The somatic nervous system provides voluntary control over skeletal muscles.
3. The autonomic nervous system provides involuntary control over smooth muscle, cardiac muscle, and glandular activity.

 POWERPOINT SLIDES

 SUGGESTION FOR CLASSROOM ACTIVITIES

• Discuss examples of voluntary control of the somatic nervous system and involuntary control of the autonomic nervous system.

LEARNING OUTCOME 3

Compare and contrast the actions of the sympathetic and parasympathetic divisions of the autonomic nervous system.

Concepts for Lecture

1. The sympathetic and parasympathetic divisions for the most part have opposite actions to maintain body homeostasis.
2. The sympathetic nervous system is activated under conditions of stress and produces the fight-or-flight response. It will ready the body for an immediate response to a potential threat.
3. The parasympathetic nervous system is activated under nonstressful conditions and produces the rest-and-digest response.

 POWERPOINT SLIDES

 SUGGESTION FOR CLASSROOM ACTIVITIES

• Discuss how the sympathetic and parasympathetic nervous systems regulate the heart, digestive tract, respiratory tract, reproductive tracts, arteries, salivary and sweat glands, and portions of the eye.

LEARNING OUTCOME 4

Explain the process of synaptic transmission and the neurotransmitters important to the autonomic nervous system.

Concepts for Lecture

1. The synaptic transmission involves the connection of two neurons outside the CNS, in series. This connection is called the ganglionic

 POWERPOINT SLIDES

synapse. The preganglionic neuron carries the impulse from the spinal cord to the ganglionic synapse. The postganglionic neuron carries the impulse from the ganglionic synapse to the second synapse at the target tissue.

2. The two primary neurotransmitters of the autonomic nervous system are norepinephrine (NE) and acetylcholine (Ach). In the sympathetic nervous system, norepinephrine is released at almost all postganglionic nerves and binds with adrenergic receptors, which involve the alpha- or beta-receptors on the effector organ. Acetylocholine is released by presynaptic nerves in the parasympathetic nervous system and binds with cholinergic receptors, which involve the muscarinic or nicotinic receptors.

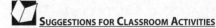

SUGGESTIONS FOR CLASSROOM ACTIVITIES

- Ask students to trace a nerve impulse in the autonomic nervous system.
- Discuss how norepinephrine and acetylcholine are formed and destroyed.

LEARNING OUTCOME 5

Compare and contrast the types of responses that occur when drugs activate alpha$_1$-, alpha$_2$-, beta$_1$-, or beta$_2$-adrenergic receptors, and nicotinic or muscarinic receptors.

Concepts for Lecture

1. Activation of alpha$_1$-adrenergic receptors, which are located in all sympathetic target organs except the heart, cause constriction of blood vessels and dilation of the pupils.
2. Activation of alpha$_2$-adrenergic receptors, which are located at presynaptic adrenergic neuron terminals, inhibits the release of norepinephrine.
3. Activation of beta$_1$-adrenergic receptors, which are located in the heart and kidneys, increase the heart rate and the force of contraction of the heart and the release of renin from the kidneys.
4. Activation of beta$_2$-adrenergic receptors, which are located in all sympathetic target organs except the heart, inhibits smooth muscle.
5. Activation of nicotinic receptors, which are located in cell bodies of sympathetic and parasympathetic postganglionic neurons, stimulates smooth muscle and secretion of glands.
6. Activation of muscarinic receptors, which are located in parasympathetic target organs except the heart, stimulates smooth muscle and secretion from glands.

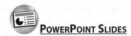

POWERPOINT SLIDES

Prototype Drug
- phenylephrine (Neo-Synephrine)

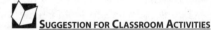

SUGGESTION FOR CLASSROOM ACTIVITIES

- Design a matching quiz for the different receptors, location of receptors, and response when activated.

LEARNING OUTCOME 6

Discuss the classification and naming of autonomic drugs based on four possible actions.

Concepts for Lecture

1. Autonomic drugs are classified based on four possible actions that can occur in the sympathetic and parasympathetic nervous systems.
2. Drugs that stimulate the sympathetic nervous system are called adrenergic agents or sympathomimetics.
3. Drugs that inhibit the sympathetic nervous system are called adrenergic-blocking agents, adrenergic antagonists, or sympatholytics.
4. Drugs that stimulate the parasympathetic nervous system are called cholinergic agents or parasympathomimetics.
5. Drugs that inhibit the parasympathetic nervous system are called cholinergic-blocking agents, anticholinergics, parasympatholytics, or muscarinic blockers.

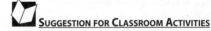

POWERPOINT SLIDES

Table 13.1 Types of Autonomic Receptors

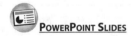

SUGGESTION FOR CLASSROOM ACTIVITIES

- Divide the class into four groups. Have each group present to the rest of the class the expected responses for the four actions of the autonomic nervous system.

LEARNING OUTCOME 7

Describe the nurse's role in the pharmacological management of patients receiving drugs affecting the autonomic nervous system.

Concepts for Lecture

1. The nurse's role in the pharmacologic management of patients receiving any type of autonomic drug involves careful monitoring of the patient's condition, providing education as it relates to the prescribed drug treatment, and noting adverse effects of the drug therapy. In addition, the nurse should identify the current drugs and/or herbal supplements for possible interactions or contraindications for the drug.

2. Parasympathomimetics: Monitor for adverse effects such as abdominal cramping, diarrhea, excessive salivation, difficulty breathing, and muscle cramping. Monitor liver enzymes with initiation of therapy and weekly for six weeks. Assess and monitor for appropriate self-care administration to prevent complications. Direct acting: Monitor intake and output ratio. Monitor for blurred vision. Monitor for orthostatic hypotension. Indirect acting: Monitor muscle strength and neuromuscular status, ptosis, diplopia, and chewing. Schedule medication around mealtimes. Schedule activities to avoid fatigue. Monitor for muscle weakness.

3. Anticholinergic: Monitor for signs of anticholinergic crisis. Report significant changes in heart rate, blood pressure, or the development of dysrhythmias. Provide comfort measures for dryness of mucous membranes. Minimize exposure to heat or cold or strenuous exercise. Monitor I & O. Monitor patient for abdominal distension, and auscultate for bowel sounds

4. Adrenergic Antagonist: For prostate hypertrophy, monitor urinary hesitancy/feeling of incomplete bladder emptying, interrupted urinary stream. Monitor for syncope. Monitor vital signs, level of consciousness, and mood. Monitor for dizziness, drowsiness, or light-headedness. Observe for side effects, which may include blurred vision, tinnitus, epistaxis, and edema. Monitor liver function.

5. Sympathomimetic: Closely monitor IV insertion sites for extravasation with IV administration. Monitor breathing patterns, shortness of breath, and/or audible wheezing. Observe patient's responsiveness to light. Monitor for rhinorrhea and epistaxis.

LEARNING OUTCOME 8

For each of the drug classes listed in "Drugs at a Glance," explain the mechanism of drug action, primary actions, and important adverse effects.

Concepts for Lecture

1. Adrenergic agents (sympathomimetics). The prototype drug is phenylephrine (Neo-Synephrine). The mechanism of action is to stimulate the sympathetic nervous system either directly, by binding to and activating adrenergic receptors, or indirectly, by causing the release of norepinephrine from the presynaptic neuron or by inhibiting the reuptake or destruction of norepinephrine. The primary use depends on which receptors are activated. The following are examples of primary actions for the different adrenergic receptors: alpha$_1$-receptors: treatment of nasal congestion or hypotension—causes dilation of pupils during ophthalmic examinations; alpha$_2$-receptors: treatment of hypertension; beta$_1$-receptors: treatment of cardiac arrest, heart failure, and shock; beta$_2$-receptors: treatment of asthma and premature-labor contractions.

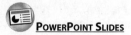

POWERPOINT SLIDES

POWERPOINT SLIDES

Table 13.2 Adrenergic Agents (Sympathomimetics)

NURSING PROCESS FOCUS

- Patients Receiving Adrenergic (Sympathomimetic) Therapy
- Patients Receiving Parasympathomimetic Therapy

SUGGESTION FOR CLASSROOM ACTIVITIES

- Discuss the uses, adverse effects, contraindications, and special considerations for the four types of autonomic-nervous-system drugs.

SUGGESTION FOR CLINICAL ACTIVITIES

- Assign students patients receiving autonomic-nervous-system drugs, and have them note the use of the drugs, any adverse effects, and the therapeutic effects.

POWERPOINT SLIDES

Prototype Drug
- prazosin (Minipress)

SUGGESTIONS FOR CLASSROOM ACTIVITIES

- Discuss why patients would have the possible adverse effects of each of the autonomic drugs.
- Discuss why blocking the parasympathetic nervous system stimulates the sympathetic nervous system.
- Have students prepare a drug card for each classification of autonomic drugs. Cards should include mechanism of action, primary use, adverse effects, and examples of drugs.

© 2011 Pearson Education, Inc.

Adverse effects are tachycardia, hypertension, dysrhythmias, CNS excitation and seizures, dry mouth, nausea, vomiting, and anorexia.

2. Adrenergic-blocking agents. The prototype drug is prazosin (Minipress). The mechanism of action inhibits the sympathetic nervous system and produces many of the same rest-and-digest symptoms of the parasympathomimetics. The primary use is in the treatment of hypertension, dysrhythmias, angina, heart failure, benign prostatic hypertrophy, and narrow-angle glaucoma. Adverse effects are dizziness, drowsiness, headache, loss of energy and strength, palpitations, and dry mouth.

3. Cholinergic agents (parasympathomimetics). The prototype drug is bethanechol (Urecholine). The mechanism of action is to activate the parasympathetic nervous system either directly by binding to cholinergic receptors or indirectly by inhibiting the action of AchE, which prevents the destruction of endogenous Ach so it remains on the cholinergic receptors longer and prolongs its action. Primary use of the drugs is in the treatment of glaucoma, urinary retention, myasthenia gravis, and Alzheimer's disease. Adverse effects are profuse salivation, increased muscle tone, urinary frequency, bronchoconstriction, and bradycardia.

4. Cholinergic-blocking agents. The prototype drug is atropine (Atropair, Atropisol). The mechanism of action is to inhibit the parasympathetic nervous system by competing with acetylcholine for binding muscarinic receptors. Primary uses of cholinergic-blocking agents are treatment of peptic ulcers and irritable bowel syndrome; to cause mydriasis or cycloplegia during eye examinations; to increase the heart rate in patients experiencing bradycardia; as a preanesthetic; and for treatment of asthma. Adverse effects are tachycardia, CNS stimulation, urinary retention in men with prostate disorders, dry mouth, dry eyes, decreased sweat, and photophobia.

LEARNING OUTCOME 9

Use the nursing process to care for patients receiving adrenergic agents, adrenergic-blocking agents, cholinergic agents, and cholinergic-blocking agents.

Concepts for Lecture

1. Assessment occurs prior to administration of the drug and includes potential nursing diagnoses, reason for drug, monitoring vital signs, doing a complete health history, cautions and contraindications for drug, allergies, drug history, possible drug interactions, and evaluating lab findings.
2. Nursing diagnosis: knowledge deficient, related to drug therapy; risk for injury, related to side effect of drug therapy; disturbed sleep pattern.
3. Planning patient goals and expectation outcomes such as that the patient will exhibit a decrease in the symptoms for which the drug is being given, demonstrate an understanding of the drug's activity, accurately describe the drug's side effects and precautions, and demonstrate proper administration technique.
4. Implementation involves interventions—such as administration of the drug and observing for adverse effects—and patient education and discharge planning. Encourage compliance with medication regimen. Provide additional education regarding medication regimen, such as a consultation with a clinical pharmacist, written and/or visual educational material, and home-health visits to ensure patient's ability to follow prescribed therapy.
5. Evaluation of outcome criteria includes evaluating the effectiveness of drug therapy by confirming that patient goals and expected outcomes have been met (see "Planning" above).

SUGGESTION FOR CLINICAL ACTIVITIES

- Assign students patients receiving autonomic-system drugs. Have students note reason for the drug, the therapeutic effect of the drug, and any adverse effects of the drug.

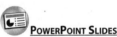
POWERPOINT SLIDES

Table 13.4 Cholinergic Agents (Parasympathomimetics)

Prototype Drug
- bethanechol (Urecholine)
- atropine (Atro-Pen, Atropair, Atropisol)

NURSING PROCESS FOCUS

- Patients Receiving Adrenergic-blocking Therapy
- Patients Receiving Anticholinergic Therapy

SUGGESTION FOR CLASSROOM ACTIVITIES

- Divide class into four groups. Assign one of the four autonomic-drug classifications to each group and have the group develop a nursing care plan for that drug classification using the nursing process.

SUGGESTION FOR CLINICAL ACTIVITIES

- Assign students patients receiving an autonomic-nervous-system drug, and have each student develop a patient education plan for that drug using the nursing process.

General Chapter Considerations

1. Have students study and learn key terms listed at the beginning of the chapter.
2. Have students complete end-of-chapter exercises either in their book or on the MyNursingKit website.
3. Use the Classroom Response Questions provided in PowerPoint to assess students prior to lecture.

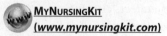

MyNursingKit
(*www.mynursingkit.com*)

- Websites
- NCLEX® questions
- Critical Thinking Questions
- Case Studies
- Animations and Videos
- Drug Prototype Questions

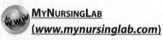

MyNursingLab
(*www.mynursinglab.com*)

- Knowledge Quick Check
- Pre/Posttests
- Customized study plans
- *Separate purchase*

Student Workbook and Resource Guide

- Chapter 13 activities
- *Separate purchase*

Pearson Nurse's Drug Guide

- *Separate purchase*

Pearson eText

- Students can search, highlight, take notes, and more all in electronic format.
- *Separate purchase*

Classroom Response Question PowerPoints

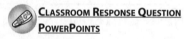

Testbank

© 2011 Pearson Education, Inc.

CHAPTER 14
DRUGS FOR ANXIETY AND INSOMNIA

LEARNING OUTCOME 1

Identify the major types of anxiety disorders.

Concepts for Lecture

1. The major types of anxiety disorders are situational anxiety, generalized anxiety disorder (GAD), panic disorder, phobias, obsessive-compulsive disorder, and post-traumatic stress disorder.
2. There is a model of anxiety that indicates when stressful events or changing mental conditions can produce the feelings of anxiety.

POWERPOINT SLIDES

Figure 14.1 A Model of Anxiety in Which Stressful Events or a Changing Mental Condition can Produce Unfavorable Symptoms, Some of Which May Be Controlled by Medication

NURSING PROCESS FOCUS

- Patients Receiving Benzodiazepine and Nonbenzodiazepine Antianxiety Therapy

SUGGESTION FOR CLASSROOM ACTIVITIES

- Divide students into six groups. Assign one of the major types of anxiety disorders to each group. Have the group define and give examples of the anxiety disorder to the class.

SUGGESTION FOR CLINICAL ACTIVITIES

- Arrange for students to attend a support group that deals with anxiety disorders and the types of anxiety disorders the group members have.

REFERENCE

- Mental Health Topics: *www.nimh.nih.gov/health/topics/index.shtml*

LEARNING OUTCOME 2

Discuss factors contributing to anxiety and explain some nonpharmacologic therapies used to cope with this disorder.

Concepts for Lecture

1. The most common factors or causes of anxiety are phobias, post-traumatic stress, generalized anxiety, obsessive-compulsive feelings, and panic disorders.
2. Some nonpharmacologic therapies used to cope with stress are cognitive behavioral therapy, counseling, biofeedback techniques, and meditation. These may help individuals change the way they think and eliminate the cause of the anxiety.

POWERPOINT SLIDES

SUGGESTION FOR CLASSROOM ACTIVITIES

- Arrange to have a mental health worker speak to the class about nonpharmacologic therapies to deal with stress.

SUGGESTION FOR CLINICAL ACTIVITIES

- Arrange for students to observe the use of nonpharmacologic therapies to cope with anxiety.

REFERENCE

- National Institute of Mental Health: *www.nimh.nih.gov/index.shtml*

LEARNING OUTCOME 3

Identify the regions of the brain associated with anxiety, sleep, and wakefulness.

Concepts for Lecture

1. The limbic system is in the middle of the brain and is responsible for emotional expression, learning, and memory. Signals pass through the limbic system and connect with the hypothalamus. This connection is associated with emotional states, anxiety, fear, anger, aggression, remorse, depression, sexual drive, and euphoria. See Figure 14.1.
2. The hypothalamus is responsible for unconscious responses to extreme stress, such as high blood pressure, elevated breathing rate, and dilated pupils. The hypothalamus connects with the reticular formation.
3. The reticular formation is a network of neurons along the length of the brainstem. Stimulation causes heightened awareness and arousal. Inhibition causes general drowsiness and the induction of sleep.
4. The reticular activating system (RAS) projects from the reticular formation in the brainstem to the thalamus. The RAS is responsible for sleeping and wakefulness. Signals from the hypothalamus pass through the RAS and on to higher brain centers.

POWERPOINT SLIDES

Pharmacotherapy Illustrated 14.1 The reticular activating system and related regions in the brain are important areas to focus for drugs used to treat anxiety and anxiety-related symptoms.

SUGGESTION FOR CLASSROOM ACTIVITIES

- Provide a blank diagram of the brain, and have students label the limbic system, reticular formation, hypothalamus, and reticular activating system.

SUGGESTION FOR CLINICAL ACTIVITIES

- On assigned patients, have students note if the patient is receiving an antidepressant, benzodiazepine, and/or barbiturate; the reason for ordering the medication; and its effectiveness.

REFERENCE

- National Institute of Mental Health: *www.nimh.nih.gov/index.shtml*

LEARNING OUTCOME 4

Identify the three classes of medications used to treat anxiety and sleep disorders.

Concepts for Lecture

Antidepressants, benzodiazepines, and barbiturates are three classes of medications used to treat anxiety and sleep disorders.

POWERPOINT SLIDES

SUGGESTION FOR CLASSROOM ACTIVITIES

- Divide students into three groups. Assign each group a different class of medications (antidepressants, benzodiazepines, barbiturates) used to treat anxiety and sleep disorders, and have each group present to the class the effects of these medications on the brain and give examples of the medications.

SUGGESTION FOR CLINICAL ACTIVITIES

- On assigned patients, have students note if the patient is receiving an antidepressant, benzodiazepine, and/or barbiturate; the reason for ordering the medication; and its effectiveness.

LEARNING OUTCOME 5

Explain the pharmacological management of anxiety and insomnia.

Concepts for Lecture

1. Antidepressants are used to treat anxiety and reduce symptoms associated with panic, obsessive-compulsive behavior, and phobia.

POWERPOINT SLIDES

SUGGESTION FOR CLASSROOM ACTIVITIES

- Ask students to give benefits and hazards of pharmacologic management of anxiety and insomnia.

© 2011 Pearson Education, Inc.

2. Benzodiazepines used to treat short-term insomnia are different from those used to treat generalized anxiety disorders.
3. Low doses of barbiturates reduce anxiety, and moderate doses promote sleep.

SUGGESTION FOR CLINICAL ACTIVITIES

- On their assigned patients, have students indicate if the patient is experiencing an anxiety or a sleep disorder and the pharmacologic agent that has been prescribed to manage the disorder.

LEARNING OUTCOME 6

Describe the nurse's role in the pharmacologic management of anxiety and insomnia.

POWERPOINT SLIDES

Concepts for Lecture

1. The nurse should monitor the patient's condition and provide education as it relates to the prescribed drug treatment. Obtain baseline vital signs, medical and drug history, lifestyle and dietary habits, and what activities the patient was involved in at the onset of the symptoms.
2. The nurse should assess patient needs for antianxiety or insomnia drugs, including intensity and duration of symptoms. Identify factors that precipitate anxiety or insomnia. Identify coping mechanisms used in managing stress, anxiety, and insomnia. Assess for a primary sleep disorder.
3. Obtain a drug history, including hypersensitivity and the use of alcohol and other CNS depressants. Assess for drug abuse and dependence.
4. Use benzodiazepines cautiously in the elderly and in patients with a suicidal potential or impaired renal or liver function.
5. Benzodiazepine and nonbenzodiazepine: Assess for common side effects related to CNS depression; neurological status; level of consciousness. Monitor vital signs. Observe respiratory patterns particularly during sleep. Monitor the patient's intake of stimulants, such as caffeine and nicotine. Monitor affect and emotional status.

SUGGESTION FOR CLASSROOM ACTIVITIES

- Divide students into pairs. Have students role-play the nurse and patient and obtain a drug history, then have students switch roles and assess the patient for need for antianxiety or insomnia drug.

SUGGESTION FOR CLINICAL ACTIVITIES

- Have students design and implement a plan to educate a patient who has been ordered an antianxiety or insomnia drug.

LEARNING OUTCOME 7

Identify normal sleep patterns and explain how these might be affected by anxiety and stress.

POWERPOINT SLIDES

Table 14.1 Stages of Sleep

Concepts for Lecture

1. People with normal sleep patterns move from nonrapid eye movement (NREM) to rapid eye movement (REM) sleep about every 90 minutes. There are four progressive stages of NREM sleep; then the sequence goes into reverse. After returning to stage I of NREM, REM sleep occurs. During REM sleep, dreaming occurs. See Table 14.1 for the stages of sleep.
2. Stress interrupts normal sleeping patterns because the patient's mind is too active.

SUGGESTION FOR CLASSROOM ACTIVITIES

- Display EEG showing waves that occur during NREM and REM sleep.

SUGGESTION FOR CLINICAL ACTIVITIES

- Arrange for students to observe in a sleep lab.

REFERENCE

- Sleep Disorders: *www.sleepnet.com/wwwboard/wwwboard.html*

LEARNING OUTCOME 8

Categorize drugs used for anxiety and insomnia based on their classification and mechanism of action.

Concepts for Lecture

1. Benzodiazepines act by binding to the gamma-aminobutyric acid (GABA) receptor-chloride channel molecule, intensifying the effects of GABA. Additional examples: Xanax, Librium, Tranxene.
2. Barbiturates act by binding to GABA receptor-chloride channel molecules, intensifying the effect of GABA throughout the brain. Additional examples: Nembutal, Seconal, Amytal.
3. Nonbenzodiazepines, nonbarbiturates (CNS depressants) act by binding to the GABA receptor, preserving sleep stages III and IV and offering minor effects of REM sleep. Additional examples: Buspar, Noctec, Placidyl.

LEARNING OUTCOME 9

For each of the classes listed in Drugs at a Glance, know representative drugs and explain their mechanisms of action, primary actions, and important adverse effects.

Concepts for Lecture

1. Benzodiazepines: The prototype drug is lorazepam (Ativan). The mechanism of action is to bind with the GABA receptor-chloride channel molecule, which intensifies the GABA effect. The primary use is to reduce anxiety disorders and insomnia. The important adverse effects include drowsiness, dizziness, and respiratory depression.
2. Barbiturates: The prototype drug is diazepam (Valium). Its mechanism of action is to bind to GABA receptor-chloride molecules, intensifying the effect of GABA throughout the brain; it also inhibits brain impulses from traveling through the limbic system and the reticular activating system, thereby calming without strong sedation. Its primary use is as a sedative and a hypnotic. The important adverse effects include tolerance, respiratory depression, and psychological and physical dependence.
3. Nonbenzodiazepines, nonbarbiturates (CNS depressants): The prototype drug is zolpidem (Ambien). The mechanism of action is to bind to GABA receptors, thereby preserving sleep stages III and IV and offering minor effects of REM sleep. The primary use is as a hypnotic. The important adverse effects include mild nausea, dizziness, diarrhea, daytime drowsiness, amnesia, sleepwalking, and ingesting carbohydrates while sleepwalking.

LEARNING OUTCOME 10

Use the nursing process to care for patients receiving drug therapy for anxiety and insomnia.

Concepts for Lecture

1. Assessment occurs prior to the administration of the drug and includes potential nursing diagnoses, reason for the drug, taking vital

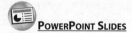

POWERPOINT SLIDES

Table 14.2 Antidepressants for Treatment of Anxiety Symptoms
Table 14.4 Benzodiazepines for Anxiety and Insomnia

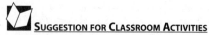

SUGGESTION FOR CLASSROOM ACTIVITIES

- Discuss the use of benzodiazepines and barbiturates as sedatives, hypnotics, and anticonvulsants.

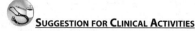

SUGGESTION FOR CLINICAL ACTIVITIES

- Have students look at charts of patients who are receiving antidepressants, benzodiazepines, or barbiturates and determine the reason for prescribing the drug.

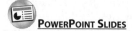

POWERPOINT SLIDES

Table 14.5 Barbiturates for Sedation and Insomnia
Table 14.6 Miscellaneous Drugs for Anxiety and Insomnia

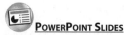

POWERPOINT SLIDES

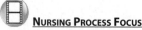

NURSING PROCESS FOCUS

- Patients Receiving Benzodiazepine and Nonbenzodiazepine Antianxiety Therapy

© 2011 Pearson Education, Inc.

signs, cautions and contraindications of the drug, possible drug inter-actions, taking a complete health history including allergies, drug his-tory, and evaluation of lab findings.

2. Nursing diagnosis: risk for injury, knowledge deficient, related to drug therapy, and ineffective individual coping.

3. Planning includes patient goals and expected outcome. The patient will exhibit a decrease in symptoms of anxiety and insomnia, demonstrate an understanding of the drug's activity, accurately describe drug side effects and precautions, and demonstrate proper administration technique.

4. Implementation of drug therapy includes interventions and rationales, administration of the drug, observing for adverse effects, and patient education and discharge planning.

5. Evaluate the effectiveness of the drug therapy by confirming that the pa-tient's goals and expected outcomes have been met (see Planning above).

GENERAL CHAPTER CONSIDERATIONS

1. Have students study and learn key terms listed at the beginning of the chapter.
2. Have students complete end-of-chapter exercises either in their book or on the MyNursingKit website.
3. Use the Classroom Response Questions provided in PowerPoint to assess students prior to lecture.

SUGGESTION FOR CLASSROOM ACTIVITIES

- Divide students into three groups. Assign each group one of the drugs in Drugs at a Glance. Have the groups develop a nursing care plan for the assigned drug using the nursing process.

SUGGESTION FOR CLINICAL ACTIVITIES

- Assign students patients who are receiving drugs for anxiety or insomnia, and have each student develop a teaching plan for that drug using the nursing process.

MYNURSINGKIT
(**www.mynursingkit.com**)

- Websites
- NCLEX® questions
- Critical Thinking Questions
- Case Studies
- Animations and Videos
- Drug Prototype Questions

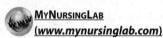

MYNURSINGLAB
(**www.mynursinglab.com**)

- Knowledge Quick Check
- Pre/Posttests
- Customized study plans
- *Separate purchase*

STUDENT WORKBOOK AND RESOURCE GUIDE

- Chapter 14 activities
- *Separate purchase*

PEARSON NURSE'S DRUG GUIDE

- *Separate purchase*

PEARSON eTEXT

- Students can search, highlight, take notes, and more all in electronic format.
- *Separate purchase*

CLASSROOM RESPONSE QUESTION POWERPOINTS

TESTBANK

CHAPTER 15
DRUGS FOR SEIZURES

LEARNING OUTCOME 1

Compare and contrast the terms *seizures, convulsions,* and *epilepsy*.

Concepts for Lecture

1. A seizure results from abnormal or uncontrolled neuronal discharges in the brain, which may affect consciousness, motor activity, and sensation. An electroencephalogram (EEG) can measure the abnormalities. See Figure 15.1 for examples of EEG recordings. A seizure is considered a symptom of an underlying disorder, not a disease itself. Known causes of seizures include infectious diseases, trauma, metabolic disorders, vascular diseases, pediatric disorders, and neoplastic disease. Seizures may also result from medications, high doses of local anesthesia causing increased stimulation of neurotransmitter or toxicity, eclampsia during pregnancy, drug abuse, and during withdrawal from alcohol or sedative-hypnotic drugs.
2. A convulsion refers to involuntary, violent spasms of the large skeletal muscles of the face, neck, arms, and legs. The term convulsion is not synonymous with seizure.
3. Epilepsy is a disorder characterized by seizures occurring on a chronic basis and is classified by the International Classification of Epileptic Seizures as partial (focal), generalized, and special epileptic syndromes.

LEARNING OUTCOME 2

Recognize possible causes of epilepsy.

Concepts for Lecture

1. Known causes of seizures include infectious diseases, trauma, metabolic disorders, vascular diseases, pediatric disorders, and neoplastic disease. Seizures may also result from medications, high doses of local anesthesia causing increased stimulation of neurotransmitter or toxicity, eclampsia during pregnancy, drug abuse, and during withdrawal from alcohol or sedative-hypnotic drugs.
2. Seizures can also have unknown etiology. Lower tolerance to environmental triggers may cause seizures when the patient is exposed to sleep deprivation, flickering lights, or fluid and electrolyte imbalances.
3. Congenital abnormalities of the CNS, perinatal brain injury, and metabolic imbalances are usually related to seizures in neonates, infants, and children.
4. Later-childhood onset of seizures is commonly related to CNS infections or neurological degenerative disorders.

 POWERPOINT SLIDES

 SUGGESTIONS FOR CLASSROOM ACTIVITIES

- Present sample EEG recordings, and have students identify the different types of seizures.
- Have students identify the nomenclature for classification of epilepsy that was commonly used in the past.

 SUGGESTION FOR CLINICAL ACTIVITIES

- Have students identify the classification of assigned client's epilepsy utilizing the health record.

 REFERENCE

- **National Institute of Neurological Disorders and Stroke:** *http://www.ninds.nih.gov/*
- **American Parkinsons Association:** *http://www.apdaparkinson.org/userND/index.asp*

 POWERPOINT SLIDES

   © 2011 Pearson Education, Inc.

5. In adults, common causes of the onset of the disorder are cerebral trauma or neoplasm and cerebrovascular disorders.

LEARNING OUTCOME 3

Relate signs and symptoms to specific types of seizures.

Concepts for Lecture

1. Signs and symptoms of seizures are directly related to the area of the brain where the abnormal activity is occurring. As discussed in the Concepts for Lecture for Learning Objective 1, the International Classification of Epileptic Seizures identifies types of seizures.
2. Partial (focal) seizures arise in a limited portion of the brain, with the point of origin of abnormal electrical activity referred to as the abnormal focus or foci. Patients experiencing simple partial seizures often briefly feel that their current location is vague, and they may hear, see, feel, or smell things that are not present. Some patients feel very emotional, and some experience arms, legs, or face twitching. Complex partial seizures result in altered levels of consciousness and symptoms involving sensory, motor, and autonomic systems. An aura usually precedes the seizure, and patients usually do not follow verbal commands during the seizure. They often do not remember the seizure.
3. Generalized seizures travel throughout the entire brain. Absence seizures are common in children and last a few seconds. Symptoms may include staring, transient loss of consciousness, and slight eyelid fluttering or myoclonic jerks. Symptoms are usually subtle and may be mistaken for daydreaming or attention deficit disorder. Atonic seizures usually last only a few seconds and are characterized by stumbling or falling for no apparent reason. Tonic-clonic seizures are the most common type of seizure in every age group and are usually preceded by an aura. Characteristics of these seizures during the tonic phase include intense muscle contractions, a hoarse cry at the onset from air being forced out of the lungs, loss of bowel or bladder control, and shallow breathing or brief periods of apnea. During the clonic phase, patients experience alternating contraction and relaxation of muscles. Tonic-clonic seizures typically last one to two minutes and are followed by drowsiness, disorientation, and deep sleep. This postseizure period is called the postictal state.
4. Special epileptic syndromes include febrile seizures, myoclonic seizures, and status epilepticus. Febrile seizures usually last one to two

SUGGESTIONS FOR CLASSROOM ACTIVITIES

- Have students list specific examples of the diseases and disorders that cause seizures.
- Divide the students into small groups, and have the groups discuss and present the ramifications that a client may experience as a result of epilepsy.

SUGGESTIONS FOR CLINICAL ACTIVITIES

- Arrange for the students to attend an epilepsy support group.
- Have the students identify the possible etiology of epilepsy in assigned clients through the client interview and health record.

REFERENCE

- *epilepsyfoundation.org*

POWERPOINT SLIDES

Table 15.1 Classification of Seizures and Symptoms

SUGGESTION FOR CLASSROOM ACTIVITIES

- Divide students into small groups and assign a type of seizure to each group. Have each group prepare a poster presentation for each of the types of epilepsy, including signs and symptoms.

SUGGESTION FOR CLINICAL ACTIVITIES

- Rotate students through neurologists' offices, and have them interview clients with epilepsy to assess the specific signs and symptoms that they experience.

minutes with tonic-clonic motor activity and occur in the 3- to 5-year age group in conjunction with a rapid rise in body temperature. Five percent of all children experience these seizures. Myoclonic seizures involve large, jerking body movements with major muscle groups contracting quickly, causing the patient to stumble or fall. These seizures can occur in infants and are not noticed because the movements are similar to the normal infantile Moro (startle) reflex. Status epilepticus is a medical emergency that can occur with any type of seizure that is repeated continuously but is most commonly exhibited with generalized tonic-clonic seizures. The continuous muscle contraction may result in a compromised airway or hypoxia, hypoglycemia, acidosis, hypothermia, and lactic acid production.

LEARNING OUTCOME 4

Describe the nurse's role in the pharmacologic management of seizures of an acute nature and epilepsy.

Concepts for Lecture

1. The role of the nurse is to obtain the previous medical history, diagnostic studies, and pathologic process that is causing the seizures, because the type of drug the patient is prescribed for control of epilepsy depends on the type of seizures she is experiencing.

2. Nursing considerations for patients taking **barbiturates and miscellaneous GABA agents** requires careful monitoring of the patient's condition and patient education regarding the medication regimen. Liver and kidney function should be closely monitored due to the drug's being metabolized in the liver and excreted in urine. Patients should be warned that these drugs are pregnancy category D. Depletion of nutrients such as vitamins D and K is common, especially in the elderly; therefore, the patient should be monitored for reduced bone density and bleeding disorders. Common side effects include drowsiness, dizziness, and postural hypotension. Alcohol and gingko biloba may decrease the antiseizure effect. Patient teaching should include using reliable contraception; immediate notification if pregnancy occurs; and reporting any signs of excessive bleeding, such as nosebleeds, black stools, heavy periods, or blood in the urine. In addition, patients should immediately report severe drowsiness and bone pain. Alcohol should be avoided, as well as gingko biloba, since they decrease the effects of barbiturates.

3. Nursing considerations for **benzodiazepines** also involve careful monitoring of the patient's condition and education of medication regimen. Benzodiazepines are a Schedule IV drug, so the patient should be assessed for drug-abuse potential and dependence. These drugs are a pregnancy-risk category D. Since benzodiazepines change intraocular pressure, patients with narrow-angle glaucoma should not receive these drugs. Liver and kidney function should also be monitored, and respiratory depression may result if the patient is taking other CNS depressants. Common side effects include drowsiness and dizziness. If a patient receives an overdose of benzodiazepines, flumazenil (Romazicon) should be administered to reverse the CNS depression. IV Valium and Ativan are given for status epilepticus, and oxygen and resuscitation equipment should be nearby to treat respiratory depression, since flumazenil (Romazicon) should not be given because of the need to stop the seizures. Do not mix these drugs with others because they tend to precipitate and are irritating to the veins. Patient teaching should include avoiding alcohol, OTC drugs, and herbal medications without notifying the prescriber, due to CNS depression. All forms of

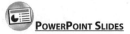
POWERPOINT SLIDES

Table 15.2 Traditional and Newer Antiseizure Drugs with Indications*

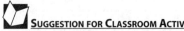
SUGGESTION FOR CLASSROOM ACTIVITIES

• Have students develop a teaching plan for each of the medications discussed in Learning Objective 4.

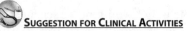
SUGGESTION FOR CLINICAL ACTIVITIES

• Have students prepare drug cards for the medications discussed in Learning Objective 4.

© 2011 Pearson Education, Inc.

nicotine should be avoided because they can decrease the effectiveness of benzodiazepines. Patients should avoid driving or hazardous activities until they know how they respond to the drug. Rebound seizures may result if the drug is abruptly stopped. The drug should be taken with food to prevent GI disturbances. patients should be aware that these drugs are often used illegally as a recreational drug.

4. **Hydantoin and phenytoin-like drugs** require serum-drug levels to be monitored to prevent toxicity. Dizziness, ataxia, diplopia, and lethargy are symptoms of toxicity. Blood dyscrasias and bleeding disorders should be watched for due to the effect of these drugs on vitamin K metabolism. Hydantoins may increase blood-glucose levels and cause hematuria. Liver and kidney function may also be affected. Fatal hepatotoxicity has recently occurred in patients taking valproic acid (Depakene, Depakote) who are also taking multiple antiseizure drugs, who have existing liver or organic brain disease, or who are under the age of 2. A history of heart block and seizures due to hypoglycemia are contraindications for hydantoins. They are pregnancy-risk category D and C drugs. Patient teaching should include ensuring patients understand the need for routine labs for serum level and liver- and kidney-function tests. Patients should immediately report signs of toxicity and unusual bleeding and diagnoses of liver or brain disease, heart block, hypoglycemia, or pregnancy.

5. Nursing consideration for patients taking succinimides includes monitoring of liver and kidney function due to metabolism and excretion. A health history should assess for other antiseizure medication, phenothiazines, and antidepressants because these medications may interact with succinimides and result in a lower seizure threshold and decreased effectiveness of succinimides. Several common adverse reactions that the patient may experience are drowsiness, headache, fatigue, dizziness, depression or euphoria, nausea and vomiting, diarrhea, weight loss, and abdominal pain. Life-threatening reactions that occur with these drugs include severe mental depression with suicide intent, Stevens-Johnson syndrome, and blood dyscrasias such as leukopenia and agranulocytosis. Symptoms of overdose that the nurse should watch for are CNS depression, stupor, ataxia, and coma. Serum levels should be monitored. Succinimides are a pregnancy-risk category C drug. Patient teaching should ensure that the patient understands the need to immediately report changes in mood, mental depression, or suicidal thoughts. Patients should avoid driving or hazardous activities and never stop the medication suddenly due to increased chance of rebound seizures. Succinimides are better tolerated when taken with food to avoid GI effects. Patients should also report symptoms of fever, sore throat, weight loss, or anorexia.

LEARNING OUTCOME 5

Explain the importance of patient drug compliance in the pharmacotherapy of epilepsy and seizures.

Concepts for Lecture

1. Seizure medications are gradually increased from the smallest initial dose possible to control seizure activity. Additional seizure medications can be added if necessary. The nurse must ensure drug compatibility prior to administration. Serum-drug levels are necessary to determine therapeutic levels of medication.

2. If a patient is seizure free for at least three years while on an antiseizure medication, the prescriber may attempt to withdraw a seizure medication, under close medical supervision. Medications

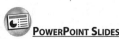
POWERPOINT SLIDES

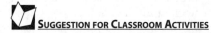
SUGGESTION FOR CLASSROOM ACTIVITIES

• Have students develop a teaching plan for a client whose antiseizure medication is being withdrawn.

are withdrawn slowly, over several months, and if any seizure activity occurs, the drug is resumed. The nurse must ensure that patients understand that abrupt withdrawal of an antiseizure medication may result in rebound seizures.

LEARNING OUTCOME 6

For each of the drug classes listed in Drugs at a Glance, know representative drug examples and explain their mechanism of drug action, primary actions, and important adverse effects.

Concepts for Lecture

1. Drugs that potentiate GABA action include barbiturates, benzodiazepines, and miscellaneous GABA agents. **Barbiturates:** The prototype drug is phenobarbital (Luminal). The mechanism of action is to change the action of GABA, which is the primary neurotransmitter in the brain, by stimulating the influx of chloride ions. This suppresses the firing ability of neurons. The primary use is to control seizures. The adverse effects include dependence, drowsiness, vitamin deficiencies, and laryngospasm. **Benzodiazepines:** The prototype drug is diazepam (Valium). The mechanism of action is similar to that of barbiturates but safer. The primary use is for short-term seizure control with absence and myoclonic seizures. IV administration is used to terminate status epilepticus. The adverse effects include drowsiness and dizziness. **Miscellaneous GABA agents:** The prototype drug is valproic acid (Depakene). The mechanism of action is similar to that of barbiturates and benzodiazepines in relation to GABA. The primary use is most often as an adjunct therapy, and information on these drugs is minimal due to limited use in clinical experience. The adverse effects include sedation; drowsiness, GI upset, and prolonged bleeding time.
2. Hydantoins and phenytoin-like drugs suppress sodium influx by dampening CNS activity, thus delaying an influx of sodium ions across neuronal membranes. **Hydantoins:** The prototype drug is phenytoin (Dilantin). The mechanism of action is to desensitize sodium channels. The primary use is treating all types of epilepsy except absence seizures. The adverse effects include CNS depression with excessive dosages, gingival hyperplasia (which occurs in about 20 percent of patients), skin rash, cardiac dysrhythmias, and hypotension. **Phenytoin-like drugs:** The prototype drug is valproic acid (Depakene). The mechanism of action is to desensitize sodium channels. The primary use is for absence seizures. The adverse effects include limited CNS depression, visual disturbances, ataxia, vertigo, and headache. Additional adverse reactions include gastrointestinal effects, hepatotoxicity, and pancreatitis.
3. **Succinimides:** The prototype drug is ethosuximide (Zarontin). The mechanism of action is to suppress calcium influx; it works by delaying calcium influx into neurons, which raises the seizure threshold and thereby suppresses the seizure. The primary use is for absence seizures. The adverse effects are rare, but drowsiness, dizziness, and lethargy may occur initially. Administering with food can reduce nausea and vomiting. Very rare but serious side effects include systemic lupus erythematosus, leukopenia, aplastic anemia, and Stevens-Johnson syndrome.

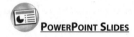

POWERPOINT SLIDES

Prototype Drug
- Diazepam (Valium)
- Phenobarbital (Luminal)
- Phenytoin (Dilantin)
- Valproic Acid (Depakane)
- Ethosuximide (Zarontin)

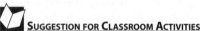

SUGGESTION FOR CLASSROOM ACTIVITIES

- Have students prepare drug cards for all of the drugs listed in Drugs at a Glance.

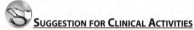

SUGGESTION FOR CLINICAL ACTIVITIES

- Have students obtain the drug list from assigned clients with seizure disorders and assess current or past adverse effects that their client has experienced.

© 2011 Pearson Education, Inc.

Learning Outcome 7

Categorize drugs used in the treatment of seizures based on their classification and mechanism of action.

Concepts for Lecture

1. Drugs that potentiate GABA action include barbiturates, benzodiazepines, and miscellaneous GABA agents. These medications work by changing the action of GABA, which is the primary neurotransmitter in the brain, by stimulating the influx of chloride ions. This suppresses the firing ability of neurons. Barbiturates include phenobarbital (Luminal), amobarbital (Amytal), secobarbital (Seconal), and pentobarbital (Nembutal). Benzodiazepines given for epilepsy include clonazepam (Klonopin), clorazepate (Tranxene), lorazepam (Ativan), and diazepam (Valium). Miscellaneous GABA agents are a newer class of antiseizure drugs and include gabapentin (Neurontin), primidone (Mysoline), tiagabine (Gabitril), and topiramate (Topamax).

2. Hydantoins and phenytoin-like drugs suppress sodium influx by delaying an influx of sodium ions across neuronal membranes, thereby dampening CNS activity. These drugs desensitize sodium channels. Sodium movement is the major factor that determines whether a neuron will undergo an action potential. Hydantoins in this class include phenytoin (Dilantin) (most common) and fosphenytoin (Cerebyx). Phenytoin-like drugs include carbamazepine (Tegretol), commonly used for tonic-clonic and partial seizures, felbamate (Felbatol), lamotrigine (Lamictal), valproic acid (Depakene, Depakote) for absence seizures and zonisamide (Zonegran).

3. Drugs that suppress calcium influx are succinimides and work by delaying calcium influx into neurons, thereby suppressing seizures. This raises the seizure threshold. Drugs in this class include ethosuximide (Zarontin), methsuximide (Celontin), and phensuximide (Milontin).

Learning Outcome 8

Use the nursing process to care for patients receiving drug therapy for epilepsy and seizures.

Concepts for Lecture

1. Assessment: Data that the nurse should collect in the assessment phase includes history of seizure activity, allergies, and drug use in order to avoid interactions; knowledge of disease process and drug therapy; and lifestyle of the patient.

2. Nursing diagnoses: Possible nursing diagnoses for the patient receiving drug therapy include disturbed sensory perception related to seizure activity; risk for injury related to seizure activity; deficient knowledge related to drug therapy and disease process; and noncompliance related to drug, regimen, and necessary serum lab testing.

3. Planning: During the planning phase of the nursing process, the nurse and patient will set goals for therapy. Goals that would be included in the care plan include absence of or reduction in the number of seizures; no injury during seizure activity; understanding of the disease and drug regimen; and compliance with necessary serum lab testing.

4. Implementation: Implementation by the nurse for the patient would include monitoring neurological status; ensuring that lab values of organ function and therapeutic levels of medications are within normal

PowerPoint Slides

Table 15.3 Antiseizure Drugs that Potentiate GABA Action
Table 15.4 Hydantoins and Related Drugs
Table 15.5 Succinimides

Suggestion for Classroom Activities

- Prepare a crossword puzzle to assist students to learn and review drug classes and mechanism of action for drugs used to treat epilepsy.

PowerPoint Slides

Nursing Process Focus

- Patients Receiving Antiseizure Drug Therapy

Suggestion for Classroom Activities

- Divide the students into small groups. Assign each group a medication for epilepsy, and have them develop a care plan for each.

Suggestions for Clinical Activities

- Have students develop a teaching care plan for a client with epilepsy.
- Have students shadow a clinical pharmacist who is teaching a client about his epilepsy medication(s).

range; teaching the patient and family about the disease and drug regimen, including possible side effects; and teaching care during seizure activity.

5. Evaluation of outcome criteria includes evaluating the effectiveness of drug therapy through evaluation of patient goals.

GENERAL CHAPTER CONSIDERATIONS

1. Have students study and learn key terms listed at the beginning of the chapter.
2. Have students complete end-of-chapter exercises either in their book or on the MyNursingKit website.
3. Use the Classroom Response Questions provided in PowerPoint to assess students prior to lecture.

 MYNURSINGKIT
(www.mynursingkit.com)
- Websites
- NCLEX® questions
- Critical Thinking Questions
- Case Studies
- Animations and Videos
- Drug Prototype Questions

 MYNURSINGLAB
(www.mynursinglab.com)
- Knowledge Quick Check
- Pre/Posttests
- Customized study plans
- *Separate purchase*

 STUDENT WORKBOOK AND RESOURCE GUIDE
- Chapter 15 activities
- *Separate purchase*

PEARSON NURSE'S DRUG GUIDE
- *Separate purchase*

 PEARSON ETEXT
- Students can search, highlight, take notes, and more all in electronic format
- *Separate purchase*

 CLASSROOM RESPONSE QUESTION POWERPOINTS

 TESTBANK

© 2011 Pearson Education, Inc.

CHAPTER 16
DRUGS FOR EMOTIONAL AND MOOD DISORDERS

LEARNING OUTCOME 1

Identify the two major categories of mood disorders and their symptoms.

Concepts for Lecture

1. Depression is a disorder characterized by a sad or despondent mood. Many symptoms are associated with depression, including lack of energy; sleep disturbances; abnormal eating patterns; and feelings of despair, guilt, and hopelessness. Depression is the most common form of mental illness in the United States.
2. Bipolar disorder, once known as manic depression or bipolar depression is characterized by extreme and opposite moods, episodes of depression that alternate with episodes of mania. Patients may oscillate rapidly between both extremes, or there may be prolonged periods when their mood is normal. Depressive symptoms are the same as defined earlier. Mania is characterized by excessive CNS stimulation that results in agitation, excessive talking, elevated mood, grandiose thoughts, flight of ideas, constant movement, impulsive behavior, inflated self-esteem, racing thoughts, and short attention span. These symptoms must be present for at least one week.

LEARNING OUTCOME 2

Identify the symptoms of attention deficit-hyperactivity disorder.

Concepts for Lecture

Attention deficit/hyperactivity disorder (ADHD) is a condition characterized by poor attention span, behavior control issues, and/or hyperactivity. Although normally diagnosed in childhood, ADHD may extend into adulthood. The symptoms may include developmentally inappropriate behaviors involving difficulty in paying attention or focusing on tasks. ADHD may be diagnosed when the child's hyperactive behaviors significantly interfere with normal play, sleep, or learning activities. Increased motor activity is manifested by a tendency to be fidgety and impulsive and to interrupt and talk excessively. Children with this disorder may not be able to interact with others appropriately.

POWERPOINT SLIDES

SUGGESTION FOR CLASSROOM ACTIVITIES

- Have a psychiatrist or psychologist speak to the students about depression and bipolar disorder.

SUGGESTION FOR CLINICAL ACTIVITIES

- Arrange for students to observe at a mental health facility that deals with patients diagnosed with depression or bipolar depression.

REFERENCE

- Depression: *www.nimb.nib.gov/ health/publications/depression/ complete-index.shtml*

POWERPOINT SLIDES

SUGGESTION FOR CLASSROOM ACTIVITIES

- Have students discuss specific behaviors of an individual diagnosed with ADHD.

REFERENCE

- Attention Deficit Hyperactivity Disorder: *www.nimb.nib.gov/health/publications/ attention-deficit-hyperactivity-disorder/ complete-index.shtml*

LEARNING OUTCOME 3

Explain the etiology of major depressive disorder.

Concepts for Lecture

Depression is associated with dysfunction of neurotransmitters in certain regions of the brain. Some women experience intense mood shifts associated with hormonal changes during the menstrual cycle, pregnancy, childbirth, and menopause. Seasonal affective disorder (SAD) is a type of depression that is associated with a reduced release of the brain neurohormone melatonin.

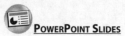
POWERPOINT SLIDES

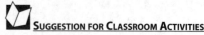
SUGGESTION FOR CLASSROOM ACTIVITIES

- Define seasonal affective disorder and its causes and treatment.

LEARNING OUTCOME 4

Discuss the nurse's role in the pharmacologic management of patients with depression, bipolar disorder, or attention deficit-hyperactivity disorder.

Concepts for Lecture

1. The role of the nurse with patients on medication for emotional and mood disorders involves careful monitoring of a patient's condition and providing education as it relates to the prescribed drug treatment. Assessing previous health history is essential, as conditions such as epilepsy, urinary retention, narrow angle glaucoma, and prostatic hypertrophy may be affected. Assess the patient's needs for antidepressant therapy by noting the intensity and duration of the patient's symptoms and identifying factors that lead to depression, such as life events and health changes. Obtain a careful drug history, including the use of CNS depressants, alcohol, and other antidepressants. Ask the patient about suicidal ideation, because the medication may take several weeks before full therapeutic benefit is obtained. Obtain a history of any disorders of sexual function and eating disorders. The patient may suffer from sexual dysfunction and weight gain. Obtain baseline vital signs, liver- and renal-function tests, cardiovascular status, and baseline body weight, as well as therapeutic blood levels as treatment continues. Information should include diet education related to foods that contain tyramine and information on signs and symptoms of lithium toxicity.
2. Antidepressants: Monitor vital signs. Monitor for dizziness, headache, tremor, nausea/vomiting, anxiety, disorientation, hyperreflexia, diaphoresis, and fever. These are signs of serotonin syndrome. Monitor neurologic and cardiovascular status. Monitor mental and emotional status. Monitor for underlying psychoses. Monitor sleep–wake cycle. Monitor renal and gastrointestinal status. Monitor liver function and hematologic status. Monitor visual acuity. Ensure patient safety.
3. Mood stabilizers: Monitor mental and emotional status. Monitor electrolyte balance, fluid balance, and I & O. Monitor renal and cardiovascular, as well as gastrointestinal, status.
4. Attention deficit/hyperactivity disorder: Monitor mental status. Monitor vital signs and gastrointestinal and nutritional status. Monitor laboratory tests as well as the effectiveness of drug therapy. Monitor growth and development and sleep–wake cycle.

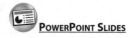
POWERPOINT SLIDES

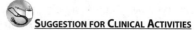
SUGGESTIONS FOR CLASSROOM ACTIVITIES

- Have students discuss the common foods that contain tyramines.
- Have students discuss the signs and symptoms of lithium toxicity.

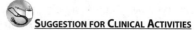
SUGGESTION FOR CLINICAL ACTIVITIES

- Have students prepare a care plan for a patient with an emotional or mood disorder.

© 2011 Pearson Education, Inc.

Learning Outcome 5

For each of the drug classes listed in Drugs at a Glance, recognize representative drug examples, and explain their mechanism of action, primary actions, and important adverse effects.

Concepts for Lecture

1. Antidepressants: Tricyclic antidepressants (TCA): The prototype drug is imipramine (Trofranil). The mechanism of action is inhibiting the reuptake of both norepinephrine and serotonins into presynaptic nerve terminals. The primary use is mainly for major depression and occasionally for milder situational depression. The adverse effects observed are orthostatic hypotension and rarely seen cardiac dysrhythmias. Sedation and anticholinergic effect are a common complaint but are generally more tolerable after several weeks of treatment. Selective serotonin reuptake inhibitors (SSRIs): The prototype drug is sertralline (Zoloft). The mechanism of action is to slow the reuptake of serotonin into presynaptic nerve terminals so that postsynaptic receptors become more sensitive. The primary use is in the treatment of depression because of their improved side effects. The most common side effects are sexual dysfunction, nausea, headache, weight gain, anxiety, and insomnia. Less common adverse effects include sedation, anticholinergic effects, and sympathomimetic effects.
2. Atypical antidepressants: Serotonin-norepinephrine reuptake inhibitors (SNRIs). The prototype drug is bupropion (Wellbutrin). The mechanism of action is to inhibit the reuptake of serotonin and affect the activity of norepinephrine and dopamine. The primary use is for depression. Adverse effects include sexual dysfunction, nausea, headache, weight gain, anxiety, and insomnia.
3. MAO inhibitors (MAOI): The prototype drug is phenelzine (Nardil). The mechanism of action is to decrease the effectiveness of the enzyme monoamine oxidase. The MAOIs limit the breakdown of norepinephrine, dopamine, and serotonin in CNS neurons. The primary use is to reduce the symptoms of depression. Common adverse effects of the MAOIs include orthostatic hypotension, headache, insomnia, and diarrhea. A primary concern is that these agents interact with a large number of foods and other medications, sometimes with serious effects.
4. Mood stabilizers: The prototype drug is lithium carbonate (Eskalith). The mechanism of action is sodium transport across cell membranes. The primary use is for bipolar disorder. The side effect may be excessive loss of sodium.
5. CNS stimulants: The prototype drug is methylphenidate hydrochloride (Ritalin). The mechanism of action is to stimulate specific areas of the CNS that heighten awareness and increase focus. The primary use is for ADHD. The adverse effects include insomnia, nervousness, anorexia, and weight loss.

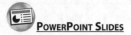

PowerPoint Slides

Prototype Drug
- sertraline (Zoloft)

Suggestion for Classroom Activities

- Divide students into groups and prepare a teaching plan for each type of medication discussed.

Suggestion for Clinical Activities

- Arrange for students to be involved with teaching a patient who has been recently placed on an antidepressant agent.

LEARNING OUTCOME 6

Categorize drugs used for mood and emotional disorders based on their classification and drug action.

Concepts for Lecture

1. Antidepressants: Tricyclic antidepressants are used mainly for major depression and affect the reuptake of norepinephrine and serotonin. Examples are Elavil, Ludiomil, and Asendin. Selective serotonin reuptake inhibitors are used for depression and slow the reuptake of serotonin. Examples are Celexa, Lexapro, and Paxil.
2. Atypical antidepressants are used for depression; they inhibit the reuptake of serotonin and affect the activity of norepinephrine and dopamine. Examples are Remeron, Serzone, and Effexor.
3. MAO inhibitors reduce the symptoms of depression, by decreasing the effectiveness of the enzyme monoamine oxidase; the MAOIs limit the breakdown of norepinephrine, dopamine, and serotonin in CNS neurons. Examples are Marplan, Nardil, and Parnate.
4. Mood stabilizers are used for bipolar disorder and transport sodium across cell membranes. An example is lithium carbonate.
5. CNS stimulants are used for ADHD and stimulate specific areas of the CNS that heighten awareness and increase focus. Examples are Adderall, Dexedrine, and Desoxyn.

LEARNING OUTCOME 7

Use the nursing process to care for patients receiving drug therapy for mood and emotional disorders.

Concepts for Lecture

1. Assessment: Assess previous health history. Assess the patient's need for antidepressant therapy by noting the intensity and duration of the patient's symptoms and identifying factors that led to depression. Obtain a careful drug history. Ask the patient about suicidal ideation. Obtain a history of any disorders of sexual function and eating disorders. Obtain laboratory tests as ordered by the physician, including baseline V/S and body weight; monitor therapeutic blood levels as treatment continues.
2. Nursing diagnoses: ineffective coping, disturbed thought processes related to side effects of the drug, and knowledge deficient, related to drug therapy.
3. Planning: Goals for patients receiving antidepressants include the patient's ability to explain depression and the medications needed to treat the condition.
4. Implementation: Encourage compliance with the medication regimen. Provide additional education regarding medication regimen with a clinical pharmacist and dietician.
5. Evaluation: Ideal outcome criteria for evaluation of the plan of care are to control the symptoms of emotional and mood disorders with limited side effects and no organ damage or injury. Patients are able to verbalize the importance of taking the prescribed medications.

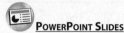 **POWERPOINT SLIDES**

Table 16.1 Antidepressants
Table 16.3 Drugs for Bipolar Disorder
Table 16.4 Drugs for Attention Deficit/ Hyperactivity Disorder

Prototype Drug
- imipramine (Tofranil)
- lithium (Eskalith)
- methylphenidate (Ritalin)

 NURSING PROCESS FOCUS
- Patients Receiving Lithium (Eskalith)
- Patients Receiving Methylphenidate (Ritalin)

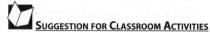 **REFERENCE**
- Information on Antidepressants: *www.nlm.nih.gov*

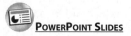 **SUGGESTION FOR CLASSROOM ACTIVITIES**
- Have students prepare drug cards for each of the classifications.

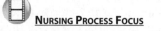 **POWERPOINT SLIDES**

Table 16.2 Foods Containing Tyramine

NURSING PROCESS FOCUS

Patients Receiving Antidepressant Therapy

Prototype Drug
- phenelzine (Nardil)

SUGGESTION FOR CLASSROOM ACTIVITIES
- Have students divide into groups to identify additional potential nursing diagnoses and document interventions and rationale for each diagnosis.

© 2011 Pearson Education, Inc.

GENERAL CHAPTER CONSIDERATIONS

1. Have students study and learn key terms listed at the beginning of the chapter.
2. Have students complete end-of-chapter exercises either in their book or on the MyNursingKit website.
3. Use the Classroom Response Questions provided in PowerPoint to assess students prior to lecture.

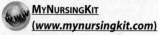

MyNursingKit
(www.mynursingkit.com)

- Websites
- NCLEX® questions
- Critical Thinking Questions
- Case Studies
- Animations and Videos
- Drug Prototype Questions

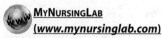

MyNursingLab
(www.mynursinglab.com)

- Knowledge Quick Check
- Pre/Posttests
- Customized study plans
- *Separate purchase*

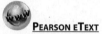

Student Workbook and Resource Guide

- Chapter 16 activities
- *Separate purchase*

Pearson Nurse's Drug Guide

- *Separate purchase*

Pearson eText

- Students can search, highlight, take notes, and more all in electronic format.
- *Separate purchase*

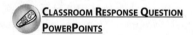

Classroom Response Question PowerPoints

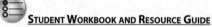

Testbank

CHAPTER 17
DRUGS FOR PSYCHOSES

LEARNING OUTCOME 1

Explain theories for the etiology of schizophrenia.

Concepts for Lecture

1. The nature of psychoses may be acute or chronic and can include such things as delusions, hallucinations, illusions, or paranoia. Delusions are firm ideas and beliefs not founded in reality. Hallucinations are seeing, hearing, or feeling something that is not there. Illusions are distorted perceptions of actual sensory stimuli. Paranoia is an extreme suspicion and delusion that individuals are being followed and that others are trying to harm them. Generally, an individual has disorganized behavior and difficulty relating to others.
2. Psychoses may be classified as an acute psychotic episode, which may occur over hours or days. Chronic psychoses develop over months or years.
3. Psychoses may be attributed to genetic, neurological, and environmental factors. Family members may have been afflicted. An individual may have imbalances in the neurotransmitters in specific areas of the brain, which may be the cause of this disorder. Environmental factors may include brain damage, overdoses of certain medications, chronic alcoholism, and drug addiction.
4. Schizophrenia is a type of psychosis characterized by abnormal thoughts and thought processes, disordered communication, withdrawal from other people and the outside environment, and severe depression. Individuals are at a high risk for suicide.

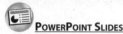

 POWERPOINT SLIDES

 SUGGESTIONS FOR CLASSROOM ACTIVITIES

- Define illusion, hallucination, and delusion, and give an example of each.
- Invite a psychiatrist to class to speak on the subject of psychoses and the most current pharmacological treatment.

 SUGGESTION FOR CLINICAL ACTIVITIES

- Develop a clinical rotation to a psychiatric facility where the student can observe the patient in an acute or chronic episode of psychoses and what pharmacological treatment is given to treat the psychoses.

LEARNING OUTCOME 2

Compare and contrast the positive and negative symptoms of schizophrenia.

Concepts for Lecture

1. Schizophrenia is the most common psychotic disorder, with symptoms first appearing in early adulthood. For men, those symptoms peak between age 15 and age 24; for women, between 25 and 34 years.
2. Many symptoms will appear, with some seemingly sudden and others developing over time. These symptoms can include hallucinations, delusions, or paranoia. Also, the patient exhibits strange and irrational behavior; severe depression, alternating rapidly between extreme hyperactivity and stupor; and attitudes of indifference or detachment toward life activities. Deterioration of personal hygiene and/or job or academic performance is seen. Withdrawal from social and interpersonal relationships is also observed.
3. Schizophrenia is characterized by positive and negative symptoms, and proper diagnosis of these symptoms is important for selection of the appropriate antipsychotic drug. Positive symptoms add on to normal behavior and include hallucinations, delusions, and a disorganized thought or speech pattern. Negative symptoms subtract from normal behavior

 POWERPOINT SLIDES

 SUGGESTIONS FOR CLASSROOM ACTIVITIES

- Describe major symptoms related to psychosis and particularly to schizophrenia.
- Define what distinguishes a positive symptom from a negative symptom.

SUGGESTION FOR CLINICAL ACTIVITIES

- From clinical rotation to a psychiatric facility, have the student observe a patient with acute schizophrenia and identify the positive and negative symptoms observed.

© 2011 Pearson Education, Inc.

and include lack of interest, motivation, responsiveness, and pleasure in daily activities. Many schizophrenics exhibit an indifferent personality. Symptoms of schizophrenia seem to be associated with the dopamine type 2 receptor. The antipsychotic medication attaches to the dopamine type 2 receptor site and reduces the symptoms of schizophrenia.

4. There is a condition known as schizoaffective disorder. The patient with this condition exhibits symptoms of both schizophrenia and mood disorder. The symptoms include distorted perceptions, hallucinations, and delusions and may be followed by extreme depression.

LEARNING OUTCOME 3

Discuss the rationale for selecting a specific antipsychotic drug for the treatment of schizophrenia.

Concepts for Lecture

1. An accurate diagnosis of schizophrenia must be made, as other conditions related to drug use, brain neoplasm, infections, or hemorrhage can cause psychotic-like symptoms.
2. The antipsychotic agents do not cure mental illness, and the patient's symptoms remain in remission only as long as the patient chooses to take the drug. There is no single drug of choice for schizophrenia. Two basic categories of drugs for psychoses are conventional antipsychotic and atypical antipsychotic. The conventional antipsychotic agents include the phenothiazines and phenothiazine-like drugs. The conventional antipsychotic is sometimes called first-generation or typical antipsychotic. They work to treat the positive signs of schizophrenia, such as hallucinations and delusions. They have been used in treatment of psychoses for 50 years. Atypical antipsychotic agents are newer alternatives to phenothiazines and control both positive and negative symptoms of schizophrenia. Antipsychotic drugs are sometimes referred to as neuroleptics.

LEARNING OUTCOME 4

Explain the importance of patient drug compliance in the pharmacotherapy of schizophrenia.

Concepts for Lecture

Management of severe mental illness is difficult. Antipsychotic medications control the symptoms but do not cure the disease. Patients with schizophrenia do not see themselves as abnormal and have difficulty understanding the need for medication. Symptoms of psychosis can be controlled by specific antipsychotic medications. The patient's symptoms can be controlled as long as the patient takes the medication. Many undesirable side effects are produced. The patient then does not want to comply with the medication regimen, causing more agitation, distrust, and frustration. Selection of the appropriate medication is based on clinician experience, the occurrence of side effects, and the needs of the patient.

  POWERPOINT SLIDES

Table 17.1 Conventional Antipsychotic Drugs: Phenothiazines
Table 17.2 Adverse Effects of Conventional Antipsychotic Drugs
Table 17.3 Conventional Antipsychotic Drugs: Nonphenothiazines

Prototype Drug
- chlorpromazine (Thorazine)
- haloperidol (Haldol)

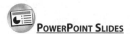 **REFERENCE**
- Mental Health Medications: *www.nimh.nih.gov/...medications/complete-index.shtm*

 POWERPOINT SLIDES

SUGGESTION FOR CLASSROOM ACTIVITIES
- Discuss reasons the patient may stop taking the antipsychotic medication.

LEARNING OUTCOME 5

Describe the nurse's role in the pharmacologic management of schizophrenia.

Concepts for Lecture

1. The role of the nurse in treatment using any type of antipsychotic medications involves careful monitoring of the patient's condition and providing education as it relates to the prescribed drug treatment. Many body systems are affected and can interact with drugs and alcohol. The nurse must obtain a complete health history, including any long-term physical problems (e.g., seizure disorders, cardiovascular disease), medication use, allergies, and lifestyle information, such as whether the patient smokes or uses alcohol, illegal drugs, caffeine, or herbal preparations. This allows for individualized treatment and may minimize the possibility of adverse reactions. Obtain a baseline health assessment, including liver and kidney function, vision problems, and mental status and, lastly, monitor for extrapyramidal symptoms and report to the physician immediately, as the medication may need to be discontinued.

2. Conventional (typical) antipsychotics: Monitor for decrease of psychotic symptoms. Monitor for side effects such as drowsiness, dizziness, lethargy, headache, blurred vision, skin rash, diaphoresis, nausea/vomiting, anorexia, diarrhea, menstrual irregularities, depression, hypotension, or hypertension. Monitor for anticholinergic side effects. Monitor for alcohol, illegal drug, and caffeine use. Monitor for cardiovascular changes. Monitor for smoking. Monitor for seizures and patient's environment.

3. Atypical antipsychotic: Monitor RBC and WBC and hematologic side effects. Observe for side effects and anticholinergic side effects. Monitor for decrease of psychotic symptoms and alcohol or illegal drug use as well as caffeine and nicotine use. Monitor the elderly closely.

LEARNING OUTCOME 6

Explain the symptoms associated with extrapyramidal side effects of antipsychotic drugs.

Concepts for Lecture

1. Extrapyramidal symptoms (EPS) include lip smacking (tardive dyskinesia); spasms of the face, tongue, or back muscles; facial grimacing; involuntary upward eye movements; jerking motions (acute dystonias); extreme restlessness (akathisia); stooped posture; shuffling gait; and tremors at rest (Parkinsonism symptoms).

2. A possible life-threatening side effect is neuroleptic malignant syndrome (NMS). In this condition, the patient suffers a toxic reaction to therapeutic doses of an antipsychotic drug. The patient exhibits elevated temperature, unstable blood pressure, profuse sweating, dyspnea, muscle rigidity, and incontinence. Observe and report to the physician immediately.

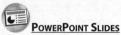

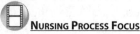

POWERPOINT SLIDES

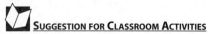

NURSING PROCESS FOCUS

- Patients Receiving Conventional Antipsychotic Therapy

SUGGESTION FOR CLASSROOM ACTIVITIES

- Discuss reasons the patient may stop taking the antipsychotic medication.

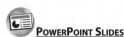

POWERPOINT SLIDES

SUGGESTIONS FOR CLASSROOM ACTIVITIES

- Define tardive dyskinesia, acute dystonia, akathisia, and Parkinsonism symptoms.
- Define the symptoms of neuroleptic malignant syndrome.

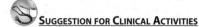

SUGGESTION FOR CLINICAL ACTIVITIES

- Identify patients in the psychiatric clinical setting with these symptoms.

© 2011 Pearson Education, Inc.

LEARNING OUTCOME 7

For each of the drug classes listed in Drugs at a Glance, know representative drug examples, and explain their mechanism of action, primary actions, and important adverse effects.

Concepts for Lecture

1. Phenothiazines: Prototype drug: phenothiazine chlorpromazine (Thorazine). The mechanism of action is thought to act by preventing dopamine and serotonin from occupying their receptor sites in certain regions of the brain. The action blocks the excitement associated with the positive symptoms of schizophrenia, although they differ in their potency and side effects. Primary use is for severe mental illness. The significant adverse effects include acute dystonia, akathisia, Parkinsonism, tardive dyskinesia, anticholinergic effects, sedation, hypotension, sexual dysfunction, and neuroleptic malignant syndrome. (See Table 17.2 for a full description of each symptom.)

2. Nonphenothiazines: Prototype drug: haloperidol (Haldol). The mechanism of action is believed to be the same as the phenothiazines; that is, by blocking of the dopamine type 2 receptor, thus reducing the symptoms. Primary use is for severe mental illness. Significant adverse effects are identical to the phenothiazines, although the degree to which a particular effect occurs depends on the specific drug. In general, the nonphenothiazine agents cause less sedation and fewer anticholinergic side effects than Thorazine but exhibit an equal or even greater incidence of extrapyramidal signs.

3. Atypical Antipsychotics: Prototype drug: clozapine (Clozaril). The mechanism of action is largely unknown, but these drugs are thought to act by blocking several different receptor types in the brain. The atypical agents block dopamine type 2 receptors as well as serotonin and alpha-adrenergic receptors. The primary use is for severe mental illness. This classification treats both the positive and negative symptoms of schizophrenia. The adverse effects are fewer with this type of medication, but the obesity and the risk factors associated with it need to be monitored.

LEARNING OUTCOME 8

Categorize drugs used for psychoses based on their classification and drug action.

Concepts for Lecture

1. Conventional (Typical) Antipsychotic Agents: Phenothiazines are thought to act by preventing dopamine and serotonin from occupying their receptor sites in certain regions of the brain. The action blocks the excitement associated with the positive side effect. Examples are Mellaril, Serentil, and Prolixin. Nonphenothiazines are believed to act by the same mechanism as the phenothiazines; that is, by blocking of the dopamine type 2 receptor, thus reducing the symptoms. Examples are Taractan, Loxitane, and Navane.

 POWERPOINT SLIDES

Table 17.1 Conventional Antipsychotic Drugs: Phenothiazines
Table 17.2 Adverse Effects of Conventional Antipsychotic Drugs
Table 17.3 Conventional Antipsychotic Drugs: Nonphenothiazines
Table 17.4 Atypical Antipsychotic Drugs

Prototype Drug
- chlorpromazine (Thorazine)
- haloperidol (Haldol)
- risperidone (Risperdal)

 SUGGESTION FOR CLASSROOM ACTIVITIES

- Prepare a classroom activity such as a crossword puzzle to help students review the actions, use, and side effects of the antipsychotic drugs.

 SUGGESTION FOR CLINICAL ACTIVITIES

- Have the students complete drug cards that will help them review the actions, use, and side effects of antipsychotic drugs.

 POWERPOINT SLIDES

2. Atypical Antipsychotics: The action is largely unknown, but they are thought to act by blocking several different receptor types in the brain. The atypical agents block dopamine type 2 receptors as well as serotonin and alpha-adrenergic receptors. This classification treats both the positive and negative symptoms of schizophrenia. Examples are Seroquel, Risperdal, and Zyprexa.

LEARNING OUTCOME 9

Use the nursing process to care for patients receiving drug therapy for psychoses.

Concepts for Lecture

1. Assessment: Monitor patients' condition, noting the positive and negative symptoms associated with schizophrenia and other behaviors associated with mental illness. Obtain baseline health assessment including vital signs, height and weight, history of past mental illness, and lifestyle information on smoking and use of illegal drugs, alcohol, and caffeine. Also include current medications and dietary habits. Obtain baseline blood and urine samples as ordered by the physician. Assess the patient's and the family's knowledge of psychoses and the medication regimen.
2. Nursing diagnosis: *Anxiety* related to symptoms of psychosis, side effects of medication; *Knowledge Deficit* related to new medication regimen; *Noncompliance* related to lack of understanding and continued use of alcohol and caffeine-containing products.
3. Planning: Goal for patients receiving antipsychotic therapy is to remain compliant with medication regimen and remain free of psychotic symptoms.
4. Implementation: Encourage compliance with medication regimen. Provide additional education regarding medication regimen, such as consultation with clinical pharmacist, written and/or visual education material, and follow-up in local outpatient psychiatric clinics.
5. Evaluation: An ideal outcome criterion for evaluation of the plan of care is the patient to remain free of symptoms related to psychoses. Patients verbalize the importance of taking prescribed medications to assist them in their continued management of the disease.

 POWERPOINT SLIDES

 NURSING PROCESS FOCUS
- Patients Receiving Atypical Antipsychotic Therapy

 SUGGESTION FOR CLASSROOM ACTIVITIES
- With the above-listed nursing diagnoses, have students list various interventions and rationale to support the diagnosis.

 SUGGESTION FOR CLINICAL ACTIVITIES
- Write a care plan for a patient receiving antipsychotic medications.

© 2011 Pearson Education, Inc.

GENERAL CHAPTER CONSIDERATIONS

1. Have students study and learn key terms listed at the beginning of the chapter.
2. Have students complete end-of-chapter exercises either in their book or on the MyNursingKit website.
3. Use the Classroom Response Questions provided in PowerPoint to assess students prior to lecture.

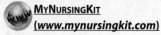

MYNURSINGKIT (*www.mynursingkit.com*)

- Websites
- NCLEX® questions
- Critical Thinking Questions
- Case Studies
- Animations and Videos
- Drug Prototype Questions

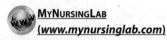

MYNURSINGLAB (*www.mynursinglab.com*)

- Knowledge Quick Check
- Pre/Posttests
- Customized study plans
- *Separate purchase*

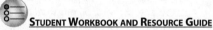

STUDENT WORKBOOK AND RESOURCE GUIDE

- Chapter 17 activities
- *Separate purchase*

PEARSON NURSE'S DRUG GUIDE

- *Separate purchase*

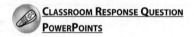

PEARSON ETEXT

- Students can search, highlight, take notes, and more all in electronic format.
- *Separate purchase*

CLASSROOM RESPONSE QUESTION POWERPOINTS

TESTBANK

CHAPTER 18
DRUGS FOR THE CONTROL OF PAIN

LEARNING OUTCOME 1

Relate the importance of pain assessment to effective pharmacotherapy.

Concepts for Lecture

1. Pain is a subjective experience in that patients may describe the same degree and type of pain differently. Health care workers are assisted in the assessment of pain with the use of numerical scales and survey instruments. Effective pharmacotherapy pain management is dependent on accurate assessment of the degree of pain and on determining underlying disorders that may be causing the pain.
2. Pain may be classified as either acute or chronic. Acute pain is usually an intense pain lasting for a defined period of time, whereas chronic pain lasts longer than six months and may interfere with daily activities.
3. Sources of pain are classified as nociceptor pain, which is due to injury to tissues, and neuropathic pain, which is caused by injury to nerves. Nociceptor pain is usually exhibited as sharp, localized pain or dull, throbbing, aching pain. Burning, shooting, or numbing pain characterizes neuropathic pain.

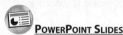
POWERPOINT SLIDES

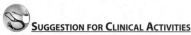
SUGGESTIONS FOR CLASSROOM ACTIVITIES

- Have students research different scales of pain assessment.
- Develop critical thinking questions that address identification of types of pain.

SUGGESTION FOR CLINICAL ACTIVITIES

- Have students assess pain level of patients using the accepted pain scale in their clinical facility and identify the type of pain.

LEARNING OUTCOME 2

Explain the neural mechanisms at the level of the spinal cord responsible for pain.

Concepts for Lecture

Pain transmission begins when nociceptors are stimulated. Nociceptors are pain receptors found throughout the body. The spinal cord receives the pain impulse along two types of sensory neurons, the A ≠ fibers, which are wrapped in myelin, and the C fibers, which are unmyelinated. A ≠ fibers signal sharp, well-defined pain, and C fibers signal dull, poorly localized pain. Since pain signals begin at the level of nociceptors in peripheral tissues and travel through the CNS, there are several target areas for pharmacological and nonpharmacological interruption of the pain transmission. Pain interruption may act at the peripheral level or at the CNS level.

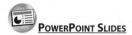
POWERPOINT SLIDES

SUGGESTION FOR CLASSROOM ACTIVITIES

- Have students diagram the transmission of pain to the level of the spinal neurotransmitters.

LEARNING OUTCOME 3

Explain how pain can be controlled by inhibiting the release of spinal neurotransmitters.

Concepts for Lecture

Neurotransmitters are responsible for passing the message of pain on to neurons once the pain impulse reaches the spinal cord. The neurotransmitter called substance P is responsible for continuing the pain message to the brain and can be affected by other neurons released

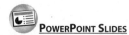
POWERPOINT SLIDES

SUGGESTION FOR CLASSROOM ACTIVITIES

- Invite a pain specialist or neurologist to speak on the topic of spinal neurotransmitters and pain control at this level.

© 2011 Pearson Education, Inc.

from the CNS. Examples of the neurons that can affect substance P are endogenous opioids, which include endorphins, dynorphins, and enkaphalins. Endogenous opioids may modify sensory information at the level of the spinal cord, interrupting the transmission of pain.

LEARNING OUTCOME 4

Describe the role of nonpharmacologic therapies in pain management.

Concepts for Lecture

1. Due to the side effects of medications for pain, some patients choose nonpharmacological pain management over pharmacological management. These therapies may be used in place or as an adjunct to medications. If used as an adjunct, lower doses of pain medications are needed. Nonpharmacological therapies include acupuncture, massage, heat or cold, relaxation, chiropractic manipulation, and transcutaneous electrical nerve stimulation (TENS).
2. Patients with intractable cancer pain may require more invasive therapy, such as radiation or chemotherapy, to reduce tumor size; relieving nerve stimulation; or surgery to remove the tumor completely. Nerve blocks are also used on patients with intractable pain.

LEARNING OUTCOME 5

Compare and contrast the types of opioid receptors and their importance in effective management of pain.

Concepts for Lecture

Opioid medications interact with opioid receptors to control pain. Opioid agonists are drugs that stimulate certain receptors, and opioid antagonists block certain receptors. The opioid receptors include mu, kappa, sigma, delta, and epsilon. Examples of the pharmacology involved includes morphine, which activates mu and kappa receptors; pentazocine (Talwin), which is a mixed agonist–antagonist since it activates the kappa receptor but blocks the mu receptor; and naloxone (Narcan), which inhibits both the kappa and mu receptors.

LEARNING OUTCOME 6

Explain the role of opioid antagonists in the diagnosis and treatment of acute opioid toxicity.

Concepts for Lecture

Acute opioid toxicity causes severe respiratory depression and is a medical emergency. Naloxone (Narcan) is an opioid antagonist that inhibits mu and kappa; therefore, it is used to reverse respiratory depression and other symptoms of opioid toxicity. If the patient is unconscious from apparent opioid toxicity and information is not available as to the drug that has been taken, opioid antagonists aid in diagnosing the overdose. If the patient's symptoms do not reverse rapidly, the overdose was most likely not due to an opioid substance.

SUGGESTION FOR CLINICAL ACTIVITIES
- Have students rotate through a neurologist's office or pain-control clinic to observe pain assessment and pain-control measures.

POWERPOINT SLIDES

SUGGESTION FOR CLASSROOM ACTIVITIES
- Invite a massage therapist, acupuncturist, and/or chiropractor to discuss nonpharmacological methods of pain management.

SUGGESTION FOR CLINICAL ACTIVITIES
- Have students rotate through a pain facility for observation of techniques.

POWERPOINT SLIDES

Table 18.1 Responses Produced by Activation of Specific Opioid Receptors

SUGGESTION FOR CLASSROOM ACTIVITIES
- Prepare questions regarding the opioid receptors and the actions of the medications on the receptor.

SUGGESTION FOR CLINICAL ACTIVITIES
- Have students monitor pain control on patients receiving opioids for pain control.

POWERPOINT SLIDES

Prototype Drug
- morphine (Astrmorph PF, Duramorph, others)
- naloxone (Narcan)

Table 18.2 Opioids for Pain Management
Table 18.3 Nonopioid Analgesics

SUGGESTION FOR CLASSROOM ACTIVITIES

- Invite an emergency room or surgery nurse to discuss his or her experiences with using naloxone (Narcan) on patients for treatment or diagnostic purposes.

LEARNING OUTCOME 7

Describe the long-term treatment of opioid dependence.

Concepts for Lecture

1. Although effective at relieving pain, the opioids have a greater risk for dependence than almost any other class of medications; tolerance develops relatively quickly. One common method of treating opioid dependence is to switch the patient from IV and inhalation forms of illegal drugs to methadone (Dolophine). Although an opioid, oral methadone does not cause the euphoria of injectable opioids. Methadone does not cure the dependence; however, the patient must continue taking the drug to avoid withdrawal symptoms. This therapy, called methadone maintenance, may continue for many months or years, until the patient decides to enter a total withdrawal treatment program.

2. A newer treatment option is to administer buprenorphine (Subutex), a mixed opioid agonist–antagonist, by the sublingual route. This drug is used early in opioid abuse therapy to prevent opioid-withdrawal symptoms. Suboxone, a combination agent, is used later in the maintenance of opioid addiction.

POWERPOINT SLIDES

SUGGESTION FOR CLASSROOM ACTIVITIES

- Have an addiction counselor speak to the students about long-term treatment for opioid addiction.

LEARNING OUTCOME 8

Compare the pharmacotherapeutic approaches of preventing migraines to those of aborting migraines.

Concepts for Lecture

1. There are two primary goals for the pharmacological therapy of migraines (see Table 18.4). The first is to stop migraines in progress, and the second is to prevent migraines from occurring. The drugs used to abort migraines are different from those used for prophylaxis. Drug therapy is most effective if begun before a migraine has reached severe level.

2. There are two major drug classes that stop migraines in progress: triptans and ergot alkaloids. Both stimulate serotonin (5-HT).

3. Triptans, such as sumatriptan (Imitrex), are selective for 5-HT receptor subtype and act by constricting certain blood vessels in the brain.

4. Ergot alkaloids, such as ergotamine (Ergostat), interact with adrenergic, dopaminergic, and serotonin receptors and promote vasoconstriction, which stops ongoing migraines.

5. Drugs for migraine prophylaxis include beta-adrenergic blockers, calcium channel blockers, antidepressants, and antiseizure drugs. These drugs are started when the number of migraines is high and the patient does not respond to the drugs used to stop migraines.

POWERPOINT SLIDES

Table 18.4 Antimigraine Drugs

SUGGESTION FOR CLASSROOM ACTIVITIES

- Discuss the side effects of drugs used to stop migraines in progress and drugs for migraine prophylaxis.

SUGGESTION FOR CLINICAL ACTIVITIES

- Have students prepare drug cards for the different drug classifications.

© 2011 Pearson Education, Inc.

LEARNING OUTCOME 9

Describe the nurse's role in the pharmacologic management of patients receiving analgesics and antimigraine drugs.

Concepts for Lecture

1. The role of the nurse in opioid therapy involves careful monitoring of a patient's condition and providing education as it relates to the prescribed drug treatment. Perform an initial assessment to determine the presence or history of severe respiratory disorders, ICP, seizures, and liver or renal disease. Obtain an allergy history before administering these drugs. Complete lab work as ordered by the physician. Assess the patient's pain level before and during therapy, including the character, duration, location, and intensity of pain. Obtain a history of current medication, especially alcohol and other CNS depressants. Assess the social context of the patient's environment for the potential for opioid dependency. If giving to drug-dependent patient, monitor for signs of opioid withdrawal such as cramping, vomiting, hypertension, and anxiety. Opioids should not be administered if respirations are below 12 per minute, and narcotic antagonists such as Narcan should be readily available to reverse the effects. Assistance with activity is important. Monitor urine output for retention and patient's bowel habits for constipation.
2. With the use of opioid antagonist therapy, the nurse wants to continue the careful monitoring of the patient's condition, especially the respiratory status. Have resuscitative equipment available.
3. In the care of the patient using nonopioid analgesics, careful monitoring of a patient's condition and providing education as it relates to the prescribed drug treatment is necessary. If the patient is on high doses of these medications, complete a thorough assessment for the presence or history of hypersensitivity, bleeding disorders, gastric ulcers, severe renal or hepatic disease, and pregnancy. Obtain laboratory tests on the patient's renal and liver function as ordered by the physician during the patient's pharmacotherapy. Good pain assessment is needed, including location, character, and intensity of pain. Monitor patient for side effects.
4. Migraine therapy also involves monitoring the patient's condition and providing education regarding the medication regimen. Data collection will include the frequency and intensity of the migraine headaches and the presence or history of MI, angina, and hypertension and the presence or history of renal and liver disease, diabetes, and pregnancy. Assess vital signs and the patient's stress levels and coping mechanisms, because migraines may be associated with these factors. Assess the patient's neurological status. Provide a quiet, calm environment with decreased noised and lighting. Apply cold packs to help lessen the pain. Assess the pain level before medication administration. Monitor for side effects: dizziness, drowsiness, tingling, weakness, and GI complaints.

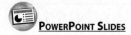

POWERPOINT SLIDES

Prototype Drug
- sumatriptan (Imitrex)

NURSING PROCESS FOCUS
- Patients Receiving NSAID Therapy
- Patients Receiving Triptan Therapy

SUGGESTIONS FOR CLASSROOM ACTIVITIES
- Have students discuss the appropriate lab to be ordered before opioid therapy and explain the rationale.
- Lead students in a discussion involving the question, when are nonopioid analgesics contraindicated and why?

SUGGESTION FOR CLINICAL ACTIVITIES
- Have student prepare a teaching plan for a patient with newly diagnosed migraine headaches.

LEARNING OUTCOME 10

For each of the drug classes listed in Drugs at a Glance, know representative drug examples, and explain the mechanisms of drug action, primary actions, and important adverse effects.

Concepts for Lecture

1. **Opioid (narcotic) analgesic:** Prototype drug: opioid agonists (morphine). The mechanism of action is to exert the effects by interacting with specific receptors. The primary use is for moderate to severe pain that cannot be controlled with other classes of analgesics and as anesthesia. Adverse effects can include respiratory depression, sedation, nausea, and vomiting. **Opioids with mixed agonist–antagonist activity:** (example: Talwin) stimulate the opioid receptor; thus, they cause analgesia. However, the withdrawal symptoms or side effects are not as intense.

2. **Opioid antagonists:** Prototype drug: naloxone (Narcan). The mechanism of action is to interact with at least six types of receptors. The primary use may be to reverse the respiratory depression and other acute symptoms. Adverse effects may include overdose as a result of overly aggressive pain therapy or as a result of substance abuse. This is a medical emergency, with respiratory depression being the most serious problem.

3. **Nonopioid analgesics:** Prototype drug: acetaminophen (Tylenol). The mechanism of action to treat fever is at the level of the hypothalamus and causes dilation of peripheral blood vessels enabling sweating and dissipation of heat. The primary use is for the treatment of fever and to relieve pain. Adverse effects are uncommon with therapeutic doses. **Nonsteroidal anti-inflammatory drugs (NSAIDs):** Prototype drug: ibuprofen (Motrin). The mechanism of action is to inhibit cyclooxygenase, an enzyme responsible for the formation of prostaglandins. With the enzyme inhibited, inflammation and pain are reduced. Primary use is for mild or moderate pain, especially for pain associated with inflammation. Adverse effects may include GI upset, such as gastric ulcers and bleeding and acute renal failure. **Salicylates:** Prototype drug: aspirin (ASA). The mechanism of action has anticoagulant, antipyretic, anti-inflammatory, and analgesic abilities. The adverse effects are possible GI distress and bleeding in high doses. Aspirin may increase the action of oral hypoglycemic agents. **Selective Cox-2 inhibitors:** Prototype drug: celecoxib (Celebrex). The mechanism of action is similar to the NSAIDs. The primary use is for relief of pain, fever, and inflammation. Adverse effects are mild and related to the GI system. **Centrally acting agents:** Prototype drug: tramadol (Ultram). The mechanism of action is weak opioid activity. The primary use is as centrally acting analgesics. Adverse effects can include: CNS, GI, CV, and dermatologic effects.

4. **Antimigraine agents:** Two drug classes—(1) the Tripans: Prototype drug: sumatriptan (Imitrex) and (2) ergot alkaloids. The mechanism of action for both is to act as serotonin agonists. The Tripans are thought to act by constricting certain intracranial vessels. The primary use is to abort migraines with or without auras. Adverse effect is GI upset. The mechanism of action of the ergot alkaloids is to promote vasoconstriction. The primary use is to terminate ongoing migraines. Adverse effects can include nausea, vomiting, weakness in the legs, myalgia, numbness and tingling in fingers and toes, angina-like pain, and tachycardia.

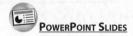

POWERPOINT SLIDES

Prototype Drug
- naloxone (Narcan)
- aspirin (Acetylsalicylic Acid, ASA)

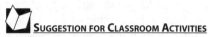

SUGGESTION FOR CLASSROOM ACTIVITIES
- Have students prepare medication cards to aid them in understanding the action, use, and side effects of each drug.

© 2011 Pearson Education, Inc.

Learning Outcome 11

Categorize drugs used in the treatment of pain based on their classification and mechanism of action.

Concepts for Lecture

1. **Opioid (narcotic) analgesic:** Opioid analgesic medications exert their effects by interacting with specific receptors. Opioids are the drugs of choice for moderate to severe pain that cannot be controlled with other classes of analgesics. Some opioids are used for anesthesia. Examples: Hydrocodone, OxyContin, Percocet.
2. **Opioids antagonists:** Overdose can occur as a result of overly aggressive pain therapy or as a result of substance abuse. This is a medical emergency, with respiratory depression being the most serious problem. The opioid antagonists may be used to reverse the respiratory depression and other acute symptoms. Examples: Revex, Narcan, Trexan.
3. **Nonopioid analgesics:** ASA is used for the treatment of fever and to relieve pain. **Nonsteroidal anti-inflammatory drugs (NSAIDs)** inhibit cyclooxygenase, an enzyme responsible for the formation of prostaglandins. With the enzyme inhibited, inflammation and pain are reduced. Use for mild or moderate pain, especially for pain associated with inflammation. **Salicylates** have anticoagulant, antipyretic, anti-inflammatory, and analgesic abilities. **Selective Cox-2 inhibitors** relieve pain, fever, and inflammation and are similar to other NSAIDs. Centrally acting agents that have weak opioid activity. Examples: Cataflam, Dolobid, Lodine, Nalfon.
4. **Antimigraine agents:** two drug classes—(1) the Tripans and (2) ergot alkaloids. Mechanism of action: They are both serotonin agonists. The Tripans are thought to act by constricting certain intracranial vessels. The ergot alkaloids promote vasoconstriction, which terminates ongoing migraines. Examples: Migranal, Axert, Relpax, Frova.

Learning Outcome 12

Use the nursing process to care for patients receiving drug therapy for pain.

Concepts for Lecture

1. Assessment of a patient on drug therapy for pain would include careful monitoring of a patient's condition. Assess vital signs, particularly respiratory status. Assess the patient's pain level before and during therapy including the character, duration, location, and intensity of pain. Obtain a history of current medication, especially alcohol and other CNS depressants. Assess for the presence or history of hypersensitivity, bleeding disorders, gastric ulcers, severe renal or hepatic disease, and pregnancy. Obtain history of the frequency and intensity of the migraine headaches. Assess the patient's stress levels and coping mechanisms, as migraines may be associated with these factors. Monitor for side effects and the potential for dependency.
2. Nursing diagnoses: *Knowledge Deficit* regarding condition, *Therapeutic Regimen*, and *Potential Side Effects of Medication*; *Risk for Dependency* related to opioid therapy.

 PowerPoint Slides

 Suggestion for Classroom Activities

- Have students prepare a teaching plan to explain the action and use of the above-listed medications.

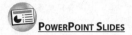 **Suggestion for Clinical Activities**

- Have the student prepare a teaching plan for an assigned patient who is being administered any of the above-listed medications.

 PowerPoint Slides

 Suggestion for Classroom Activities

- Have students discuss additional nursing diagnoses related to medication for pain control.

 Suggestion for Clinical Activities

- Have students prepare a care plan for a patient on opioid therapy.

3. Planning: The goal for patients receiving medication for pain control is to explain the proper use of medication and to be free of pain without dependency.
4. Implementation: Encourage compliance with medication regimen. Provide additional education regarding medication regimen, such as consultation with the clinical pharmacist, written and/or visual educational material, and home-health visits to ensure patient's ability to follow prescribed therapy.
5. Evaluation: An ideal outcome criterion for evaluation of the plan of care is pain control with limited side effects and no dependency. Patient is able to verbalize the importance of taking prescribed medications to assist in continued management of the disease.

GENERAL CHAPTER CONSIDERATIONS

1. Have students study and learn key terms listed at the beginning of the chapter.
2. Have students complete end-of-chapter exercises either in their book or on the MyNursingKit website.
3. Use the Classroom Response Questions provided in PowerPoint to assess students prior to lecture.

MyNursingKit (www.mynursingkit.com)

- Websites
- NCLEX® questions
- Critical Thinking Questions
- Case Studies
- Animations and Videos
- Drug Prototype Questions

MyNursingLab (www.mynursinglab.com)

- Knowledge Quick Check
- Pre/Posttests
- Customized study plans
- *Separate purchase*

STUDENT WORKBOOK AND RESOURCE GUIDE

- Chapter 18 activities
- *Separate purchase*

PEARSON NURSE'S DRUG GUIDE

- *Separate purchase*

PEARSON eTEXT

- Students can search, highlight, take notes, and more all in electronic format.
- *Separate purchase*

CLASSROOM RESPONSE QUESTION POWERPOINTS

TESTBANK

CHAPTER 19
DRUGS FOR LOCAL AND GENERAL ANESTHESIA

LEARNING OUTCOME 1

Compare and contrast the five major clinical techniques for administering local anesthetics.

Concepts for Lecture

1. Topical (surface) anesthesia is administered via creams, sprays, suppositories, drops, and lozenges. These types of anesthesia are applied to mucous membranes such as the eyes, lips, gums, nasal membranes, and throat. Topical anesthetics are generally safe unless absorbed.
2. Infiltration (field-block) anesthesia is administered by direct injection into tissue immediate to the surgical site. The drug diffuses into the tissue and blocks a specific group of nerves near the surgical site.
3. Nerve-block anesthesia is directly injected into tissues that may be distant from the surgical site. This method affects the nerve bundles supplying the surgical area and is used to block sensation in a limb or large area of the face.
4. Spinal anesthesia is injected into the cerebral spinal fluid (CSF) and affects large regional areas such as the lower abdomen and legs.
5. Epidural anesthesia is injected into the epidural space of the spinal canal and is used most often in obstetrics during labor and delivery.

LEARNING OUTCOME 2

Describe differences between the two major chemical classes of local anesthetics.

Concepts for Lecture

1. Esters are a group of local anesthetics that contain an ester chemical linkage in their structure. Incidence of allergic reactions is low, and the method of metabolism is plasma esterases.
2. Amides are a group of local anesthetics that contain an amide chemical linkage in their structure. Incidence of allergic reactions is *very* low, and the method of metabolism is hepatic enzymes. Amides have replaced most esters because amides have a longer duration of action and fewer side effects.
3. Local anesthetics work by stopping axonal conduction, thereby blocking sodium channels in the axonal membrane. This stops sodium influx, which brings conduction to a halt.

 POWERPOINT SLIDES

Table 19.1 Methods of Local Anesthetic Administration

 SUGGESTION FOR CLASSROOM ACTIVITIES

• Ask a nurse anesthetist to speak to the class regarding clinical techniques for administering local anesthesia.

 SUGGESTION FOR CLINICAL ACTIVITIES

• Rotate students through a surgery center or surgeon's office to observe local anesthetic administration.

 POWERPOINT SLIDES

Table 19.2 Selected Local Anesthetics

 SUGGESTION FOR CLASSROOM ACTIVITIES

• Have students develop review questions on the differences between esters and amides.

LEARNING OUTCOME 3

Explain why epinephrine and sodium hydroxide are sometimes included in local anesthetic cartridges.

Concepts for Lecture

1. A small amount of epinephrine is sometimes added to local anesthetics in order to constrict blood vessels in the immediate area being anesthetized. By doing this, the anesthetic is kept in the area longer, which increases the duration of the anesthetic.
2. Sodium hydroxide, an alkaline agent, is sometimes added to increase the effectiveness of an anesthetic in areas that have extensive local infection since bacteria acidifies the area. Anesthetics do not work as well in an acidic environment.

LEARNING OUTCOME 4

Identify the actions of general anesthetics on the CNS.

Concepts for Lecture

General anesthetics act by preventing the flow of sodium into neurons in the CNS. This delays nerve impulses and reduces neural activity. This action rapidly produces unconsciousness and lack of responsiveness to all painful stimuli.

LEARNING OUTCOME 5

Compare and contrast the two primary ways that general anesthesia may be induced.

Concepts for Lecture

1. General anesthesia may be administered by inhalation. These agents may be gases or volatile liquids. Gases exist in a gaseous state at atmospheric pressure. The only gas in current use is nitrous oxide. Volatile liquids exist in a liquid state at atmospheric pressure and can easily be volatilized for administration by inhalation.
2. Intravenous anesthetics are usually administered first because they act within a few seconds. These may be used alone or in combination with inhalation agents. IV agents allow dosages of inhalation agents to be reduced, and they produce effects that cannot be achieved with an inhalation agent alone. This approach is called balanced anesthesia.

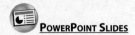 **POWERPOINT SLIDES**

Prototype Drug
• lidocaine (Xylocaine)

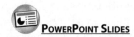 **POWERPOINT SLIDES**

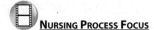 **NURSING PROCESS FOCUS**
• Patients Receiving Local Anesthesia

SUGGESTION FOR CLASSROOM ACTIVITIES
• Invite a nurse anesthetist to speak about general anesthetics.

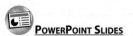 **POWERPOINT SLIDES**

Table 19.4 Inhaled General Anesthetics

Prototype Drug
• nitrous oxide
• halothane (Fluothane)

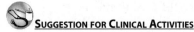 **SUGGESTION FOR CLASSROOM ACTIVITIES**
• Discuss the different types, risks, uses, and nursing care associated with anesthesia.

SUGGESTION FOR CLINICAL ACTIVITIES
• Rotate students through a surgery center or hospital to observe an anesthesiologist or nurse anesthetist administer general anesthesia to several patients.

© 2011 Pearson Education, Inc.

LEARNING OUTCOME 6

Identify the four stages of general anesthesia.

Concepts for Lecture

1. Stages of general anesthesia begin with Stage I, loss of pain—patient loses general sensation and proceeds until loss of consciousness; Stage II, excitement and hyperactivity—patient may be delirious, heart rate and breathing may be irregular, and blood pressure increases; Stage III, surgical anesthesia—skeletal muscles become relaxed, delirium and vital signs stabilize, eye movements slow, and patient is still, with surgery beginning; and Stage IV, paralysis of the medulla region in the brain, which can result in death. This stage is usually avoided.

LEARNING OUTCOME 7

For each of the drug classes listed in Drugs at a Glance, know representative drug examples, and explain their mechanisms of action, primary actions, and important adverse effects.

Concepts for Lecture

1. Local anesthetics fall, primarily, under the classes of amides and esters. **Amides:** Prototype drug: lidocaine (Xylocaine). The mechanism of action for local anesthetics is stoppage of axonal conduction by blocking sodium channels in the axonal membrane. The primary use of local anesthetics is primarily for brief medical or dental procedures. Adverse effects for local anesthetics are uncommon but may include CNS stimulation with early adverse effects, CNS depression with later adverse effects, and rash. Allergies are rare, but if they do occur, it is usually due to sulfites that are added as a preservative. **Esters:** Prototype drug: procaine (Novocain). The mechanism of action and primary use is as stated above with the amides. Amides have largely replaced the esters.

2. General anesthetics include inhalation agents. These agents are either gases or volatile liquids. Prototype drug: nitrous oxide. Mechanism of action: Inhalation agents work by preventing the flow of sodium into neurons in the CNS. This delays nerve impulses and reduces neural activity. Primary use: Inhalation agents are usually used in conjunction with IV agents to maintain loss of consciousness. The only gaseous agent is nitrous oxide, which can be given alone, most commonly used for dental procedures. Adverse effects of inhalation agents include nausea and vomiting, CNS depression, respiratory difficulty, and vital-sign changes.

3. Intravenous agents for general anesthesia include barbiturate and barbiturate-like agents, opioids, and benzodiazepines. A prototype-drug example of barbiturate and barbiturate-like agents is thiopental sodium (Penthonal). IV agents are most often used in combination with inhalation agents. The benefit of using both types of agents is that lesser amounts of each results in fewer serious side effects. IV agents are only used alone for medical procedures lasting approximately 15 minutes. These agents act rapidly to induce unconsciousness, within 10 to 20 seconds after being administered, and are then followed by inhalation agents. These agents produce unconsciousness and amnesia, and some are used for conscious sedation. Adverse reactions include allergic

POWERPOINT SLIDES

Table 19.3 Stages of General Anesthesia

SUGGESTION FOR CLASSROOM ACTIVITIES

- Ask students who have had surgery to share their experiences with anesthesia.

SUGGESTION FOR CLINICAL ACTIVITIES

- Have students interview postoperative patients regarding their experience with anesthesia.

POWERPOINT SLIDES

Table 19.5 Intravenous Anesthetics
Table 19.6 Selected Adjuncts to Anesthesia

Prototype Drug
- thipental (Pentothal)
- succinylcholine (Anectine)

SUGGESTION FOR CLASSROOM ACTIVITIES

- Have students prepare drug cards for all the classes of anesthetics.

SUGGESTION FOR CLINICAL ACTIVITIES

- Have students rotate through the recovery room (postanesthetic room) of a local hospital to observe and assess patients.

reactions, dysrhythmias, respiratory depression, CNS depression, shivering, headache, nausea and vomiting, and vital-sign changes. During the immediate postoperative period, hallucinations, confusion, and excitability may occur.

4. Adjuncts to anesthesia are medications that are given to complement the effects of general anesthesia or to treat anticipated side effects of anesthesia and may be given prior to, during, or after surgery.

LEARNING OUTCOME 8

Categorize drugs used for anesthesia based on their classification and drug action.

Concepts for Lecture

1. The local anesthetics fall under the classifications of amides and esters. These drugs work by stopping axonal conduction, thereby blocking sodium channels in the axonal membrane. This causes a rapid loss of sensation to a limited part of the body. Examples of amides: lidocaine (Xylocaine), articaine (Septodont), bupivacaine (Marcaine); examples of esters: benzocaine (Solarcaine), procaine (Novocain), chloroprocaine (Nesacaine).

2. General anesthetics are classified as either inhalation agents or intravenous agents. Inhalation agents include gaseous and volatile liquid agents. These drugs work by preventing the flow of sodium into neurons in the CNS, which delays nerve impulses and produces a reduction in neural activity. Inhaled agents are usually used in combination with intravenous agents. The only gaseous agent is nitrous oxide. Volatile liquid agents include halothane (Fluothane), enflurane (Ethrane), and isoflurane (Forane).

3. Intravenous agents for general anesthesia include the drug classes of barbiturates and barbiturate-like agents, opioids, and benzodiazepines. These drugs are usually used in combination with inhalation agents and are administered first to induce rapid unconsciousness. Barbiturate and barbiturate-like agents induce unconsciousness and include thiopental sodium (Penthonal) and methohexital sodium (Brevital). Benzodiazepines induce unconsciousness and amnesia and include diazepam (Valium), lorazepam (Ativan), and midazolam hydrochloride (Versed). Opioids, such as fentanyl citrate (Sublimaze), are often given with the antipsychotic agent droperidol (Inapsine) to produce neurolept analgesia, in which patients are conscious but insensitive to pain and unconnected to their surroundings.

LEARNING OUTCOME 9

Use the nursing process to care for patients who are receiving anesthesia.

Concepts for Lecture

1. Assessment: The nurse should collect information regarding allergies to anesthetics; obtain complete health and drug history; assess for the presence or history of any severe respiratory, cardiac, renal, or liver disorders; obtain baseline vital signs and lab results; assess patient's knowledge of procedure and level of anxiety; for local anesthetics, assess the skin for intactness, infections, or wounds.

2. Nursing diagnoses: Possible nursing diagnoses that would apply to the patient receiving a local anesthetic include *Risk for Aspiration; Risk for*

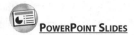
POWERPOINT SLIDES

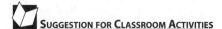
SUGGESTION FOR CLASSROOM ACTIVITIES

- Have students prepare flash cards to learn the drug classes of anesthetics.

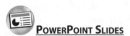
POWERPOINT SLIDES

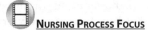
NURSING PROCESS FOCUS

- Patients Receiving General Anesthesia

© 2011 Pearson Education, Inc.

injury; and *Deficient Knowledge* related to drug use. Nursing diagnoses that could apply to the patient receiving a general anesthetic include *Anxiety* related to surgical procedure; *Impaired Gas Exchange*; *Nausea* related to drug side effect; *Disturbed Sensory Perception*; *Ineffective Breathing Pattern*; and *Decreased Cardiac Output*.

3. Planning: During the planning phase of the nursing process, possible goals for the patient receiving an anesthetic would be for the patient to experience no pain during the procedure; experience no side effects or adverse reactions to the anesthetic; and experience adequate anesthesia during the procedure.

4. Implementation: Interventions that may be implemented in order to meet the patient's needs when receiving anesthesia could include monitoring for cardiovascular and respiratory side effects; monitoring for length of anesthetic effectiveness; providing for patient safety; monitoring vital signs; and monitoring recovery from anesthesia.

5. Evaluation should ensure that the effectiveness of the drug therapy as evidenced by patient goals and expected outcomes is being met.

GENERAL CHAPTER CONSIDERATIONS

1. Have students study and learn key terms listed at the beginning of the chapter.
2. Have students complete end-of-chapter exercises either in their book or on the MyNursingKit website.
3. Use the Classroom Response Questions provided in PowerPoint to assess students prior to lecture.

SUGGESTIONS FOR CLASSROOM ACTIVITIES

- Divide students into small groups. Assign a specific nursing diagnosis to each group, and have the group develop a care plan for that diagnosis.
- Have students role-play with a classmate the assessment phase of obtaining the health history of a preoperative patient.

SUGGESTION FOR CLINICAL ACTIVITIES

- Have students complete a care plan for assigned surgical patients who have received local or general anesthesia.

MYNURSINGKIT (*www.mynursingkit.com*)

- Websites
- NCLEX® questions
- Case studies
- Making the Patient Connection

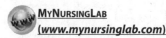

MYNURSINGLAB (*www.mynursinglab.com*)

- Knowledge Quick Check
- Pre/Posttests
- Customized study plans
- *Separate purchase*

STUDENT WORKBOOK AND RESOURCE GUIDE

- Chapter 19 activities
- *Separate purchase*

PEARSON NURSE'S DRUG GUIDE

- *Separate purchase*

PEARSON ETEXT

- Students can search, highlight, take notes, and more all in electronic format.
- *Separate purchase*

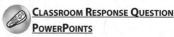

CLASSROOM RESPONSE QUESTION POWERPOINTS

TESTBANK

CHAPTER 20
DRUGS FOR DEGENERATIVE DISEASES OF THE NERVOUS SYSTEM

LEARNING OUTCOME 1

Identify the most common degenerative diseases of the central nervous system (CNS).

Concepts for Lecture

1. Alzheimer's disease is the most common type of degenerative disease of the CNS. Alzheimer's disease is a progressive loss of brain function characterized by memory loss, confusion, and dementia.
2. Amyotrophic lateral sclerosis is a progressive weakness and wasting of muscles caused by destruction of motor neurons.
3. Huntington's chorea is an autosomal dominant genetic disorder that results in progressive dementia and involuntary, spasmodic movements of limb and facial muscles.
4. Multiple sclerosis results from demyelination of neurons in the CNS, resulting in progressive weakness, visual disturbances, mood alterations, and cognitive deficits.
5. Parkinson's disease is the second most common degenerative disease of the CNS. Parkinson's is a progressive loss of dopamine in the CNS, causing tremor, muscle rigidity, and abnormal movement and posture.

 POWERPOINT SLIDES

Table 20.1 Degenerative Diseases of the Central Nervous System

 SUGGESTION FOR CLASSROOM ACTIVITIES

- Divide students into small groups, and have them prepare and present a poster identifying common degenerative CNS diseases.

 SUGGESTION FOR CLINICAL ACTIVITIES

- Have students attend support group meetings for degenerative CNS diseases.

 REFERENCES

- National Institute of Neurological Disorders and Stroke: *www.ninds.nih.gov/*
- Huntington's Disease Society of America: *www.hdsa.org*
- National Parkinson Foundation: *www.parkinson.org/Page.aspx?pid=201*

LEARNING OUTCOME 2

Describe symptoms of Parkinson's disease.

Concepts for Lecture

The symptoms of Parkinson's disease include tremors, such as shakiness of the hand and head when at rest and pin-rolling with the thumb and forefinger; muscle rigidity, characterized by stiffness and rigid facial expression; bradykinesia, characterized by a shuffling gait and difficulty chewing, swallowing, and speaking; and postural instability, exhibited by stumbling, frequently falling, and humped back.

 POWERPOINT SLIDES

 SUGGESTION FOR CLASSROOM ACTIVITIES

- Develop a word search that contains symptoms of Parkinson's disease.

 SUGGESTION FOR CLINICAL ACTIVITIES

- Rotate students through a neurologist's office for observation of patients with Parkinson's disease.

LEARNING OUTCOME 3

Explain the neurochemical basis for Parkinson's disease, focusing on the roles of dopamine and acetylcholine in the brain.

Concepts for Lecture

1. Symptoms of Parkinson's disease result from degeneration and destruction of dopamine-producing neurons in the substantia nigra portion of the brain.

 POWERPOINT SLIDES

 SUGGESTION FOR CLASSROOM ACTIVITIES

- Discuss how dopamine and acetylcholine work in the brain.

© 2011 Pearson Education, Inc.

In a healthy patient, neurons in this region of the brain supply dopamine to the corpus striatum. The corpus striatum controls unconscious muscle movement.

2. The proper balance of the neurotransmitters dopamine and acetylcholine in the corpus striatum affects balance, posture, muscle tone, and involuntary movement. Absence of dopamine allows acetylcholine to stimulate this area of the brain, resulting in Parkinson symptoms (parkinsonism). Drug therapy for parkinsonism restores dopamine function and blocks acetylcholine in the corpus striatum.

LEARNING OUTCOME 4

Describe the nurse's role in the pharmacologic management of Parkinson's disease and Alzheimer's disease.

Concepts for Lecture

1. The role of the nurse in the pharmacologic management of Parkinson's disease is based on nursing considerations for **dopaminergic** drug therapy. These drugs are contraindicated in patients with narrow-angle glaucoma. During initial treatment, the patient's vital signs should be closely monitored, since these drugs can cause hypotension and tachycardia. Muscle twitching and mood changes are signs of drug toxicity. Patient teaching should include increasing fiber and fluid to prevent constipation and avoiding drugs and foods high in pyridoxine (vitamin B_6), which includes some OTC drugs and fortified cereals. The patient should know that it may take several months before the drug is fully effective and that abruptly stopping the drug may cause a Parkinsonism crisis to occur.

2. The role of the nurse in the pharmacologic management of Parkinson's disease based on **anticholinergics,** which block the effect of acetylcholine, is similar to the nurse's role with dopaminergics, with the following differences in patient teaching. To relieve dry mouth, patients should take frequent drinks of cool liquids or suck on sugarless candy. The medication should be taken with milk or food to prevent GI upset. The patient should avoid alcohol, wear dark glasses, and avoid bright sunlight. Stopping the drug abruptly may result in tremors, insomnia, and restlessness.

3. The role of the nurse in the pharmacologic management of Alzheimer's disease based on **acetylcholinesterase (AChE) inhibitors** includes assessing baseline vital signs and monitoring for hypotension; monitoring patients for side effects or reactions such as a change in mental status, mood changes, dizziness, insomnia, and anorexia. Patients with narrow-angle glaucoma should not take revastigmine (Exelon). Patient teaching includes encouraging the patient to take the drug with food or milk to avoid GI upset, to drink cool liquids or suck on hard candy for dry mouth, and to take the drug strictly as prescribed to avoid serious side effects. Teach signs and symptoms of overdose, which include severe nausea/vomiting, sweating, salivation, hypotension, bradycardia, convulsions, and increased muscle weakness (including respiratory muscles).

 POWERPOINT SLIDES

Table 20.2 Dopaminergic Drugs Used for Parkinsonism

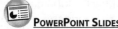 **SUGGESTION FOR CLASSROOM ACTIVITIES**

- Invite a nurse practitioner to speak to students regarding the role of the nurse in the pharmacotherapy of patients with Parkinson's disease and Alzheimer's disease.

 SUGGESTION FOR CLINICAL ACTIVITIES

- Have the students develop a drug-regimen teaching plan for assigned patients with Parkinson's disease and Alzheimer's disease.

LEARNING OUTCOME 5

Describe symptoms of Alzheimer's disease and explain theories about why these symptoms develop.

Concepts for Lecture

1. Drugs for Parkinson's disease include dopaminergics agents. The prototype drug is levodopa (Larodopa). The mechanism of action is to attempt to restore the functional balance of dopamine and acetylcholine in the corpus striatum of the brain. Combining levodopa (Laradopa) with the carbidopa (combined drug name Sinemet) increases its effectiveness. Other dopaminergics drugs are given as adjunct therapy, such as ropinirole (Requip) and bromocriptine (Parlodel). The primary use is to inhibit enzymes that destroy levodopa or directly activate the dopamine receptor in the brain. Important adverse reactions include nausea and vomiting, dyskinesias, postural hypotension, psychosis, dark urine and sweat, and activation of malignant melanoma.

2. Drugs for Parkinson's disease also include anticholinergics. The prototype drug is benztropine mesylate (Cogentin). The mechanism of action is centrally acting drugs that block the effect of the neurotransmitter acetylcholine. This inhibits the overactivity of acetylcholine that occurs with Parkinson's disease. These drugs are not as effective as dopaminergics. The primary use is in the early stages of the disease. Important adverse reactions occur because of the peripheral anticholinergic effects and include dry mouth, blurred vision, photophobia, urinary retention, constipation, tachycardia, and aggravation or precipitation of glaucoma.

3. Acetylcholinesterase (AchE) inhibitors are used in the treatment of Alzheimer's disease. The prototype drug is donepezil hydrochloride (Aricept). The mechanism of action is to prevent the breakdown of acetylcholine by AchE, which increases the availability of acetylcholine at cholinergic synapses. This enhances the transmission in the cholinergic neurons that have not been destroyed by the disease. The primary use is to slow the progression of the disease. Adverse reactions include nausea/vomiting, dizziness and headache, bronchoconstriction, and liver injury (tacrine/Cognex).

LEARNING OUTCOME 6

Explain the goals of pharmacotherapy for Alzheimer's disease and the efficacy of existing medications.

Concepts for Lecture

1. The cause of Alzheimer's disease (AD) is unknown. Theories on the cause of the disease include genetic defects on chromosome 1, 14, or 21; chronic inflammation; excess free radicals; and environmental factors. However, the structural damage in the brain consists of amyloid plaques and neurofibrillary tangles. These changes in the brain have been found during autopsies of nearly all patients with the diagnosis. These structural changes cause loss in both the number and function of neurons. Symptoms result from progressive damage to neurons in the area of the brain that is responsible for learning and memory, the hippocampus, which requires acetylcholine as the neurotransmitter.

2. Symptoms include impaired memory and judgment, confusion and disorientation, inability to recognize family or friends, aggressive behavior, depression, psychoses, and anxiety.

POWERPOINT SLIDES

Pharmacotherapy Illustrated 20.1
Antiparkinson Drugs

Prototype Drug
- levodopa (Larodopa)

NURSING PROCESS FOCUS

- Patients Receive Levodopa (Larodopa or Levodopa with Carbidopa (Sinemet)

REFERENCE

- Levodopa and Parkinson's *www.ninds.nih.gov/disorders/parkinsons_disease/detail_parkinsons_disease.htm*

SUGGESTION FOR CLASSROOM ACTIVITIES

- Have students prepare drug cards for the drugs listed in Drugs at a Glance.

SUGGESTION FOR CLINICAL ACTIVITIES

- Have students assess and present assessment information on drug side effects of assigned patients during postconference.

POWERPOINT SLIDES

SUGGESTION FOR CLASSROOM ACTIVITIES

- Discuss symptoms and theories of Alzheimer's disease (AD).

SUGGESTION FOR CLINICAL ACTIVITIES

- Have students report on their assessment of AD patients to other students during postconference discussions.

© 2011 Pearson Education, Inc.

LEARNING OUTCOME 7

Describe the signs and basis for development of multiple sclerosis symptoms.

Concepts for Lecture

The goal of pharmacotherapy for AD is to slow memory loss and other progressive symptoms of dementia and to improve functioning in three domains: activities of daily living (ADLs), behavior, and cognition. There is no cure for AD, and efficacy is only moderate for these drugs, slowing the progress of the disease by only a few months in many patients. Treatment is often ineffective in late stages of AD because many neurons have been damaged by this point and the drugs only work on functioning neurons. All of the AChE inhibitors have equal efficacy. Many new drugs are currently under investigation for the treatment of AD. Medications are also given as adjunct therapy for symptoms of depression, anxiety, and psychoses.

LEARNING OUTCOME 8

Categorize drugs used in the treatment of Alzheimer's disease, Parkinson's disease, and multiple sclerosis based on their classification and mechanism of action.

Concepts for Lecture

1. Drugs for AD include AChE inhibitors. These drugs prevent the breakdown of acetylcholine by AchE, which increases the availability of acetylcholine at cholinergic synapses. This enhances the transmission in the cholinergic neurons that have not been destroyed by the disease. These drugs do not stop the progression of Alzheimer's; they only slow the progression. Included in this class of drugs are donepezil hydrochloride (Aricept), galantamine (Reminyl), tacrine (Cognex), and rivastigmine tartrate (Exelon).

2. Dopaminergics are drugs used to treat Parkinson's disease. These drugs attempt to restore the functional balance of dopamine and acetylcholine in the corpus striatum of the brain. Levodopa (Laradopa) is the most effective drug for treatment of the disease. Combining levodopa (Laradopa) with carbidopa (combined drug name Sinemet) increases its effectiveness. Other dopaminergics drugs are given as adjunct therapy, such as ropinirole (Requip) and bromocriptine (Parlodel). These drugs have properties that inhibit enzymes that destroy levodopa or directly activate the dopamine receptor in the brain.

3. Drugs for Parkinson's disease also include anticholinergics, such as benztropine mesylate (Cogentin) and triexyphenidyl hydrochloride (Artane). These medications are centrally acting drugs that block the effect of the neurotransmitter acetylcholine. This inhibits the overactivity of acetylcholine that occurs with Parkinson's disease. These drugs are not as effective as dopaminergics; therefore, they are most beneficial in the early stages of the disease.

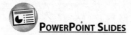
POWERPOINT SLIDES

Table 20.4 Acetylcholinesterase Inhibitors Used for Alzheimer's Disease

Prototype Drug
- bentropine (Cogentin)

SUGGESTION FOR CLASSROOM ACTIVITIES

- Have students research and report on new drugs being investigated for AD.

SUGGESTION FOR CLINICAL ACTIVITIES

- Have students assess patients and report on effectiveness of drug therapy for assigned patients.

POWERPOINT SLIDES

Table 20.4 Disease-modifying Drugs Used for Multiple Sclerosis

Prototype Drug
- donepezil (Aricept)

SUGGESTION FOR CLASSROOM ACTIVITIES

- Have students prepare drug cards for each class of drug.

LEARNING OUTCOME 9

For each of the drug classes listed in Drugs at a Glance, know representative drug examples, and explain their mechanisms of action, primary actions, and important adverse effects.

Concepts for Lecture

1. **Assessment:** During the assessment phase of the nursing process, the nurse should obtain a complete health history (including allergies and drug history, in order to help prevent interactions), baseline evaluation of the severity of the disease (including current signs and symptoms), baseline vital signs and lab tests, and the patient's and patient's family's knowledge of disease process.

2. **Nursing diagnoses:** Possible nursing diagnoses for the patient receiving drug therapy for degenerative diseases of the CNS include *Risk for Falls; Deficient Knowledge* related to drug therapy; *Deficient Knowledge* related to disease process; *Impaired Physical Mobility; Self-Care Deficit, Feeding, Bathing, Toileting; Constipation.*

3. **Planning:** Expected outcomes and patient goals include an increased ease of movement and decreased symptoms of the disease; understanding of the drug regimen; understanding of the disease process; importance of adhering to the drug regimen; and immediately reporting side effects.

4. **Implementation:** Interventions that may be implemented for the patient receiving drug therapy for degenerative diseases of the CNS include monitoring of vital signs and lab tests, providing for patient safety, and monitoring for behavior changes and symptoms of overdose. Additional interventions include monitoring the patient for improved functional status and monitoring for drug side effects.

5. Evaluation of the plan of care consists of evaluating the effectiveness of drug therapy by confirming that the patient goals and expected outcomes have been met.

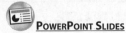

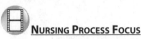

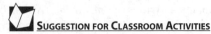

- Patients Receiving Levodopa (Larodopa) or Levodopa with Carbidopa (Sinemet)

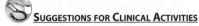

SUGGESTION FOR CLASSROOM ACTIVITIES

- Divide students into small groups and have them prepare and present a sample care plan for a patient with a degenerative CNS disease.

SUGGESTIONS FOR CLINICAL ACTIVITIES

- Have students attend a care plan meeting for assigned patients with degenerative CNS disease.
- Have students develop their own care plan on assigned patients with degenerative CNS.

© 2011 Pearson Education, Inc.

GENERAL CHAPTER CONSIDERATIONS

1. Have students study and learn key terms listed at the beginning of the chapter.
2. Have students complete end-of-chapter exercises either in their book or on the MyNursingKit website.
3. Use the Classroom Response Questions provided in PowerPoint to assess students prior to lecture.

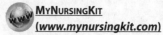

MYNURSINGKIT
(*www.mynursingkit.com*)

- Websites
- NCLEX® questions
- Critical Thinking Questions
- Case Studies
- Animations and Videos
- Drug Prototype Questions

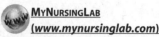

MYNURSINGLAB
(*www.mynursinglab.com*)

- Knowledge Quick Check
- Pre/Posttests
- Customized study plans
- *Separate purchase*

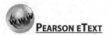

STUDENT WORKBOOK AND RESOURCE GUIDE

- Chapter 20 activities
- *Separate purchase*

PEARSON NURSE'S DRUG GUIDE

- *Separate purchase*

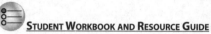

PEARSON ETEXT

- Students can search, highlight, take notes, and more all in electronic format.
- *Separate purchase*

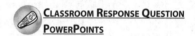

CLASSROOM RESPONSE QUESTION POWERPOINTS

TESTBANK

CHAPTER 21
DRUGS FOR NEUROMUSCULAR DISORDERS

LEARNING OUTCOME 1

Identify the different body systems contributing to muscle movement.

Concepts for Lecture

Muscle movement is dependent on several body systems, such as the nervous, muscular, endocrine, and skeletal systems. Blood levels of the minerals sodium, potassium, and calcium help determine the proper functioning of the neural pathways and functioning of the muscles, bones, and joints.

 POWERPOINT SLIDES

 SUGGESTION FOR CLASSROOM ACTIVITIES

• Review the anatomy and physiology of the musculoskeletal system.

LEARNING OUTCOME 2

Discuss nonpharmacologic therapies used to treat muscle spasms and spasticity.

Concepts for Lecture

1. Muscle spasms are involuntary contractions of a muscle or group of muscles, which result in a diminished level of functioning.
2. Spasticity is a condition that often results from damage to the CNS in which certain muscle groups remain in a continuous state of contraction. These muscles become stiff with increased muscle tone.
3. Nonpharmacologic treatment of muscle spasms is commonly used in conjunction with medications. Treatment includes performing a history and a physical exam to determine the etiology and then immobilization of the affected muscle, application of heat or cold, hydrotherapy, ultrasound, supervised exercise, massage, and manipulation.
4. Nonpharmacologic treatment of muscle spasticity includes regular and consistent physical therapy, muscle stretching, muscle-group-strengthening exercises, and repetitive-motion exercises. In extreme cases, surgery for tendon release or severing of a nerve-muscle pathway may be performed.

 POWERPOINT SLIDES

 SUGGESTION FOR CLASSROOM ACTIVITIES

• Invite a physical therapist and a massage therapist to speak to students regarding nonpharmacotherapy of patients experiencing muscle spasms or spasticity.

 SUGGESTION FOR CLINICAL ACTIVITIES

• Rotate students through a rehabilitation unit or hospital to observe patients receiving therapy for muscle spasms or spasticity.

 REFERENCE

• Muscle Spasms: *www.medicinenet.com/muscle_spasms/article.htm*

LEARNING OUTCOME 3

Explain the goals of pharmacotherapy with skeletal muscle relaxants.

Concepts for Lecture

1. The therapeutic goals of pharmacotherapy with skeletal-muscle relaxants are aimed at minimizing discomfort, increasing range of motion, and improving the patient's ability to function independently.
2. Pharmacotherapy for muscle spasms includes analgesics, anti-inflammatory agents, and centrally acting muscle relaxants.

 POWERPOINT SLIDES

 SUGGESTION FOR CLASSROOM ACTIVITIES

• Invite a clinical pharmacist to speak to students regarding the goals of pharmacotherapy for muscle relaxants.

 SUGGESTION FOR CLINICAL ACTIVITIES

• Have students monitor the effects of muscle relaxants on assigned patients.

© 2011 Pearson Education, Inc.

LEARNING OUTCOME 4

Describe the nurse's role in the pharmacologic management of muscle spasms.

Concepts for Lecture

The role of the nurse in the pharmacological management of muscle spasms includes obtaining a complete health history, including allergies, drug history, and possible drug interactions. Establish a baseline level of consciousness and vital signs. Assessing for drowsiness and dizziness is important, since these are common side effects due to the CNS-depression effect of the drugs. Monitor pain, including its location, duration, and precipitating factors. Monitor for withdrawal reactions. Monitor muscle tone, range of motion, and degree of muscle spasm. Provide additional pain-relief measures, such as positioning and gentle massage. Monitor for side effects, which can include drowsiness, dry mouth, dizziness, muscle weakness, nausea, and diarrhea. Educate the patients who have liver disease, or pulmonary and/or cardiac dysfunction that they should not take these drugs. Patients should be warned against drinking alcohol or taking any drug that depresses the CNS, since these practices would intensify the CNS-depressant effects of these drugs. Abruptly stopping these drugs can result in seizures.

LEARNING OUTCOME 5

Compare and contrast the roles of the following drug categories in treating muscle spasms and spasticity: centrally acting skeletal-muscle relaxants, direct-acting antispasmodics, and skeletal muscle relaxants for short medical procedures.

Concepts for Lecture

1. Skeletal-muscle relaxants are used to treat local spasms resulting from muscular injury. These drugs decrease localized pain and tenderness, which often result in increased range of motion.
2. The direct-acting antispasmodics produce an antispasmodic effect at the neuromuscular junction and skeletal muscle to suppress hyperactive reflexes. These drugs are typically used for spasms resulting from CNS disorders.

LEARNING OUTCOME 6

For each of the drug classes listed in Drugs at a Glance, know representative drugs, and explain their mechanisms of action, primary actions, and important adverse effects.

Concepts for Lecture

1. Centrally acting muscle relaxants act at various levels of the CNS. The prototype drug is cyclobenzaprine (Flexeril). The mechanism of action works by inhibiting upper-motor-neuron activity within the brain

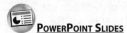

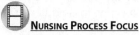 **POWERPOINT SLIDES**

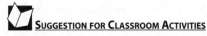 **NURSING PROCESS FOCUS**

- Patients Receiving Drugs for Muscle Spasms or Spasticity

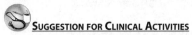 **SUGGESTION FOR CLASSROOM ACTIVITIES**

- Prepare critical-thinking questions that are specific to the nurse's role in the pharmacological management of muscle spasms. Review answers in discussion with entire class.

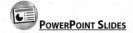 **SUGGESTION FOR CLINICAL ACTIVITIES**

- Prepare a teaching plan for patients receiving medications for muscle spasms.

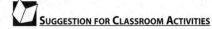 **POWERPOINT SLIDES**

Table 21.1 Centrally Acting Skeletal Muscle Relaxants
Table 21.2 Direct-acting Antispasmodic Drugs

Prototype Drug
- cyclobenzaprine (Flexeril, Cycoflex)

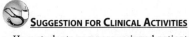 **SUGGESTION FOR CLASSROOM ACTIVITIES**

- Divide students into two groups to discuss the roles of the two categories.

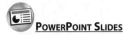 **SUGGESTION FOR CLINICAL ACTIVITIES**

- Have students compare assigned patients' drug regimen during postconference.

POWERPOINT SLIDES

Table 21.3 Neuromuscular Blocking Agents

Prototype Drug
- dantrolene sodium (Dantrium)

© 2011 Pearson Education, Inc.

and/or spinal cord, which causes CNS depression and/or alterations in simple spinal reflexes. The primary use is to treat localized spasms. Adverse reactions include CNS depression, hepatic toxicity, physical dependence, and anticholinergic effects.

2. Direct-acting antispasmodics. The prototype drug is dantrolene (Dantrium). The mechanism of action is to work at the neuromuscular junction, which interferes with the release of calcium ions in skeletal muscle. The primary use is to relieve symptoms of dystonias and to relieve leg cramps. Adverse effects include hepatic toxicity, muscle weakness, drowsiness, and diarrhea.

LEARNING OUTCOME 7

Use the nursing process to care for patients who are receiving drug therapy for muscle spasms.

Concepts for Lecture

1. Assessment of the patient receiving drug therapy for muscle spasms includes obtaining a complete health history (including allergies and drug history to determine possible interactions), physical examination, baseline vital signs and lab tests, and baseline level of consciousness (LOC), since these drugs often cause CNS depression.

2. Nursing diagnoses may include *Pain,* related to the muscle spasms; *Impaired Physical Mobility; Risk for Injury,* related to the drug side effects; *Deficient Knowledge,* related to drug-treatment regimen.

3. Planning: Patient goals and expected outcomes for the patient receiving drug therapy for muscle spasms include the patient's reporting a decrease in pain, an increase in range of motion, and a reduction of the muscle spasm; having no adverse effects from drug therapy; and demonstrating an understanding of the drug regimen.

4. Implementation: Possible interventions for the patient include monitoring LOC and vital signs; monitoring pain; monitoring muscle tone, range of motion, degree of muscle spasm; and provide adjunct therapy for pain; e.g., position changes, hot or cold applications.

5. Evaluation of the effectiveness of drug therapy is evidenced by patient goals and outcomes being met.

SUGGESTION FOR CLASSROOM ACTIVITIES

- Have students prepare drug cards for the drugs in the classes found in Drugs at a Glance.

SUGGESTION FOR CLINICAL ACTIVITIES

- Have students share in postconference adverse reactions they have assessed in assigned patients.

POWERPOINT SLIDES

NURSING PROCESS FOCUS

- Patients Receiving Drugs for Muscle Spasms or Spasticity

SUGGESTION FOR CLASSROOM ACTIVITIES

- Divide students into small groups and have them prepare a sample care plan for patients receiving drug therapy for muscle spasms.

SUGGESTION FOR CLINICAL ACTIVITIES

- Have students prepare care plans for assigned patients receiving drug therapy for muscle spasms.

© 2011 Pearson Education, Inc.

GENERAL CHAPTER CONSIDERATIONS

1. Have students study and learn key terms listed at the beginning of the chapter.
2. Have students complete end-of-chapter exercises either in their book or on the MyNursingKit website.
3. Use the Classroom Response Questions provided in PowerPoint to assess students prior to lecture.

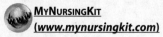

MYNURSINGKIT
(*www.mynursingkit.com*)

- Websites
- NCLEX® questions
- Case studies
- Making the Patient Connection

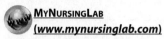

MYNURSINGLAB
(*www.mynursinglab.com*)

- Knowledge Quick Check
- Pre/Posttests
- Customized study plans
- *Separate purchase*

STUDENT WORKBOOK AND RESOURCE GUIDE

- Chapter 21 activities
- *Separate purchase*

PEARSON NURSE'S DRUG GUIDE

- *Separate purchase*

PEARSON ETEXT

- Students can search, highlight, take notes, and more all in electronic format.
- *Separate purchase*

CLASSROOM RESPONSE QUESTION POWERPOINTS

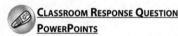

TESTBANK

CHAPTER 22
DRUGS FOR LIPID DISORDERS

LEARNING OUTCOME 1

Summarize the link between high blood cholesterol, LDL levels, and cardiovascular disease.

Concepts for Lecture

Lipids and cardiovascular disease: Research during the 1960s and 1970s brought about a nutritional revolution as new knowledge about lipids and their relationship to obesity and cardiovascular disease allowed people to make more intelligent lifestyle choices. Advances in the diagnosis of lipid disorders have helped to identify those patients at greatest risk for cardiovascular disease and those most likely to benefit from pharmacologic intervention. Research in pharmacology has led to safe, effective drugs for lowering lipid levels, thus decreasing the risk of cardiovascular-related diseases. As a result of this knowledge and from advancements in pharmacology, the incidence of death due to most cardiovascular diseases has been declining.

LEARNING OUTCOME 2

Compare and contrast the different types of lipids.

Concepts for Lecture

1. The three types of lipids are triglycerides, phospholipids, and steroids. (See Figure 22.1.)
2. The most common are the triglycerides, or neutral fats, which form a large family of different lipids, all having three fatty acids attached to a chemical backbone of glycerol. They are the major storage forms of fat in the body and serve as an energy source; they account for 90% of total lipids in the body.
3. The second type is the phospholipids, which are formed when a phosphorous group replaces one of the fatty acids in a triglyceride. This class is essential to building plasma membranes. The best known phospholipids are **lecithins,** found in high concentration in egg yolks and soybeans.
4. The third type are the steroids, which have a common chemical structure called the sterol nucleus or ring. Cholesterol is the most widely known of the steroids, and its role in promoting atherosclerosis has been clearly demonstrated. Cholesterol serves as the building block for a number of essential biochemicals, including vitamin D, bile acids, cortisol, estrogen, and testosterone, and is a natural and vital component of plasma membranes. While cholesterol is clearly essential for life, the body only needs minute amounts of it, which it makes for itself—it is not necessary to provide additional cholesterol in the diet.

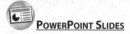

POWERPOINT SLIDES

Table 22.1 Standard Laboratory Lipid Profiles

SUGGESTION FOR CLASSROOM ACTIVITIES

- Have students question family members about their cholesterol levels.

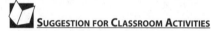

REFERENCE

- American Heart Association:
  www.americanheart.org

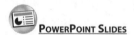

POWERPOINT SLIDES

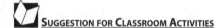

SUGGESTION FOR CLASSROOM ACTIVITIES

- Have students discuss the consequences of poorly managed cholesterol, triglycerides, and HDL and LDL levels in the blood.

© 2011 Pearson Education, Inc.

LEARNING OUTCOME 3

Illustrate how lipids are transported through the blood.

Concepts for Lecture

Lipid molecules are not soluble in plasma; they must be specially packaged for transport through the blood. The body forms complexes called lipoproteins that consist of various amounts of cholesterol, triglycerides, and phospholipids, along with a protein carrier. The protein carrier is known as apoprotein. Each type varies in lipid and apoprotein makeup and serves a different function in transporting lipids from sites of synthesis and absorption to sites of utilization. The three lipoproteins are high-density lipoprotein (HDL), low-density lipoprotein (LDL), and very low-density lipoprotein (VLDL).

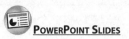
POWERPOINT SLIDES

LEARNING OUTCOME 4

Compare and contrast the different types of lipoproteins.

Concepts for Lecture

1. LDL carries the highest amount of cholesterol. LDL transports cholesterol from the liver to the tissues and organs, where it is used to build plasma membranes or to synthesize other steroids. It is stored in the tissue for later use. Storage of cholesterol in the blood vessels is not desirable, so LDL is known as "bad" cholesterol.
2. VLDL is the primary carrier of triglycerides in the blood.
3. HDL is manufactured in the liver and small intestine and assists in the transport of cholesterol away from the body tissues and back to the liver in a process called reverse cholesterol transport. The cholesterol component of the HDL is then broken down to unite with bile that is subsequently excreted in the feces. Excretion via bile is the only route the body uses to remove cholesterol. Because HDL transports cholesterol for destruction and removes it from the body, it is considered "good" cholesterol.

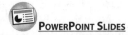
POWERPOINT SLIDES

SUGGESTIONS FOR CLASSROOM ACTIVITIES
- Discuss the different types of lipoproteins; differentiate between HDL, VLDL, and LDL.
- Have students define hyperlipidemia, hypercholesterolemia, and dyslipidemia.

LEARNING OUTCOME 5

Give examples of how cholesterol and LDL levels can be controlled through nonpharmacologic means.

Concepts for Lecture

Lifestyle changes should always be included in any treatment plan for reducing blood-lipid levels. Many patients with borderline laboratory values can control their dyslipidemia entirely through nonpharmacologic means. To emphasize the importance of lifestyle changes, patients should be taught that all drugs used for hyperlipidemia have side effects and that, to the extent possible, maintaining normal lipid values without pharmacotherapy should be a therapeutic goal. The most important lipid-reduction lifestyle interventions include monitoring blood-lipid levels regularly; maintaining weight at an optimum level; implementing a medically supervised exercise plan; reducing dietary saturated fats and cholesterol; increasing soluble fiber in the diet, as found in oat bran, apples, beans, grapefruit, and broccoli; and reducing or eliminating tobacco use.

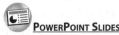
POWERPOINT SLIDES

SUGGESTION FOR CLASSROOM ACTIVITIES
- Have students identify which therapeutic lifestyle changes they could make in their own lives.

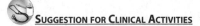
SUGGESTION FOR CLINICAL ACTIVITIES
- Have the students develop patient education material for one of the lifestyle changes.

Learning Outcome 6

For each of the drug classes listed in Drugs at a Glance, know representative drug examples, and explain their mechanisms of action, primary actions, and important adverse effects.

Concepts for Lecture

1. HMG-CoA reductase inhibitors/statins. The prototype drug is atorvastatin (Lipitor). Statins are the first drugs of choice in reducing blood-lipid levels. The mechanism of action is to inhibit HMG-CoA reductase, which results in less cholesterol biosynthesis. Statins can reduce the LDL-cholesterol levels by 20 to 40%. They can also lower triglyceride and VLDL levels and raise the level of "good" HDL cholesterol. The primary use is to reduce serum-lipid levels. (See Pharmacology Illustrated 22.1 for more detail.) Adverse effects can include headache, fatigue, muscle or joint pain, and heartburn.

2. Bile-acid resins. The prototype drug is cholestyramine (Questran). The mechanism of action is to bind with bile acids, thus increasing the excretion of cholesterol in the stool. Bile-acid resins are sometimes used in combination with the statins and are capable of producing a 20% drop in LDL. The primary use is to lower serum-lipid levels. Adverse effects are more frequent than those with statins and are limited to the GI tract, such as bloating and constipation. These agents can also bind other drugs, such as digoxin and warfarin, thus increasing the potential for drug-drug interactions.

3. Nicotinic acid. Prototype drug: Niacin, a B-complex vitamin. The mechanism of action is to decrease VLDL levels, and, because LDL is synthesized from VLDL, the patient experiences a reduction in LDL levels. The primary use is to reduce triglycerides and increase HDL levels. Adverse effects are more pronounced. Flushing and hot flashes occur in almost every patient. A variety of uncomfortable intestinal effects such as nausea, excess gas, and diarrhea are commonly reported.

4. Fibric-acid agents. The prototype drug is gemfibrozil (Lopid). Once widely used, they have been largely replaced by the statins. The mechanism of action is unknown. Combining a fibric-acid agent with statins results in greater decreases in triglyceride levels than the use of either drug used alone. The primary use is for treating severe hypertriglyceridemia. An adverse effect is GI distress, and if patient is on anticoagulant therapy, watch for signs of bleeding.

5. Cholesterol absorption inhibitor. The prototype drug is ezetimibe (Vytorin). The mechanism of action is to inhibit the absorption of cholesterol, causing less cholesterol to enter the blood. Unfortunately, the body responds by synthesizing more cholesterol; thus, a statin may be administered concurrently. The primary use: given alone, it produces a modest reduction in the LDL. No side effects have been noted.

Learning Outcome 7

Explain the nurse's role in the pharmacologic management of lipid disorders.

Concepts for Lecture

1. The role of the nurse in the therapy for hyperlipidemia, no matter what pharmacological treatment is chosen, involves careful monitoring of the patient's condition and providing education as it relates to the

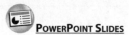
PowerPoint Slides

Table 22.2 Drugs for Dyslipidemias

Prototype Drug
- atorvastatin (Lipitor)
- cholestyramine (Questran)
- gemfibrozil (Lopid)

Reference
- Lipid Lowering Drugs: *www.ncbi.nlm.nih.gov:80/pmc/articles*

PowerPoint Slides

Suggestions for Clinical Activities
- Have the students prepare a teaching plan for a newly diagnosed patient with hyperlipidemia.
- Have a clinical pharmacist speak with the students about patient education related to the agents given for hyperlipidemia.

© 2011 Pearson Education, Inc.

prescribed drug treatment. First, assess the patient's laboratory tests for triglyceride, total cholesterol, LDL, and HDL levels.

2. **Statins:** Monitor the side effects, as they can be serious. Liver dysfunction can occur, monitor liver-function tests before and during the first few months of therapy. Do not use with those who wish to be pregnant or are pregnant or breast-feeding. Watch for signs of GI upset, as this is a common but less serious side effect.

3. **Bile-acid resins:** Monitor for the significant GI effects such as constipation, abdominal pain, bloating, nausea, vomiting, diarrhea, and steatorrhea. Take a careful history for past GI disorders such as peptic ulcer disease, hemorrhoids, inflammatory bowel disease, or chronic constipation. Bile-acid resins may worsen these conditions.

4. **Nicotinic acid (niacin):** Monitor carefully the patient's liver function prior to and during therapy for risk of liver toxicity. Patients with a history of liver disease, elevated liver enzymes, or peptic ulcer disease should not take niacin. In patients predisposed to gout, nicotinic acid may increase uric-acid levels and precipitate acute gout. If a diabetic, monitor blood-sugar levels. Nicotinic acid can affect glycemic control.

5. **Fibric-acid agents:** Assess the patient for complaints of abdominal pain, nausea, and vomiting. These are common side effects of the medication, so knowing baseline complaints will enable you to determine if later complaints are a result of drug therapy or an underlying problem. Using these agents with warfarin (Coumadin) may potentiate the effects of the anticoagulant, so lower warfarin doses may be needed. Monitor prothrombin time and international normalized ration (PT/INR).

LEARNING OUTCOME 8

Use the nursing process to care for patients receiving drug therapy for lipid disorders.

Concepts for Lecture

1. Assessment: Obtain blood samples as ordered by the physician. Assess the patient's laboratory tests for triglyceride, total cholesterol, LDL, and HDL levels. Collect the patient's height and weight. Obtain the nursing history, including lifestyle, current medications, and dietary habits. Assess the patient's and family's knowledge of hyperlipidemia and medication regimen.

2. Nursing diagnoses: *Knowledge Deficit* regarding condition, therapeutic regimen, and potential side effects of medications; *Ineffective Therapeutic Regimen Management* related to complexity of therapy and cost of medications; *Risk for Bleeding,* as agent may potentiate the effects of the anticoagulant the patient may be taking.

3. Planning: Goals for the patient receiving medication to reduce serum-lipid levels include the ability to explain hyperlipidemia and needed lifestyle changes and medications and to verbalize the ability to follow the prescribed therapy.

4. Implementation: Encourage compliance with medication regimen. Provide additional education regarding the medication regimen, such as consultation with the clinical pharmacist, written and/or visual educational material, and home-health visits to ensure patient's ability to follow prescribed therapy.

5. Evaluation: Ideal outcome criteria for evaluation of the plan of care are lowered serum-lipid levels with limited side effects, no organ damage, and no injury. Patients verbalize the importance of taking prescribed medications to assist them in their continued management of the disease.

 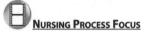 **POWERPOINT SLIDES**

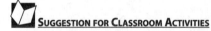 **NURSING PROCESS FOCUS**

- Patients Receiving Lipid-Lowering Therapy

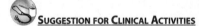 **SUGGESTION FOR CLASSROOM ACTIVITIES**

- Have students role-play the teaching plans they have created in another class period.

SUGGESTION FOR CLINICAL ACTIVITIES

- Have students witness lipid-disorder education given to a patient by a nurse, dietician, or clinical pharmacist.

GENERAL CHAPTER CONSIDERATIONS

1. Have students study and learn key terms listed at the beginning of the chapter.
2. Have students complete end-of-chapter exercises either in their book or on the MyNursingKit website.
3. Use the Classroom Response Questions provided in PowerPoint to assess students prior to lecture.

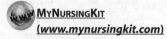

MyNursingKit
(www.mynursingkit.com)

- Websites
- NCLEX® questions
- Critical Thinking Questions
- Case Studies
- Animations and Videos
- Drug Prototype Questions

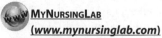

MyNursingLab
(www.mynursinglab.com)

- Knowledge Quick Check
- Pre/Posttests
- Customized study plans
- *Separate purchase*

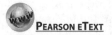

Student Workbook and Resource Guide

- Chapter 22 activities
- *Separate purchase*

Pearson Nurse's Drug Guide

- *Separate purchase*

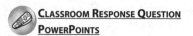

Pearson eText

- Students can search, highlight, take notes, and more all in electronic format.
- *Separate purchase*

Classroom Response Question PowerPoints

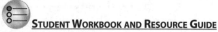

Testbank

CHAPTER 23
DRUGS FOR HYPERTENSION

LEARNING OUTCOME 1

Explain how hypertension is classified.

Concepts for Lecture

1. Cardiovascular disease (CVD) includes conditions of the heart and blood vessels, and hypertension is the most common form of CVD. It is the most frequent cause of death in the United States. Hypertension is the consistent elevation of systemic arterial blood pressure. Multiple measurements of the blood pressure (B/P) are taken over several visits to the physician to make an accurate diagnosis. Sustained systolic B/P of greater than 140 mmHg or diastolic pressure greater than 90–99 mmHg constitutes a diagnosis of hypertension. (See Table 23.1.)
2. Hypertension is classified into three categories: prehypertension, Stage 1, and Stage 2. There are key elements that identify one stage from another: Prehypertension is classified as 120 to 139 mmHg/80 to 89 mmHg; Stage 1 hypertension as 140 to 159 mmHg/90 to 99 mmHg; and Stage 2 hypertension as 160 or higher/100 or higher.
3. Blood pressure changes throughout the lifespan. What is considered normal blood pressure at one age can be considered abnormal as we age.

 POWERPOINT SLIDES

Table 23.1 Classification and Management of Hypertension in Adults

 SUGGESTION FOR CLASSROOM ACTIVITIES

• Demonstrate the proper technique of assessment of blood pressure, and have students return a demonstration of blood pressure assessment.

 SUGGESTION FOR CLINICAL ACTIVITIES

• Have students assess the blood pressure of five patients on their assigned unit.

 REFERENCE

• Understanding Hypertension: *www.clevelandclinicmeded.com*
• National High Blood Pressure Education Program: *www.nhlbi.nih.gov*

LEARNING OUTCOME 2

Summarize the long-term consequences of untreated hypertension.

Concepts for Lecture

1. Untreated hypertension affects four target organs: the heart, brain, kidneys, and retina.
2. The workload of the heart is increased due to untreated hypertension, resulting in heart failure. Blood vessel damage occurs from untreated hypertension resulting in decreased blood and oxygen to the brain, potentially resulting in transient ischemic attack or cerebral vascular accident. Vessels damaged in the kidneys from untreated hypertension lead to progressive loss of function of the renal system. Visual impairment and blindness result from damage to the vessels supplying blood to the retina.

 POWERPOINT SLIDES

 SUGGESTION FOR CLASSROOM ACTIVITIES

• Break students into groups, and have them list signs and symptoms of heart failure, transient ischemic attack or cerebral vascular accident, renal failure, and retinal damage.

 SUGGESTION FOR CLINICAL ACTIVITIES

• Have students review assigned patients' medical record for diagnoses related to untreated hypertension and identify patients' signs and symptoms of these diseases.

LEARNING OUTCOME 3

Explain the effects of cardiac output, peripheral resistance, and blood volume on blood pressure.

Concepts for Lecture

1. The three factors responsible for creating blood pressure are cardiac output, peripheral resistance, and blood volume. Cardiac output is the volume of blood pumped per minute. Higher cardiac output yields higher blood pressure. Stroke volume (amount of blood pumped by contraction of the ventricles) and heart rate determine cardiac output. Medications that affect cardiac output, stroke volume, and heart rate will influence the patient's blood pressure.
2. Peripheral resistance is the friction in the arteries as blood flows through the vascular system. Greater resistance in the arteries yields higher blood pressure. Medications that affect vascular smooth muscles may lower or raise the blood pressure. The autonomic nervous system also plays a role in controlling peripheral resistance. Refer to Chapter 13.
3. Blood volume is the total amount of blood in the vascular system. Increased blood volume (i.e., intravenous fluids) yields higher blood pressure. Medications that affect blood volume may lower or raise the blood pressure.

LEARNING OUTCOME 4

Discuss how the vasomotor center, baroreceptors, chemoreceptors, emotions, and hormones influence blood pressure.

Concepts for Lecture

1. The central and autonomic nervous systems are involved in regulating blood pressure. (See Figure 23.3.) In the medulla oblongata, the vasomotor center sends nerve impulses to smooth muscle in arteries to either constrict or relax, thereby constantly regulating blood pressure. Baroreceptors in the aorta and carotid arteries sense pressure changes in these arteries and relay this information to the vasomotor center. Chemoreceptors detect oxygen, carbon dioxide, and pH levels in the blood and relay this information to the vasomotor center. The vasomotor center reacts by raising or lowering blood pressure according to the information received.
2. Emotions are involved in regulating blood pressure. Blood pressure is increased by anger and stress and is decreased by depression and lethargy.
3. The endocrine system is involved in regulating blood pressure. (See Figure 23.3.) Natural hormones affect blood pressure on a daily basis. Epinephrine and norepinephrine injections cause vasoconstriction and raise blood pressure. Antidiuretic hormone causes vasoconstriction and raises blood pressure by raising blood volume.

LEARNING OUTCOME 5

Discuss the role of therapeutic lifestyle changes in the management of hypertension.

Concepts for Lecture

1. Assessment of patient's lifestyle to identify any personal habits that may be affecting the patient's blood pressure is needed to give proper

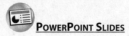
POWERPOINT SLIDES

REFERENCE
- How Blood Pressure Works: *health.howstuffworks.com*

SUGGESTION FOR CLASSROOM ACTIVITIES
- Discuss conditions that could influence cardiac output, peripheral resistance, and blood volume and how these would affect blood pressure.

SUGGESTIONS FOR CLINICAL ACTIVITIES
- Identify assigned patients' hypertensive medications and how these medications may affect cardiac output, peripheral resistance, and blood volume.
- Evaluate effectiveness of antihypertensive medications on assigned patients.

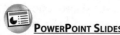
POWERPOINT SLIDES

Figure 23.3 Nervous and Hormonal Factors Influencing Blood Pressure

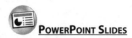
POWERPOINT SLIDES

© 2011 Pearson Education, Inc.

education on the treatment and/or prevention of hypertension. Personal habits may include the patient's dietary habits and exercise/activity regimen, as well as use of any medication.

2. Genetics as well as environmental factors may contribute to the patient's risk for hypertension. Our race, gender, and family history of hypertension may contribute to a diagnosis of hypertension. Environmental factors that may contribute to the patient's risk for hypertension are tobacco use, high-fat diets, obesity, excessive sodium intake or alcohol consumption, and a sedentary lifestyle.

3. Losing weight can help control or prevent hypertension. The loss of only ten to twenty pounds may significantly lower blood pressure. Limiting foods high in fat and cholesterol can reduce serum-lipid levels, resulting in decreasing body weight and blood pressure. Limiting sodium, tobacco, and alcohol to recommended levels or stopping the intake of any of the above may help reduce the risk of hypertension and/or lower the patient's present blood pressure. Beginning an exercise program will also help.

SUGGESTIONS FOR CLASSROOM ACTIVITIES
- Identify personal therapeutic and nontherapeutic lifestyle habits that may positively or negatively affect the student's blood pressure.
- Identify personal lifestyle changes that could impact blood pressure.

SUGGESTION FOR CLINICAL ACTIVITIES
- Prepare a teaching plan for a newly diagnosed patient with hypertension, emphasizing non-pharmacological methods.

LEARNING OUTCOME 6

Differentiate between drug classes used for the primary treatment of hypertension and those secondary agents reserved for persistent hypertension.

Concepts for Lecture

1. **Primary antihypertensive agents:**
   Diuretics: These are the first drug of choice; they have few side effects and are effective in treating mild and moderate hypertension as well as heart failure.
   Angiotensin-converting enzyme (ACE) inhibitors: These medications, with the angiotensin II receptor blockers, assist the body's own mechanism to control blood pressure and fluid balance. ACE inhibitors cause intense vasoconstriction and lower the blood pressure.
   Angiotensin II receptor blockers: This class of medication also affects the hormone aldosterone from the adrenal cortex. This increases sodium reabsorption in the kidneys and aids in retention of fluid in the blood vessels, thereby increasing blood pressure.
   Beta-adrenergic antagonists: These affect the vasomotor center and the sympathetic nervous system to control blood pressure.
   Calcium channel blockers: These drugs have emerged as a primary choice in the treatment of hypertension and other cardiovascular diseases. They are used for individuals who do not respond well to other pharmacological choices.
2. **Secondary antihypertensive agents:**
   Alpha$_1$-adrenergic antagonists: These affect the sympathetic nervous system's control of the blood pressure by blocking the sympathetic receptors in the arterioles, thereby causing the vessels to dilate.
   Alpha$_2$-adrenergic agonists: These drugs decrease the outflow of sympathetic nerve impulses from the central nervous system to the heart and arterioles. This has the same effect as the alpha$_1$.
   Direct-acting vasodilators: These directly affect vascular smooth muscle, which lowers blood pressure. This class has many side effects and is used for the hypertensive crisis.

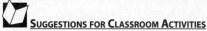

POWERPOINT SLIDES

Table 23.2 Combination Drugs for Hypertension

SUGGESTION FOR CLINICAL ACTIVITIES
- Identify primary and secondary antihypertensive agents of assigned patients.

LEARNING OUTCOME 7

Describe the nurse's role in the pharmacologic management of patients receiving drugs for hypertension.

Concepts for Lecture

1. The role of the nurse in managing a patient with hypertension is to obtain a complete health history, including allergies, drug history, and possible drug interactions. Obtain vital signs for a baseline and to compare with previously obtained vital signs. A good physical assessment should be done, and blood and urine specimens need to be obtained for analysis.

2. **Diuretics:** Key areas for the nurse to monitor with the use of nonpotassium-sparing diuretics include orthostatic hypotension; laboratory electrolyte values and daily weights; potassium levels; increased weight of more than two pounds in 24 hours; intake and output assessment of edema and heart and lung sounds for signs of fluid overload. The patient's ability to safely ambulate to the bathroom should be assessed, since diuretics increase urination. The patient should also be aware of the side effect of photosensitivity and of the possible need to increase potassium in the diet or with supplements.

    For a potassium-sparing diuretic, teach the patient to limit the use of salt substitutes and potassium-rich foods. Also, pregnant and lactating women should not take these types of diuretics. Patients with a history of gout and kidney stones should be monitored closely. Key areas for the nurse to monitor include uric acid levels and gynecomastia and hirsutism for spironolactone (Aldactone). With the use of thiazide-like diuretics, key areas to monitor include laboratory values (potassium, sodium, calcium, magnesium, CBC, BUN, creatinine, and serum lipids); blood-glucose levels in diabetics, since these drugs may cause hyperglycemia; uric-acid levels. Patients should increase potassium because these are not potassium-sparing drugs. The nurse should assess the patient for pregnancy and lactation, systemic lupus erythematosus, and the use of digoxin; these medications should be avoided in patients with these conditions, or patients should be monitored more closely. For loop diuretics, the nurse should monitor these key areas: severe potassium loss; hypovolemia; hypotension; hearing loss (these drugs are ototoxic); glucose and uric acid levels.

3. **Calcium channel blockers (CCBs):** Key areas for the nurse to assess include the following: ECG, heart rate, and blood pressure prior to therapy, since CCBs affect the coronary arteries and myocardial contractility; during therapy the nurse should monitor heart rate and blood pressure regularly; health history specific for heart dysrhythmias, because these drugs are contraindicated with some dysrhythmias; assess for signs of CHF and reflex tachycardia since some CCBs reduce myocardial contractility; with IV administration, tachycardia and hypotension are more pronounced; assess for pregnancy since CCBs are a category C for pregnancy; dizziness, headache, and flushing are minor side effects. The nurse should teach the patient to avoid drinking grapefruit juice because it increases the absorption of these drugs.

4. **Renin-angiotensins:** Key areas for the nurse to assess and monitor include the following: baseline vital signs; hypotension, because ACE inhibitors given for the first time or by the IV route can cause a severe drop in blood pressure; angiodema, a serious side effect of ACE inhibitors, which can cause laryngeal swelling, leading to asphyxia; lab values and signs of infection for the serious side effect of neutropenia or agranulocytosis; potassium levels for hypokalemia, especially in patients with CHF, impaired kidney function, and diabetes. Less serious side

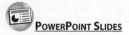

POWERPOINT SLIDES

SUGGESTION FOR CLASSROOM ACTIVITIES
- Have students prepare drug cards for the drug classes discussed.

SUGGESTION FOR CLINICAL ACTIVITIES
- Have students prepare a teaching plan for any assigned patients taking these medications.

effects to monitor for include dizziness, light-headedness, headache, and a tickling nonproductive cough; pregnancy-risk category D.

5. **Adrenergic antagonists:** Key areas for the nurse to assess and monitor include the following: baseline vital signs and blood pressure response; hold the medication for pulse below 60 beats per minute and B/P below 90/60; monitor cardiac response through ECG, heart rate, and rhythm; assess for bradycardia, which may be an indication of heart block; orthostatic hypertension and other minor side effects, such as dizziness, nausea, and dry mouth. In order to avoid the complication of rebound hypertension, administration of adrenergic antagonists should not be stopped abruptly. Diabetic patients taking these drugs may experience hypoglycemia without exhibiting signs or symptoms, so fingerstick blood-sugar levels should be assessed regularly. Patients taking alpha$_1$ drugs should be monitored specifically for GI complaints, and elderly patients should be assessed for hypothermic effects related to the vasodilation of these drugs. The pregnancy-risk categories for these drugs are B and C. Patients with hypertension that is not controlled by other medications are candidates for alpha$_2$ therapy, since these drugs are centrally acting and have multiple side effects. The nurse should assess these patients for the following: orthostatic hypotension; sedation; decreased libido; impotence; sodium/water retention and dry mouth; pregnancy-risk category C. Specific nursing considerations for beta-adrenergic drugs include monitoring for effects of vasoconstriction, evidenced by any respiratory distress, including wheezing and shortness of breath.

6. **Direct vasodilators:** Key areas for the nurse to assess and monitor include the following: Since these drugs are used primarily for emergency situations to reduce blood pressure quickly, the vital signs, ECG, and pulse oximetry should be continuously monitored; assess the health history specifically for hypersensitivity, coronary artery disease, rheumatic mitral-valve disease, cerebrovascular disease, renal insufficiency, and systemic lupus erythematosus, since these conditions are contraindicated with these drugs. Additional nursing considerations are monitoring for priapism; signs of fluid retention with repeated IV diazoxide (Hyperstat); body-hair changes and orthohypotension with administration of minoxidil (Loniten) that reverse when drug is stopped. Nurses should only mix nitroprusside IV administration with 5% dextrose in water, and know that this drug is extremely light sensitive (container should be wrapped in an opaque substance), is brown in color, and is only stable for 24 hours. This drug can be used for hypertensive emergencies during labor and delivery.

LEARNING OUTCOME 8

For each of the drug classes listed in Drugs at a Glance, know representative drug examples, and explain their mechanisms of drug action, primary actions, and important adverse effects.

Concepts for Lecture

1. **Diuretics:** The prototype drug is hydrochlorothiazide (HydroDiuril). The mechanism of action is to decrease blood pressure by increasing the amount of urine produced and excreted. Primary use is for mild to moderate hypertension. Adverse effects include electrolyte imbalances, especially loss of potassium.

2. **Calcium channel blockers:** The prototype drug is nifedipine (Procardia). The mechanism of action is to cause vasodilation in the arteriole,

 POWERPOINT SLIDES

Table 23.3 Diuretics for Hypertension
Table 23.4 Calcium Channel Blockers for Hypertension
Table 23.5 ACE Inhibitors and Angiotensin II Receptor Blockers for Hypertension
Table 23.6 Adrenergic Antagonists for Hypertension
Table 23.7 Direct-acting Vasodilators for Hypertension

which decreases blood pressure by blocking calcium channels in the plasma membrane. Primary use is for hypertension and angina. Adverse effects include dizziness, headache, and flushing.

3. **Drugs affecting the renin-angiotensin system:** Angiotensin-converting enzyme (ACE) inhibitors. The prototype drug is enalapril (Vasotec). The mechanism of action is to decrease blood pressure by decreasing blood volume through blocking of the angiotensin-converting enzyme (ACE). This blocks formation of angiotensin II, causing vasodilation and decreased reabsorption of sodium by the kidneys with increased urine excretion. The primary use is for hypertension, with some significant adverse effects being persistent cough and hypotension. An example of angiotensin-receptor blockers (ARBs) is the prototype drug losartan potassium (Cozaar). The mechanism of action is to decrease blood pressure by blocking angiotensin receptors in arterial smooth muscle and adrenal glands, causing arterial dilation and increased renal sodium excretion. The primary use is for hypertension; an adverse effect is hypotension.

4. **Adrenergic antagonists:** The prototype drugs are the alpha-adrenergic blocker doxazosin (Cardura) and the beta-adrenergic blocker metoprolol (Lopressor). The mechanism of action is to decrease blood pressure by blocking alpha and beta receptors or stimulation of alpha$_2$ in the vasomotor center (brain stem), which blocks effects of the sympathetic nervous system leading to vasodilation. Its primary use is to treat hypertension, with significant adverse effects such as orthostatic hypotension, dizziness, nausea, bradycardia, and dry mouth.

5. **Direct vasodilators:** The prototype drug is hydralazine (Apresoline). The mechanism of action is to decrease blood pressure through direct relaxation of arterial smooth muscle, causing vasodilation. Its primary use is for severe hypertension and hypertensive crisis. The adverse effects would include reflex tachycardia and sodium and fluid retention.

LEARNING OUTCOME 9

Use the nursing process to care for patients receiving antihypertensive drugs.

Concepts for Lecture

1. Assessment process will include taking the patient's blood pressure in each arm for baseline; assessing the patient's height and weight, and obtaining blood and urine samples as ordered by the physician; obtaining a nursing history, including lifestyle, current medications, and dietary habits. Assess the patient's and family's knowledge of hypertension and medication regimen.

2. **Nursing diagnoses:** Possible nursing diagnoses for various antihypertensive drugs: *Decreased Cardiac Output* related to excessive or prolonged systemic vascular resistance; *Knowledge Deficit* regarding condition, therapeutic regimen, and potential side effects of medications; *Ineffective Therapeutic-Regimen Management* related to complexity of therapy and cost of medications; *Risk for Sexual Dysfunction* related to side effects of medications.

3. **Planning:** Goals for patients receiving antihypertensive drugs include a reduction in systolic/diastolic blood pressure and the patient's ability to explain hypertension and needed medications and to verbalize the ability to follow prescribed therapy.

4. **Implementation:** Encourage compliance with medication regimen, and provide additional education regarding medication regimen, such as consultation with the clinical pharmacist, written and/or visual

Prototype Drug
- hydrochlorothiazide (Microzide)
- nifedipine (Adalat, Procardia, others)
- enalapril (Vasotec)
- doxazosin (Cardura)
- hydralazine (Apresoline)

SUGGESTION FOR CLASSROOM ACTIVITIES

- Prepare classroom games similar to *Jeopardy* or create crossword puzzles to help students review the actions, use, and side effects of antihypertensive drugs.

SUGGESTION FOR CLINICAL ACTIVITIES

- Students will prepare medication cards for each class of antihypertensive drugs.

POWERPOINT SLIDES

NURSING PROCESS FOCUS

- Patients Receiving Diuretic Therapy
- Patients Receiving Calcium Channel Blocker Therapy
- Patients Receiving ACEI (Angiotension-Converting Enzyme Inhibitor) and ARB (Angiotension Receptor Blocker) Therapy
- Patients Receiving Adrenergic Antagonist Therapy
- Patients Receiving Direct Vasodilator Therapy

SUGGESTION FOR CLASSROOM ACTIVITIES

- With the above-listed nursing diagnoses, have students list various interventions and rationales to support the diagnoses. Students will list additional possible diagnoses with intervention and rationale.

SUGGESTION FOR CLINICAL ACTIVITIES

- Write a care plan for a patient receiving antihypertensive drugs.

© 2011 Pearson Education, Inc.

educational material, and home-health visits to ensure patient's ability to follow prescribed therapy.

5. **Evaluation:** Ideal outcome criteria for evaluation of the plan of care are a lowered blood pressure with limited side effects, no organ damage, and no injury. Patients should be able to verbalize the importance of taking prescribed medications to assist them in their continued management of the disease.

GENERAL CHAPTER CONSIDERATIONS

1. Have students study and learn key terms listed at the beginning of the chapter.
2. Have students complete end-of-chapter exercises either in their book or on the MyNursingKit website.
3. Use the Classroom Response Questions provided in PowerPoint to assess students prior to lecture.

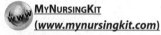

MYNURSINGKIT
(www.mynursingkit.com)

- Websites
- NCLEX® questions
- Critical Thinking Questions
- Case Studies
- Animations and Videos
- Drug Prototype Questions

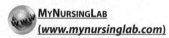

MYNURSINGLAB
(www.mynursinglab.com)

- Knowledge Quick Check
- Pre/Posttests
- Customized study plans
- *Separate purchase*

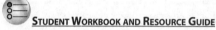

STUDENT WORKBOOK AND RESOURCE GUIDE

- Chapter 23 activities
- *Separate purchase*

PEARSON NURSE'S DRUG GUIDE

- *Separate purchase*

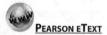

PEARSON eTEXT

- Students can search, highlight, take notes, and more all in electronic format.
- *Separate purchase*

CLASSROOM RESPONSE QUESTION POWERPOINTS

TESTBANK

CHAPTER 24
DRUGS FOR HEART FAILURE

LEARNING OUTCOME 1

Identify the major diseases that accelerate the progression of heart failure.

Concepts for Lecture

Heart failure (HF) is defined as the inability of the ventricles to pump enough blood to meet the body's metabolic demands. Weakening of the heart muscle occurs with aging; however, the following diseases may cause or accelerate HF: mitral stenosis, myocardial infarction (MI), chronic hypertension (HTN), coronary artery disease (CAD), and diabetes mellitus. There is no cure, only prevention and slowing the progression of HF.

LEARNING OUTCOME 2

Relate how the symptoms associated with heart failure may be caused by weakened heart muscle and diminished cardiac output.

Concepts for Lecture

1. In left-sided HF, excess blood accumulates in the left ventricle, causing it to thicken and enlarge (hypertrophy) in order to compensate for the increased workload. Blood eventually backs up into the lungs, resulting in the classic symptoms of cough and shortness of breath.
2. In right-sided HF, excess blood backs up into veins, resulting in peripheral edema and engorgement of organs, such as the liver. Right-sided heart failure is less common than left-sided HF.

LEARNING OUTCOME 3

Explain how preload and afterload affect cardiac function.

Concepts for Learning

1. Cardiac output is affected by preload; that is, the degree to which the myocardial fibers in the heart are stretched prior to contraction. This occurs just before the chambers of the heart contract as they are filling to their maximum capacity with blood.
2. Cardiac output is also affected by afterload, or the degree of pressure in the aorta that must be overcome for blood to be ejected from the left ventricle.

 POWERPOINT SLIDES

 SUGGESTION FOR CLASSROOM ACTIVITIES

- Divide students into five groups, representing each disease associated with HF. Have each group list the reason each of these diseases is a precursor to HF.

 SUGGESTION FOR CLINICAL ACTIVITIES

- Assign patients with the above-listed diseases to students, and have students assess for signs and symptoms of HF.

 POWERPOINT SLIDES

Figure 24.1 The pathophysiology of HF

 SUGGESTION FOR CLASSROOM ACTIVITIES

- Develop a word-search puzzle containing the types of heart failure and their symptoms.

 SUGGESTION FOR CLINICAL ACTIVITIES

- Rotate students through a cardiac rehabilitation facility

 POWERPOINT SLIDES

 SUGGESTION FOR CLASSROOM ACTIVITIES

- Invite a cardiologist to speak to students regarding heart failure and cardiac function.

 SUGGESTION FOR CLINICAL ACTIVITIES

- Have students shadow an ICU nurse caring for cardiac patients.

© 2011 Pearson Education, Inc.

LEARNING OUTCOME 4

Describe the nurse's role in the pharmacologic management of heart failure.

Concepts for Lecture

1. The role of the nurse is to obtain a complete health history, including allergies, drug history, and possible drug interactions. Assess vital signs, urinary output, and cardiac output, initially and throughout therapy. Drugs are used to treat the symptoms of HF by mechanisms such as slowing the heart rate, increasing contractility, and reducing the heart's workload.

2. The nurse's role in the pharmacological management of HF with **ACE-inhibitor therapy** includes monitoring the CBC, since these drugs can cause neutropenia; assessing for severe hypotension (especially with initial doses); and using with caution in patients who have impaired kidney function, hyperkalemia, and autoimmune diseases. Patient teaching should include notifying the patient that it may take weeks or months for the maximum therapeutic response, noting sodium and potassium restrictions, and cautioning patient to not take any other medications, OTCs, herbals, or vitamins without notifying the prescriber.

3. The nurse's role in **diuretic therapy** for HF includes assessing renal function, because these drugs are contraindicated for kidney diseases, and monitoring electrolyte levels and for weakness, hypotension, and confusion. Additionally, the nurse should monitor vital signs, intake and output, and blood glucose and blood-urea nitrogen (BUN). Patient teaching includes instructing patients to monitor their sodium intake in order to not exceed 4,000 mg daily; to report a weight loss of more than two pounds per week and any fatigue or muscle cramping; and to change position slowly to avoid dizziness.

4. The nurse's role in **beta-adrenergic blockers** (antagonists) includes monitoring for worsening of symptoms, hepatic toxicity, and liver function. These drugs are contraindicated in patients with chronic obstructive pulmonary disease (COPD), bradycardia, heart block, and decompensated heart failure. Patient teaching should include monitoring for blood pressure and pulse (notify health care provider if the pulse is below 50 beats/minute); reporting signs and symptoms of worsening HF, such as shortness of breath, edema, and chest pain; and being warned to not stop taking the drug without notifying the prescriber.

5. The nurse's roles in **cardiac glycoside** therapy includes evaluating the patient for ventricular dysrhythmias not associated with HF and assessing renal function, since this drug is excreted by the kidneys. Monitor for drug interactions, and do not give the medication within two hours of giving antidiarrheal medications or antacids, because this decreases the absorption of digoxin. Patient teaching includes having lab tests to monitor therapeutic range, knowing the signs and symptoms of toxicity (nausea, vomiting, anorexia, and visual disturbances), and counting the pulse for one full minute and notifying the prescriber if the pulse is below 60 or above 100. The patient should report a weight gain of two or more pounds per day and should eat foods high in potassium.

6. The nurse's role in **phosphodiesterase inhibitors** and **other inotropic agents** involves assessment of potassium levels for hypokalemia, monitoring for hypotension, and assessing for renal impairment and dysrhythmias. If given an IV, the patient should be continuously monitored for ventricular dysrhythmias, such as premature

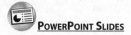
POWERPOINT SLIDES

SUGGESTION FOR CLASSROOM ACTIVITIES

- Invite a nurse practitioner to speak to students regarding pharmacotherapy for HF.

SUGGESTION FOR CLINICAL ACTIVITIES

- Assign students to care for patients and do a medication pass on a cardiac unit.

ventricular contractions (PVCs), ectopic beats, ventricular tachycardia, and fibrillation. Patient teaching includes ensuring the patient immediately reports irregular or rapid heart rate, a fever of 101 degrees or higher, or an increase in chest pain. If given an IV, the patient should be monitored for a fever of 101 degrees or higher or pain or swelling at the infusion site.

LEARNING OUTCOME 5

For each of the drug classes listed in Drugs at a Glance, know representative drug examples and explain their mechanisms of action, primary actions, and important adverse effects.

Concepts for Lecture

1. **ACE inhibitors:** The prototype drug is lisinopril (Prinivil, Zestril). The mechanism of action is to reduce the afterload on the heart and lower blood pressure by enhancing the excretion of sodium and water, which lowers peripheral resistance and reduces blood volume. These are drugs of choice for HF. The primary use is to lower the blood pressure and the risk of heart failure. Important adverse reactions include first-dose hypotension, cough, hyperkalemia, and renal failure.

2. **Diuretics:** The prototype drug is furosemide (Lasix). The mechanism of action increases urine flow, which reduces blood volume and cardiac workload and also reduces edema and pulmonary congestion. The primary uses are to reduce blood pressure, reduce blood volume, and reduce the workload of the heart. Important adverse reactions include dehydration, electrolyte imbalances, hypotension, and ototoxicity.

3. **Beta-adrenergic blocker:** The prototype drug is carvedilol (Coreg). The mechanism of action works by slowing the heart and reducing blood pressure, which reduces the workload of the heart by exhibiting a negative inotropic effect. The primary use is to reduce symptoms of heart failure and slow the progression of the disease. Important adverse reactions include fluid retention and worsening of HF, fatigue, hypotension, bradycardia, and heart block.

4. **Vasodilators:** The prototype drug: isosorbide dinitrate (Isordil). The mechanism of action is to directly relax blood vessels. The primary use is to lower the blood pressure. These drugs are usually only used for patients who cannot take ACE inhibitors. Important adverse reactions include reflex tachycardia and orthostatic hypotension.

5. **Cardiac glycosides:** The prototype drug is digoxin (Lanoxin). The mechanism of action is to cause the heart to beat more forcefully and more slowly, which improves cardiac output. The primary use is to increase the contractility or strength of myocardial contraction. These drugs are now considered second-line treatment for heart failure. Adverse effects include neutropenia, dysrhythmias, and digitalis toxicity.

6. **Phosphodiesterase inhibitors and other inotropic agents:** The prototype drug is milrinone (Primacor). The mechanism of action is to block the enzyme phosphodiesterase in cardiac and smooth muscle, which increases the amount of calcium available for myocardial contraction. This causes a positive inotropic response and vasodilation, thus increasing cardiac output by increasing the contractility and decreasing afterload. These drugs are usually only used for very short periods of time—2 to 3 days—when ACE inhibitors are not effective. The primary use is for short-term treatment of heart failure. Important adverse reactions are hypokalemia, hypotension, and ventricular dysrhythmias.

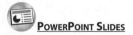

POWERPOINT SLIDES

Table 24.1 Drugs for Heart Failure

Prototype Drug
- lisinopril (Prinivil, Zestril)
- furosemide (Lasix)
- digoxin (Lanoxin)
- metoprolol (Lopressor)
- milrinone (Primacor)

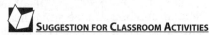

SUGGESTION FOR CLASSROOM ACTIVITIES
- Have students prepare drug cards for the drugs listed in Drugs at a Glance.

SUGGESTION FOR CLINICAL ACTIVITIES
- Have students note any adverse reactions that they see in their assigned patients and discuss at postconference.

© 2011 Pearson Education, Inc.

LEARNING OUTCOME 6

Use the nursing process to care for patients who are receiving drug therapy for heart failure.

Concepts for Lecture

1. Assessment of the patient who is receiving drug therapy for heart failure should include obtaining a complete health history (including allergies and drug history for possible interactions); assessing vital signs, urinary output, and cardiac output; determining the reason the medication is being administered; and assessing the patient's knowledge of the disease process.

2. **Nursing diagnoses:** Possible nursing diagnoses would include *Ineffective Tissue Perfusion,* related to impaired cardiac status; *Decreased Cardiac Output; Excess Fluid Volume;* and *Deficient Knowledge,* related to drug regimen and disease process.

3. **Planning:** Patient goals and expected outcomes for the patient receiving drug therapy for heart failure include the patient's reporting decreased symptoms of cardiac decompensation related to fluid overload, exhibiting signs of improved organ perfusion, demonstrating an understanding of the drug regimen, and immediately reporting important side effects.

4. **Implementation:** Interventions that the nurse may implement include monitoring the patient's ECG, observing for drug side effects, weighing the patient for drug effectiveness or signs of fluid overload, monitoring serum-drug levels of medication and for signs of drug toxicity, and monitoring electrolyte levels.

5. Evaluation of the effectiveness of drug therapy is evidenced by patient goals and outcomes being met.

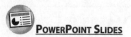
POWERPOINT SLIDES

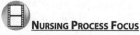
NURSING PROCESS FOCUS
- Patients Receiving Digoxin Therapy

GENERAL CHAPTER CONSIDERATIONS

1. Have students study and learn key terms listed at the beginning of the chapter.
2. Have students complete end-of-chapter exercises either in their book or on the MyNursingKit website.
3. Use the Classroom Response Questions provided in PowerPoint to assess students prior to lecture.

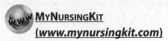

MyNursingKit (www.mynursingkit.com)

- Websites
- NCLEX® questions
- Critical Thinking Questions
- Case Studies
- Animations and Videos
- Drug Prototype Questions

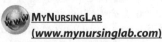

MyNursingLab (www.mynursinglab.com)

- Knowledge Quick Check
- Pre/Posttests
- Customized study plans
- *Separate purchase*

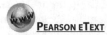

STUDENT WORKBOOK AND RESOURCE GUIDE

- Chapter 24 activities
- *Separate purchase*

PEARSON NURSE'S DRUG GUIDE

- *Separate purchase*

PEARSON eTEXT

- Students can search, highlight, take notes, and more all in electronic format.
- *Separate purchase*

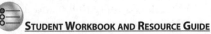

CLASSROOM RESPONSE QUESTION POWERPOINTS

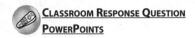

TESTBANK

© 2011 Pearson Education, Inc.

CHAPTER 25
DRUGS FOR ANGINA PECTORIS AND MYOCARDIAL INFARCTION

LEARNING OUTCOME 1

Explain the relationship between atherosclerosis and coronary artery disease.

Concepts for Lecture

1. Coronary artery disease (CAD) is one of the leading causes of mortality in the United States. The primary defining characteristic of CAD is narrowing or occlusion of a coronary artery. The narrowing deprives cells of needed oxygen and nutrients, a condition known as myocardial ischemia.
2. The most common etiology of CAD in adults is atherosclerosis, the presence of plaque, a fatty, fibrous material within the walls of the coronary arteries.

LEARNING OUTCOME 2

Describe factors that affect myocardial oxygen supply and demand.

Concepts for Lecture

1. The heart is the hardest working organ in the body, functioning continually during both activity and rest. Because the heart is a muscle, it needs a steady supply of nourishment to sustain itself and maintain the systemic circulation in a balanced state of equilibrium. Disturbances in blood flow to the vital organs or the myocardium itself—even for brief episodes—can result in life-threatening consequences.
2. The myocardium receives its blood via the right and left coronary arteries, which arise within the aortic sinuses at the base of the aorta. These arteries further diverge into smaller branches that encircle the heart, bringing the myocardium a continuous supply of oxygen and nutrients.
3. Coronary artery disease causes a narrowing of the coronary arteries that results in decreased blood flow and oxygen to the heart muscle.
4. Progressive CAD decreases the oxygen to the myocardium and places a greater demand on the heart muscle to function.

LEARNING OUTCOME 3

Explain the pathophysiology of angina pectoris and myocardial infarction.

Concepts for Lecture

1. **Angina pectoris** is acute chest pain caused by insufficient oxygen reaching a portion of the myocardium; it usually accompanies physical exertion or emotional excitement. These events cause increased myocardial oxygen demand.

 POWERPOINT SLIDES

 SUGGESTION FOR CLASSROOM ACTIVITIES
- Define myocardial ischemia, atherosclerosis, and plaque.

 REFERENCE
- Carotid Artery Disease: *www.texasheartinstitute.org/HIC/Topics/cond/CarotidArteryDisease.cfm*

 POWERPOINT SLIDES

Figure 25.1 Development of Atherosclerosis

 SUGGESTION FOR CLASSROOM ACTIVITIES
- Review the normal anatomy of the coronary arteries.

 SUGGESTION FOR CLINICAL ACTIVITIES
- Have students visit the cardiac catheterization laboratory.

 POWERPOINT SLIDES

 SUGGESTION FOR CLINICAL ACTIVITIES
- Have students review a chart(s) of patients with recent admission for angina pectoris and/or MI and identify signs and symptoms.

2. The classic presentation of angina pectoris is steady, intense pain in the anterior chest, sometimes accompanied by a crushing or constricting sensation. The discomfort radiates to the left shoulder and proceeds down the left arm. It may also extend posteriorly to the thoracic spine or move upward to the jaw. In some patients, the pain is experienced in the midepigastrium or abdominal area. Emotional distress may accompany the discomfort—a feeling of panic with fear of impending death. There is usually pallor, dyspnea with cyanosis, diaphoresis, tachycardia, and elevated blood pressure.

3. Angina pectoris episodes are usually of short duration. With physical rest and/or stress reduction, the increased demands upon the heart diminish, and the discomfort subsides within 5 to 10 minutes.

4. Angina is classified as **stable** or **unstable**. The pain associated with stable angina is usually relieved by rest. When episodes of angina arise more frequently, have added intensity, and occur during periods of rest, this condition is called unstable angina. Two other types of angina are known as **vasospastic** and **silent angina**. Vasospastic angina is caused by spasms of coronary arteries; silent angina is a form of the disease that occurs in the absence of angina pain. One or more coronary arteries are occluded, but the patient remains asymptomatic.

5. Angina pain often parallels the signs and symptoms of a heart attack. The nurse must accurately identify and differentiate the two conditions, because the pharmacological interventions related to angina differ considerably from those of **myocardial infarction (MI)**. MI, however, carries a high mortality rate if appropriate treatment is delayed.

LEARNING OUTCOME 4

Describe the nurse's role in the pharmacologic management of patients with angina and myocardial infarction.

Concepts for Lecture

1. The role of the nurse in treatment of the patient with angina pectoris or an MI will include careful monitoring of a patient's condition and providing education as it relates to the prescribed drug treatment; obtaining baseline vital signs, medical and drug history, lifestyle and dietary habits, and what activities the patient was involved with at the onset of the symptoms; and obtaining a detailed description of the symptoms and any pharmacological treatment initiated by the patient.

2. **Nitrates:** Obtain baseline blood pressure prior to administering nitrates, and continue to monitor blood pressure, because IV nitrates have the greatest risk for causing severe hypotension. Educate patient that alcohol is contraindicated with the use of nitrates. If hypotension occurs, withhold nitrates or remove topical forms of nitrate until blood pressure returns to normal.

3. **Beta-adrenergic blocker** (antagonists): Prior to administration, assess apical heart rate, especially if patient is on digoxin, because both drugs slow AV conduction. Obtain baseline blood pressure, and continue to monitor; monitor respiratory status as well. Treatment with beta blockers may mask symptoms of hypoglycemia; monitor serum-glucose levels. Educate patient not to discontinue medications abruptly, because this may exacerbate angina or cause tachycardia or MI in patients with cardiovascular disease.

4. **Calcium channel blockers** (CCB): Assess vital signs because CCB therapy affects blood pressure and heart rate. Hold medication if

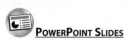
POWERPOINT SLIDES

Prototype Drug
• nitroglycerin (Nitrostat, Nitro-Bid, Nitro-Dur, others)

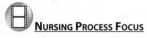
NURSING PROCESS FOCUS
• Patients Receiving Nitroglycerin

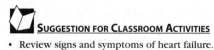
SUGGESTION FOR CLASSROOM ACTIVITIES
• Review signs and symptoms of heart failure.

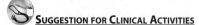
SUGGESTION FOR CLINICAL ACTIVITIES
• In the clinical setting, assign the student to the coronary-care unit to observe a patient with a recent MI or admission with angina pectoris.

© 2011 Pearson Education, Inc.

patient is hypotensive and or has a heart rate of 60 beats per minute or below. Obtain blood pressure while patient is lying, sitting, and standing. Obtain an ECG prior to administration as ordered by the physician. Assess for signs of deteriorating heart failure. Obtain daily weights. Assess bowel functions, as problems with constipation can occur.

5. **Thrombolytics:** Assess for conditions that would be contraindicated, including recent trauma, biopsies, surgery, and thrombocytopenia, because thrombolytics place the patient at increased risk for bleeding. Anyone with renal or liver disease should not be given thrombolytics. Start IV lines and arterial lines, and insert a Foley catheter prior to beginning therapy. Monitor vital signs, intake and output, and changes in laboratory values (hematocrit, hemoglobin, platelets, and coagulation studies) that may indicate bleeding. Because cerebral hemorrhage is a concern, assess for changes in mental and neurological status. Monitor cardiac function, and assess for dysrhythmia, because cardiac tissue perfusion is reestablished after MI.

LEARNING OUTCOME 5

Explain mechanisms by which drugs can be used to decrease cardiac oxygen demand and relieve angina pain.

Concepts for Lecture

Although various drug classes are used to treat disease, antianginal medications may be placed into two basic categories: those that *terminate* an acute angina episode in progress and those that decrease the *frequency* of angina episodes. The primary means by which antianginal drugs accomplish these goals is to reduce the myocardial demand for oxygen. This may be accomplished by slowing the heart rate; dilating veins so the heart receives less blood (reduced preload); causing the heart to contract with less force (reduced contractility); and lowering blood pressure, thus offering the heart less resistance when it is ejecting blood from its chambers (reduced afterload).

LEARNING OUTCOME 6

Identify classes of drugs that are given to treat the symptoms and complications of myocardial infarction.

Concepts for Lectures

1. Maintaining cardiac functioning and preventing permanent damage post MI can be achieved by the use of thrombolytic therapy to improve perfusion.
2. Glycoprotein inhibitors and nitrates improve blood flow preventing further damage.
3. Beta-adrenergic blockers and angiotensin-converting enzyme inhibitors reduce myocardial demand.

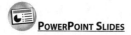

Prototype Drug
- atenolol (Tenormin)
- diltiazem (Cardizem, Cartia XT, Dilacor XR, Taztia XT, Tiazac)
- reteplase (Retavase)

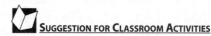

- Define preload, contractility, and afterload.

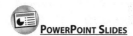

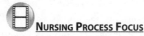

- Patients Receiving Thrombolytic Therapy

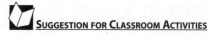

- Have students prepare a teaching plan for patients receiving glycoprotein inhibitors.

LEARNING OUTCOME 7

For each of the drug classes listed in Drugs at a Glance, know representative drug examples, and explain their mechanism of action, primary actions, and important adverse effects.

Concepts for Lecture

1. **Organic nitrates:** prototype drug: nitroglycerin (Nitrostat). The mechanism of action is to be a potent vasodilator in vascular smooth muscle. The primary use of the organic nitrates is to relax both arterial and venous smooth muscle, thus decreasing the workload on the heart and lowering myocardial oxygen demand. Adverse effects: severe hypotension, dizziness, blurred vision, dry mouth, or severe headache.
2. **Beta-adrenergic blockers:** prototype drug: atenolol (Tenormin). The mechanism of action is to reduce the cardiac workload by slowing the heart rate and reducing contractility. The primary use is for the prophylaxis of chronic angina. Adverse effects: hypotension, dizziness, fatigue during exercise.
3. **Calcium channel blockers:** prototype drug: diltiazem (Cardizem). The mechanism of action is similar to the beta blockers: reducing the cardiac workload. The primary use of CCBs is to relax arteriolar smooth muscle, thus lowering blood pressure. An additional effect is their ability to dilate the coronary arteries, bringing more oxygen to the myocardium. Adverse effects: hypotension, bradycardia, heart failure, and constipation.
4. **Thrombolytics:** prototype drug: reteplase (Retavase). When treating MI, thrombolytic therapy is administered to dissolve clots obstructing the coronary arteries. The primary use is to restore circulation to the myocardium. Adverse effects: The primary risk of thrombolytics is excessive bleeding due to interference with the normal clotting process.

LEARNING OUTCOME 8

Use the nursing process to care for patients who are receiving drug therapy for angina and myocardial infarction.

Concepts for Lecture

1. **Assessment:** careful monitoring of a patient's condition and providing education as it relates to the prescribed drug treatment; obtaining baseline vital signs, medical and drug history, lifestyle and dietary habits, and what activities the patient was involved with at the onset of the symptoms; obtaining a detailed description of the symptoms, including frequency and severity, and any pharmacological treatment initiated by the patient.
2. **Nursing diagnoses:** *Knowledge Deficit* regarding condition, *Therapeutic Regimen, and Potential Side Effects of Medications; Ineffective Therapeutic-Regimen Management* related to complexity of therapy and cost of medications; *Risk for Hypotension* related to side effects of medications.
3. **Planning:** Goals for patients receiving drugs for angina pectoris and myocardial infarction include the patient's ability to explain angina pectoris and needed medications and to verbalize the ability to follow prescribed therapy.
4. **Implementation:** Encourage compliance with medication regimen. Provide additional education regarding medication regimen, such as consultation with the clinical pharmacist, written and/or visual

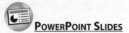
POWERPOINT SLIDES

Table 25.1 Selected Drugs for Angina and Myocardial Infarction

NURSING PROCESS FOCUS
- Patients Receiving Calcium Channel Blocker Therapy

SUGGESTION FOR CLASSROOM ACTIVITIES
- Have students prepare a teaching plan for a patient on medications for angina pectoris.

SUGGESTION FOR CLINICAL ACTIVITIES
- Have students prepare a care plan on a newly diagnosed patient with angina pectoris or MI.

POWERPOINT SLIDES

SUGGESTION FOR CLASSROOM ACTIVITIES
- Have students role-play the teaching plans they have created in another class period.

educational material, and home-health visits to ensure patient's ability to follow prescribed therapy.

5. **Evaluation:** Ideal outcome criteria for evaluation of the plan of care are that patients are free of or are having reduced episodes of angina with limited side effects and that patients are able to verbalize the importance of taking prescribed medications to assist them in their continued management of the disease.

GENERAL CHAPTER CONSIDERATIONS

1. Have students study and learn key terms listed at the beginning of the chapter.
2. Have students complete end-of-chapter exercises either in their book or on the MyNursingKit website.
3. Use the Classroom Response Questions provided in PowerPoint to assess students prior to lecture.

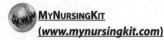 **MYNURSINGKIT** (*www.mynursingkit.com*)

- Websites
- NCLEX® questions
- Critical Thinking Questions
- Case Studies
- Animations and Videos
- Drug Prototype Questions

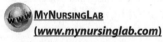 **MYNURSINGLAB** (*www.mynursinglab.com*)

- Knowledge Quick Check
- Pre/Posttests
- Customized study plans
- *Separate purchase*

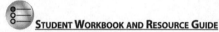 **STUDENT WORKBOOK AND RESOURCE GUIDE**

- Chapter 25 activities
- *Separate purchase*

PEARSON NURSE'S DRUG GUIDE

- *Separate purchase*

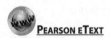 **PEARSON ETEXT**

- Students can search, highlight, take notes, and more all in electronic format.
- *Separate purchase*

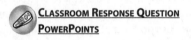 **CLASSROOM RESPONSE QUESTION POWERPOINTS**

 TESTBANK

CHAPTER 26
DRUGS FOR DYSRHYTHMIAS

LEARNING OUTCOME 1

Explain how rhythm abnormalities can affect cardiac function.

Concepts for Lecture

1. Dysrhythmias are abnormalities of electrical conduction or rhythm in the heart. Also known as *arrhythmias,* they can range from harmless to life threatening.
2. The electrocardiogram may be used to record electrophysiological events in the heart and to diagnose dysrhythmias. Proper diagnosis and pharmacotherapy can significantly affect the prognosis of a patient with dysrhythmias.
3. The frequency of dysrhythmias in the population is difficult to predict because symptoms can range from none to sudden death, though dysrhythmias are estimated to be quite common. Persistent or severe dysrhythmias increase the risk of stroke and heart failure.

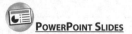

POWERPOINT SLIDES

Table 26.1 Types of Dysrthymia
Figure 26.2 Normal ECG and Its Relationship to Impulse Conduction to the Heart

SUGGESTIONS FOR CLASSROOM ACTIVITIES

- Direct students to find a website that shows the chambers of the heart.
- Direct students to complete the sudden arrhythmia death syndrome risk assessment form at *www.sads.org*

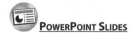

REFERENCE

- Sudden Arrhythmia Death Syndromes Foundation: *www.sads.org*

LEARNING OUTCOME 2

Illustrate the flow of electrical impulses through the normal heart.

Concepts for Lecture

1. Some myocardial cells in these regions have the property of automaticity. They are able to initiate an action potential. The electrical conduction pathway from the sinoatrial (SA) node, across both atria to the atrioventricular (AV) node through the atrioventricular bundle (bundle of His), to the right and left bundle branches and Purkinje fibers keeps the heart beating in a synchronized manner.
2. The purpose of the conduction system is to regulate the heart and maintain cardiac output. Trace the normal conduction pathway in the diagram found in Figure 26.1.

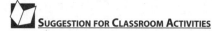

POWERPOINT SLIDES

Figure 26.1 Normal Conduction Pathway in the Heart

SUGGESTION FOR CLASSROOM ACTIVITIES

- Have students diagram the normal conduction pathway of the heart.

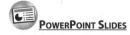

REFERENCE

- The Mysterious Human Heart: *www.pbs .org/wnet/heart/*

LEARNING OUTCOME 3

Classify dysrhythmias based on their location and type of rhythm abnormality.

Concepts for Lecture

1. Dysrhythmias can occur in both healthy and diseased hearts; they disrupt the regulation of the heart and may decrease cardiac output. The

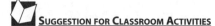

POWERPOINT SLIDES

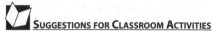

SUGGESTION FOR CLASSROOM ACTIVITIES

- Direct the student to search online to find the types of dysrhythmias common in pediatric patients.

© 2011 Pearson Education, Inc.

exact cause of dysrhythmias is elusive, but they are closely associated with certain conditions, such as heart disease and myocardial infarctions.

2. Dysrhythmias are classified by the location (atrial or ventricular) or type (flutter, fibrillation, or block) of rhythm abnormality produced. Atrial fibrillation is the most common type of dysrhythmia.

3. Types of dysrhythmias include premature atrial or premature ventricular contractions (PVCs), atrial or ventricular tachycardia, atrial or ventricular flutter and/or fibrillation, sinus bradycardia, and heart block.

Learning Outcome 4

Explain how an action potential is controlled by the flow of sodium, potassium, and calcium ions across the myocardial membrane.

Concepts for Lecture

1. Action potentials are electrical impulses that travel across the myocardium; they are found in neural and cardiac cells. Changes in extra- and intracellular ion polarization create the electrical impulse. A cell membrane is said to be polarized when it is at rest. The potential across the membrane is negative inside the cell relative to the outside, sodium and calcium are outside the cell, and potassium is inside the cell at this time.

2. Generation of the action potential begins when sodium-ion channels open and sodium ions rush in, causing depolarization. Then the calcium-ion channels open and calcium ions enter the cell, stimulating cardiac-muscle contraction. SA and AV cells depolarize in response to calcium-ion influx. After the brief period of depolarization, the sodium pump removes sodium from the cell, and potassium-ion channels allow potassium to move back into the cell. This phase is called repolarization, or a return to a polarized state.

3. Discuss the ion channels in myocardial cells as diagrammed in Figure 26.3.

4. The pharmacological strategies used to terminate dysrhythmias work in two ways: either they either block potassium-, sodium-, or calcium-ion channels; or they prolong the refractory period, a brief period in the conduction cycle during which myocardial cells cannot produce another action potential.

Learning Outcome 5

Identify the importance of nonpharmacologic therapies in the treatment of dysrhythmias.

Concepts for Lecture

Nonpharmacological therapies for dysrhythmias include cardioversion and defibrillation for serious types of dysrhythmias. These are both examples of an electrical shock that stops all electrical impulses in the heart and allows the sinoatrial node to regain control. Catheter ablation identifies and destroys aberrant cardiac cells that cause dysrhythmias. Cardiac pacemakers pace the heart at a set rate. Implantable cardioverter defibrillators (ICD) are a combination of pacemaker and defibrillator.

Suggestion for Clinical Activities

- Observe the procedure of obtaining a 12-lead ECG in the clinical area.

PowerPoint Slides

Figure 26.3 Flow of Ions During the Action Potential

Suggestion for Classroom Activities

- Have students draw a diagram of ion channels in myocardial cells and the movement of ions through the channels.

PowerPoint Slides

References

- Implantable Cardioverter Defibrillator: *www.nhlbi.nih.gov/health/dci/Diseases/icd/icd_whatis.html www.americanheart.org/presenter.jhtml?identifier=11227*

Suggestion for Classroom Activities

- Display pictures or actual equipment used in nonpharmacological treatment of dysrhythmias for students to view.

Suggestion for Clinical Activities

- Provide an opportunity in the clinical area for the students to view the equipment used in nonpharmacological treatment of dysrhythmias.

LEARNING OUTCOME 6

Identify the general mechanisms of action of antidysrhythmic drugs.

Concepts for Lecture

1. Antidysrhythmic drugs are categorized into four classes according to their mechanism of action. They act by blocking conduction (flow of ions) or altering automaticity (autonomic activity). The use of antidysrhythmic drugs is declining significantly. Although these drugs have the ability to correct dysrhythmias, they can also worsen or even create new dysrhythmias. Nonpharmacological therapies have improved and are being used more frequently to treat dysrhythmias.
2. Groups of antidysrhythmic drugs—see Table 26.2.
    Class I: sodium-ion-channel blockers—Blocking sodium-ion channels prevents depolarization; the spread of the action potential across the myocardium will slow, and areas of ectopic pacemaker activity will be suppressed.
    Class II: beta-adrenergic antagonists—Beta blockers slow the heart rate and decrease conduction velocity through the AV node.
    Class III: potassium-ion-channel blockers—Repolarization depends upon replacement of potassium inside the cell. The class III medications delay repolarization of the myocardial cells and lengthen the refractory period, which tends to stabilize dysrhythmias.
    Class IV: calcium-ion-channel blockers—A blockade of calcium-ion channels reduces automaticity in the SA node and slows impulse conduction through the AV node. This slows the heart rate and prolongs the refractory period. Miscellaneous antidysrhythmic drugs—work by slowing conduction through the AV node and/or decreasing automaticity of the SA node.

LEARNING OUTCOME 7

Describe the nurse's role in the pharmacologic management of patients with dysrhythmias.

Concepts for Lecture

1. The role of the nurse in antidysrhythmic drug therapy involves careful monitoring of a patient's condition and providing education as it relates to the prescribed drug treatment. Obtain a complete medical and drug history and physical examination, including baseline ECG, vital signs, diagnostic tests, dietary habits, and routine activity.
2. Sodium-ion-channel blockers: Monitor ECG for changes; monitor for hypotension, changes in level of consciousness, and diarrhea. Teach the patient to not skip a dose of medication, to not take two doses at one time, and to avoid the use of alcohol. This medication is contraindicated in those with heart failure or renal impairment.
3. Beta-adrenergic blockers: This medication is contraindicated in patients with heart block, severe bradycardia, AV block, and asthma. Monitor for hypotension and hypoglycemia. Elderly patients may show signs of cognitive impairment. Teach patients to take their own pulse, how to rise slowly from sitting or lying down, and to report signs of heart failure.
4. Potassium-ion-channel blockers: Use cautiously in patients with heart block; these medications are not recommended for use during pregnancy (category C or D) or lactation. Teach patients to monitor for vision changes, palpitations, jaundice, and abdominal pain and to avoid sun exposure and take with food.

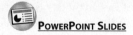
 POWERPOINT SLIDES

Table 26.2 Classification of Antidysrhythmics

 SUGGESTION FOR CLASSROOM ACTIVITIES

- Divide the students into small groups, and have them prepare questions and answers for different categories of drugs used to treat dysrhythmias. Have them include questions on each drug's classification and mechanisms of action for each type of disease.

 SUGGESTION FOR CLINICAL ACTIVITIES

- Assign students to care for patients being treated for antidysrhythmias and to analyze the clinical use of antidysrhythmic drugs.

 POWERPOINT SLIDES

 SUGGESTION FOR CLASSROOM ACTIVITIES

- Direct students to break into groups of two and role-play the parts of nurse and patient, with the nurse providing education about an antidysrhythmic and the patient asking questions.

SUGGESTION FOR CLINICAL ACTIVITIES

- Arrange for students to have a clinical/observational experience at an acute-care facility. Assign them to observe patients who have a dysrhythmia diagnosis.

© 2011 Pearson Education, Inc.

5. Calcium-ion-channel blockers: Do not use for patients with sick-sinus syndrome, heart block, severe hypotension, cardiogenic shock, and severe congestive heart failure. Monitor for hypotension, especially in the elderly; do not use during pregnancy (category C) or lactation. Teach patients to report any palpitations, blood pressure changes, edema, or shortness of breath and to rise slowly from a sitting or lying-down position.

6. Miscellaneous drugs for dysrhythmias: Monitor for heart rate and blood pressure changes. Assess those patients taking digoxin for symptoms of digoxin toxicity.

LEARNING OUTCOME 8

Know representative drug examples for each of the drug classes listed in Drugs at a Glance, and explain their mechanisms of action, primary actions, and important adverse effects.

Concepts for Lecture

1. Sodium-ion-channel blockers (Class I): prototype drug: procainamide (Pronestyl). The mechanism of action of this largest group of antidysrhythmics is to block the sodium-ion channels, which slow the rate of impulse conduction across the heart. The primary use is to correct many types of atrial and ventricular dysrhythmias. Adverse effects include the creation of new dysrhythmias or worsening of existing ones, lupus effect, nausea, vomiting, abdominal pain, and headache. High doses can produce CNS effects.

2. Beta-adrenergic blockers (Class II): prototype drug: propranolol (Inderal). The mechanism of action is to block beta receptors, which reduces automaticity and slows conduction velocity across the myocardium. The primary use is treatment of atrial dysrhythmias associated with heart failure. Adverse effects include bradycardia, hypotension with dizziness and fainting, bronchospasms, hypoglycemia, and diminished libido.

3. Potassium-ion-channel blockers (Class III): prototype drug: amiodarone (Cordarone). The mechanism of action is to block potassium-ion channels in myocardial cells, which prolongs the refractory period of the heart. The primary use is to treat resistant ventricular tachycardia and atrial dysrhythmias with heart failure. Adverse effects include blurred vision, pneumonia-like syndrome, bradycardia, and hypotension. Potassium-ion-channel blockers can create new dysrhythmias or worsen existing ones.

4. Calcium-ion-channel blockers (Class IV): prototype drug: verapamil (Calan). The mechanism of action is to block calcium channels, which reduces automaticity and slows myocardial (AV) conduction velocity. Their actions and effects are similar to those of beta blockers. The primary use is treatment of supraventricular tachycardia. Adverse effects include bradycardia, hypotension, and headache.

5. Miscellaneous antidysrhythmics: Examples of miscellaneous antidysrhythmics are digoxin (Lanoxin) and adenosine (Adenocard). The mechanism of action for both of these drugs is to decrease automaticity of the SA node and slow conduction through the AV node but not act by blocking ion channels. The primary use for digoxin is treatment of certain types of atrial dysrhythmias. Adenosine is used to treat serious atrial tachycardia. Adverse effects include creating new dysrhythmias or worsening existing ones. Specific to digoxin are nausea, vomiting, headache, and visual disturbances. Specific to adenosine are facial flushing and dyspnea.

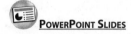 **POWERPOINT SLIDES**

Prototype Drug
- procainamide (Procanabid)
- propranolol (Inderal, InnoPran)
- amiodarone (Cordarone, Pacerone)
- verapamil (Calan, Covera-HS, Isoptin SR, Verelan)

 SUGGESTION FOR CLASSROOM ACTIVITIES

- Have each student make drug cards for each classification of drug used to treat dysrythmias. Use two different drugs for each classification. The card should include mechanisms of action, primary actions, and important adverse effects.

 SUGGESTION FOR CLINICAL ACTIVITIES

- Direct students to locate the policies for treating dysrhythmias in the ED and CCU. Have the student present information on these emergency drugs in postclinical.

Learning Outcome 9

Use the nursing process to care for patients receiving drug therapy for dysrhythmias.

Concepts for Lecture

1. Assessment: Obtain complete health history including allergies, drug history, and possible drug interactions; do assessment of cardiac output and obtain a baseline ECG to compare throughout therapy.
2. Nursing diagnoses: Ineffective tissue perfusion, knowledge deficit, risk for injury, and decreased cardiac output.
3. Planning: Goals for the patient receiving drugs for treatment of dysrhythmia include improved cardiac output, understanding of drug therapy, and prevention of adverse effects.
4. Implementation: Monitor cardiac rate and rhythm, monitor IV site, investigate possible causes of dysrhythmia, and observe for correct administration of the drugs and their adverse effects.
5. Evaluation: Ideal outcomes include improved cardiac output, patient verbalization of understanding of drug therapy, and prevention of adverse effects.

General Chapter Considerations

1. Have students study and learn key terms listed at beginning of chapter.
2. Have students complete end-of-chapter exercises either in their book or on the MyNursingKit website.
3. Use the Classroom Response Questions provided in PowerPoint to assess students prior to lecture.

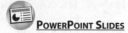 **PowerPoint Slides**

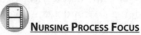 **Nursing Process Focus**
- Patients Receiving Antidysrhythmic Therapies

 Suggestion for Classroom Activities
- Divide students into small groups, and have each group develop a teaching plan for a patient receiving antidysrhythmic therapy.

 Suggestion for Clinical Activities
- Assign students to care for patients with dysrhythmias.

 MyNursingKit (*www.mynursingkit.com*)
- Websites
- NCLEX® questions
- Critical Thinking Questions
- Case Studies
- Animations and Videos
- Drug Prototype Questions

 MyNursingLab (*www.mynursinglab.com*)
- Knowledge Quick Check
- Pre/Posttests
- Customized study plans
- *Separate purchase*

 Student Workbook and Resource Guide
- Chapter 26 activities
- *Separate purchase*

Pearson Nurse's Drug Guide
- *Separate purchase*

 Pearson eText
- Students can search, highlight, take notes, and more all in electronic format.
- *Separate purchase*

 Classroom Response Question PowerPoints

Testbank

© 2011 Pearson Education, Inc.

CHAPTER 27
DRUGS FOR COAGULATION DISORDERS

LEARNING OUTCOME 1

Illustrate the major steps of hemostasis and fibrinolysis.

Concepts for Lecture

1. Hemostasis is a complex process involving a number of **clotting factors** that are activated in a series of sequential steps. The final product is a fibrin clot that stops blood loss.
2. The clotting process begins when blood-vessel injury causes vessel spasm (constriction); platelets are attracted to and adhere to the injured area. That aggregation of platelets forms a plug in which formation of insoluble fibrin strands and coagulation (*coagulation cascade*) occurs. Normal blood clotting occurs in about 6 minutes. The basic steps of hemostasis are shown in Figure 27.1.
3. The coagulation cascade includes intrinsic and extrinsic pathways that lead to formation of the fibrin clot. Near the end of the cascade, a chemical called **prothrombin activator** or prothrombinase is formed. Prothrombin activator converts the clotting factor **prothrombin** to an enzyme called **thrombin.** Thrombin then converts **fibrinogen,** a plasma protein, to long strands of **fibrin.** The fibrin strands provide a framework for the clot. Thus, two of the factors essential to clotting, thrombin and fibrin, are formed only *after* injury to the vessels. The fibrin strands form an insoluble web over the injured area to stop blood loss. The steps in each coagulation cascade are shown in Figure 27.2.
4. Fibrinolysis or clot removal involves several sequential steps. When the fibrin clot is formed, nearby blood vessel cells secrete the enzyme **tissue plasminogen activator (TPA).** TPA converts the inactive protein **plasminogen,** which is present in the fibrin clot, to its active enzymatic form, **plasmin.** Plasmin then digests the fibrin strands to remove the clot. The body normally regulates fibrinolysis such that *unwanted* fibrin clots are removed, whereas fibrin present in wounds is left to maintain hemostasis. The steps of fibrinolysis are shown in Figure 27.3.

LEARNING OUTCOME 2

Describe thromboembolic disorders that are indicators for coagulation modifiers.

Concepts for Lecture

Diseases of hemostasis include thromboembolic disorders caused by thrombi and emboli, thrombocytopenia, and bleeding disorders such as hemophilia and von Willebrand's disease.

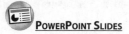
POWERPOINT SLIDES

Figure 27.1 Basic Steps in Hemostasis
Figure 27.2 Major Steps in the Coagulation Cascade: Common Pathway
Figure 27.3 Primary Steps in Fibrinolysis

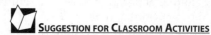
SUGGESTION FOR CLASSROOM ACTIVITIES

- Have students draw a diagram to illustrate the process of hemostasis and fibrinolysis.

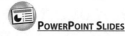
POWERPOINT SLIDES

SUGGESTION FOR CLASSROOM ACTIVITIES

- Direct students to access information on immune thrombocytopenic purpura (ITP) online and create a poster summarizing the symptoms and treatment for ITP.

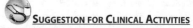
SUGGESTION FOR CLINICAL ACTIVITIES

- Direct students to access information on deep vein thrombosis (DVT) at *www.dvt.net/* and then create a patient-education pamphlet for their patients with DVT.

REFERENCE

• The Coalition to Prevent Deep-Vein
  Thrombosis: *www.dvt.net*

LEARNING OUTCOME 3

Identify the primary mechanisms by which coagulation modifier drugs act.

Concepts for Lecture

1. Drugs can modify hemostasis by four basic mechanisms. The basic mechanisms of hemostasis are shown in Table 27.2.
2. Anticoagulants prevent the formation of clots by either inhibiting specific clotting factors in the coagulation cascade or diminishing the clotting action of platelets. All anticoagulant drugs will increase the normal clotting time.
3. Antiplatelets prevent clot formation by inhibiting platelet action.
4. Thrombolytics remove an existing clot by dissolving life-threatening clots.
5. Hemostatics promote clot formation by inhibiting fibrin destruction.

POWERPOINT SLIDES

Table 27.2 Mechanisms of Action of Coagulation Modifiers

SUGGESTION FOR CLASSROOM ACTIVITIES

• Have students prepare class presentations on the uses of each of the coagulation-modifier drugs.

SUGGESTION FOR CLINICAL ACTIVITIES

• Direct students to create concept maps showing the etiology, symptoms, and treatment of coagulation disorders in their clinical patients to present during postclinical conference.

LEARNING OUTCOME 4

Explain how laboratory testing of coagulation parameters is used to monitor anticoagulant pharmacotherapy.

Concepts for Lecture

Laboratory tests are an integral part of diagnosing bleeding disorders and monitoring anticoagulant pharmacotherapy. These tests include Activated clotting time, Activated partial thromboplastin time (aPTT), Bleeding time, Heparin anti-Xa, Platelet count, Prothrombin Time (PT), Thrombin time.

POWERPOINT SLIDES

Table 27.1 Laboratory Testing for Coagulation Disorders

SUGGESTION FOR CLASSROOM ACTIVITIES

• Direct students to explain laboratory tests used to measure coagulation and their uses.

SUGGESTION FOR CLINICAL ACTIVITIES

• Arrange for students to observe the processing of lab tests that measure coagulation.

LEARNING OUTCOME 5

Describe the nurse's role in the pharmacologic management of coagulation disorders.

Concepts for Lecture

1. The role of the nurse in the pharmacologic management of coagulation disorders involves careful monitoring of patient's condition and providing education as it relates to the prescribed drug treatment. Obtain baseline medical, surgical, and drug history; lifestyle and dietary habits, including use of herbal or alternative therapies; and detailed description of symptomology and current therapies.

POWERPOINT SLIDES

SUGGESTION FOR CLASSROOM ACTIVITIES

• Assign students into small groups to create concept maps detailing the care of a patient with a coagulation disorder.

SUGGESTION FOR CLINICAL ACTIVITIES

• Direct students to create patient-education brochures explaining the lab studies associated with coagulation. Have students use the brochures when they are doing patient education.

© 2011 Pearson Education, Inc.

2. **Anticoagulants:** The most serious side effect is bleeding; monitor for signs and symptoms of excessive visible bleeding: bleeding at IV sites, wounds, excessive echhymosis, petechiae, hematuria, black/tarry stools, rectal bleeding, "coffee-ground" emesis, epistaxis, bleeding from gums, hemoptysis, prolonged and/or heavy menstrual flow; and for occult bleeding: pallor, dizziness, hypotension, tachycardia, abdominal pain, areas of abdominal wall swelling or firmness, lumbar pain, decreased level of consciousness. Risk for bleeding increases during the transition time from heparin to warfarin when both drugs are given at the same time. Do not give warfarin to pregnant patients; heparin and low-molecular-weight heparin can be given to pregnant patients. Take warfarin at the same time each day. Avoid vitamin K supplements, and protein supplement drinks (e.g., Ensure™ or Boost™), which often have vitamin K added, and limit intake of garlic. Teach patient or caregiver in proper self-administration techniques.

3. **Antiplatelets:** Monitor for signs and symptoms of bleeding: oozing at IV sites or wounds, ecchymosis, petechiae, hematuria, black/tarry stools, rectal bleeding, "coffee-ground" emesis, epistaxis, bleeding from gums, prolonged and/or heavy menstrual flow; and for occult bleeding: pallor, dizziness, hypotension, tachycardia, abdominal pain, areas of abdominal wall swelling or firmness, lumbar pain, decreased level of consciousness. Risk for bleeding; increases if given concurrently with anticoagulants. Injection or venipuncture sites will need prolonged pressure to control bleeding. Continue to monitor peripheral pulses for quality and volume, complaints of angina or chest pain, especially if new or of sudden onset or accompanied by dyspnea.

4. **Thrombolytics:** Be aware of conditions that exclude patients from receiving thrombolytics. Monitor frequently for signs and symptoms of excessive visible bleeding: bleeding at IV sites, wounds, hematuria, rectal bleeding, "coffee-ground" emesis, bleeding from gums, hemoptysis, bleeding at previous recent incisional sites; and for occult bleeding: pallor, hypotension, tachycardia, dizziness, sudden severe headache, lumbar pain, and decreased level of consciousness. Monitor vital signs and ECG every 15 minutes during first hour of infusion, and then every 30 minutes during remainder of infusion and for first 8 hours. Report any dysrhythmias immediately. Monitor baseline coagulation studies. Monitor level of consciousness, as cerebral hemorrhage is a concern. Observe for reperfusion arrhythmias. Teach patient about the increased risk of bleeding.

5. **Hemostatics:** Monitor for clotting in the peripheral vascular system, pulmonary system, nervous system, and cardiac system. Administer intravenously; monitor site closely for thrombophlebitis and extravasation. Assess for presence of myopathy and myoglobinuria (reddish-brown urine). Teach patient to report symptoms of clotting or bleeding. Do not take aspirin.

LEARNING OUTCOME 6

For each of the classes listed in Drugs at a Glance, know representative drug examples, and explain the mechanism of drug action, primary actions, and important adverse effects.

Concepts for Lecture

1. **Parenteral Anticoagulants:** prototype drug: heparin. The mechanism of action is to inhibit specific clotting factors, thereby interfering with the coagulation cascade and preventing formation or enlargement of clots. Within minutes after intravenous (IV) administration of heparin, the loss

POWERPOINT SLIDES

Table 27.3 Anticoagulants
Table 27.4 Antiplatelet Agents
Table 27.5 Thrombolytics
Table 27.6 Hemostatics

of activated clotting factors prevents the formation of fibrin clots. The primary use is to prevent formation of clots in veins and treat thromboembolic disorders. Adverse effects include abnormal bleeding.

2. The heparin molecule has been shortened and modified to create a newer class of drugs called low-molecular-weight heparins (LMWHs). The mechanism of action of these agents is similar to that of heparin, except their inhibition is more specific to active factor X (see Figure 27.2). Their duration of action is two to four times longer than that of heparin. The LMWHs also produce a more stable response than heparin; thus, fewer follow-up lab tests are needed, and family members or the patient can be trained to give the necessary SC injections at home. These anticoagulants are less likely than heparin to cause thrombocytopenia. LMWHs have become the drugs of choice for a number of clotting disorders, including the prevention of DVT following surgery.

3. **Other parenteral anticoagulants** include the direct thrombin inhibitors argatroban (Acova, Novastan), bivalirudin (Angiomax), and lepirudin (Refludan). The mechanism of action is to bind to the active site of thrombin, preventing the formation of fibrin clots. The thrombin inhibitors have limited therapeutic uses.

4. **Oral anticoagulants:** prototype drug: warfarin (Coumadin). The mechanism of action is to inhibit the hepatic synthesis of coagulation factors II, VII, IX, and X. Often, patients begin anticoagulation therapy with heparin and are switched to warfarin when their condition stabilizes. When transitioning, the two drugs are administered concurrently for 2 to 3 days because warfarin takes several days to achieve optimum effect. Pentoxifylline (Trental) is another oral anticoagulant that works by a different mechanism than heparin. Pentoxifylline reduces the viscosity of red blood cells and increases their flexibility. It is given to increase the microcirculation in patients with intermittent claudication. The most frequent, and potentially serious, adverse effect of all the anticoagulant agents is bleeding. Specific antagonists may be administered to reverse the anticoagulant effects: protamine sulfate is used for heparin, and vitamin K is administered for warfarin (see the drug prototype features in this chapter). (See Table 27.3 for a list of anticoagulants.)

5. **Antiplatelet** drugs include aspirin, ADP blockers, glycoprotein 11b/111a receptor anatagonists, and miscellaneous agents for treating intermittent claudication. The prototype drug in the antiplatelet class is (ADP receptor blocker) clopidogrel (Plavix). The mechanism of action is to prolong bleeding time by inhibiting platelet aggregation directly inhibiting ADP binding to its receptor. The primary use is to prevent thromboembolic events in patients with a recent history of MI, CVA, or peripheral artery disease. It is also approved for thrombi prophylaxis in patients with unstable angina, including those who are receiving vascular bypass procedures or angioplasty. Adverse effects include abnormal bleeding. (See Table 27.4 for a list of antiplatelets.)

6. **Thrombolytics** are used to dissolve existing intravascular clots in patients with MI and CVA. The prototype drug in this class is altepase (Activase). The mechanism of action is to convert plasminogen to plasmin, which digests the fibrin and dissolves the clot. The primary uses are treatment of acute myocardial infarction (MI), deep vein thrombosis (DVT), cerebrovscular accident (CVA), pulmonary embolism, and arterial thrombosis and to clear intravenous (IV) catheters. Adverse effects include abnormal bleeding; it is contraindicated in patients with a bleeding disorder or who have had recent trauma or surgery. (See Table 27.5 for a list of thrombolytics.)

7. **Hemostatics** or **antifibrinolytics** are used to promote the formation of clots in patients with excessive bleeding from surgical sites.

Prototype drugs
- heparin (parenteral)
- warfarin (oral)
- clopidogrel (Plavix)
- alteplase (Activase)
- aminocaproic acid (Amicar)

ANIMATIONS AND VIDEOS

- Mechanism in action: Warfarin (Coumadin)
- Mechanism in action: Heparin (Heplock)

SUGGESTION FOR CLASSROOM ACTIVITIES

- Divide students into small groups and have them prepare questions and answers for different categories of drugs used to treat coagulation disorders. Have them include questions on each drug's classification and mechanism of action.

SUGGESTION FOR CLINICAL ACTIVITIES

- Assign students to care for patients being treated for coagulation disorders and to analyze clinical use of drugs used in the treatment of coagulation disorders.

© 2011 Pearson Education, Inc.

The prototype drug for this class is aminocaproic acid (Amicar). Its mechanism of action is to prevent fibrin from dissolving. The primary use is to prevent and treat excessive bleeding from surgical sites. Adverse effects include possible hypercoagulation with concurrent use of estrogens and oral contraceptives. Aminocaproic acid is contraindicated in patients with disseminated intravascular clotting or severe renal impairment. (See Table 27.5 for a list of hemostatics.)

LEARNING OUTCOME 7

Use the nursing process to care for patients receiving drug therapy for coagulation disorders.

Concepts for Lecture

1. **Patients receiving anticoagulant therapy**—Assessment: Obtain a complete health history including any surgeries, drug therapy including herbal drugs, and dietary intake (especially note intake of vitamin K-rich foods and garlic). Assess coagulation studies initially and as therapy progresses.
2. **Patients receiving anticoagulant therapy**—Nursing Diagnoses: *Pain* (thrombosis and lessened perfusion); *Ineffective Tissue Perfusion* (decreased circulation); *Impaired Skin Integrity* (ineffective tissue perfusion); *Anxiety; Deficient Knowledge* (drug therapy); *Risk for Injury* (bleeding, related to adverse effects of anticoagulant therapy).
3. **Patients receiving anticoagulant therapy**—Planning: The patient will experience therapeutic effects dependent on the reason the drug is being given (e.g., prevention of thrombosis or limited extension of existing thrombosis); being free from, or experiencing minimal adverse effects, verbalizing an understanding of the drug's use, adverse effects and required precautions and demonstrating proper self-administration of the medication (e.g., dose, timing, when to notify provider).
4. **Patients receiving anticoagulant therapy**—Implementation: Monitor for adverse clotting reactions, skin necrosis, and cautious use in specific populations, monitoring for bleeding, monitoring of lab values, including prothrombin time (PT), international normalized ratio (INR), thrombin time, activated partial thromboplastin time (aPTT), and complete blood count (CBC).
5. **Patients receiving anticoagulant therapy**—Evaluation: The patient will experience a reduction in blood coagulation as noted in laboratory studies, be free from, or experience minimal adverse effects, demonstrate proper self-administration of the medication (e.g., dose, timing, when to notify provider). Verbalize an understanding of the drug's use, adverse effects, and required precautions, and verbalize an understanding of anticoagulant therapy.
6. **Patients receiving thrombolytic therapy**—Assessment: Obtain a complete health history, including trauma, allergies, drug history, and possible drug interactions. Obtain vital signs; assess in context of patient's baseline values. Assess lab values: prothrombin time (PT), international normalized ratio (INR), thrombin time, activated partial thromboplastin time (aPTT), and complete blood count (CBC).
7. **Patients receiving thrombolytic therapy**—Nursing diagnoses: *Pain* (thrombosis and lessened perfusion); *Ineffective Tissue Perfusion* (decreased circulation); *Impaired Gas Exchange* (pulmonary emboli); *Impaired Skin Integrity* (ineffective tissue perfusion); *Anxiety; Deficient Knowledge* (drug therapy); *Risk for Injury* (bleeding and hemorrhage, related to adverse effects of thrombolytic therapy).

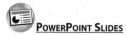

POWERPOINT SLIDES

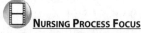

NURSING PROCESS FOCUS
- Patients Receiving Anticoagulant Therapy
- Patients Receiving Thrombolytic Therapy

SUGGESTION FOR CLASSROOM ACTIVITIES
- Divide the students into small groups and have them prepare questions and answers for different categories of drugs used to treat coagulation disorders. They should include questions on each drug's classification and mechanisms of action of each type of disease.

SUGGESTION FOR CLINICAL ACTIVITIES
- Assign students to care for patients receiving pharmacological therapy for coagulation disorders.

8. **Patients receiving thrombolytic therapy**—Planning: The patient will experience therapeutic effects dependent on the reason the drug is being given (e.g., reperfusion of coronary arteries, being free from or experiencing minimal adverse effects, verbalizing an understanding of the drug's use, adverse effects and required precautions and demonstrating proper self-administration of the medication (e.g., dose, timing, when to notify provider).

9. **Patients receiving thrombolytic therapy**—Implementation: Monitor vital signs and ECG every 15 minutes during the first hour of infusion, and then every 30 minutes during the remainder of infusion and for the first 8 hours. Report any dysrhythmias immediately. Frequently check vital signs and assess for adverse effects of the drug including hypotension and tachycardia associated with bleeding and for dysrhythmias. Maintain the patient on bedrest and with limited activity during the infusion. (Limited physical activity and bedrest decrease the chance for bruising, injury and bleeding.) Monitor neurological status frequently, especially if thrombolytics are used for CVA. Avoid invasive procedures during infusion and up to 8 hours post-infusion when possible. (Any puncture site or site of invasive procedure will create an additional site for bleeding.) Whenever an invasive procedure must be used (e.g., ABGs), the site must be maintained under pressure for 30 minutes or longer to prevent hemorrhage. Monitor vital signs frequently; prevent injury; assess neurovascular and cardiovascular status frequently; monitor lab values including prothrombin time (PT); international normalized ratio (INR); thrombin time; activated partial thromboplastin time (aPTT); and complete blood count (CBC).

10. **Patients receiving thrombolytic therapy**—Evaluation: The patient experiences therapeutic effects dependent on the reason the drug is being given (e.g., reperfusion of coronary arteries). The patient is free from, or experiences minimal adverse effects; verbalizes an understanding of the drug's use, adverse effects, and required precautions; and demonstrates proper self-administration of the medication (e.g., dose, timing, when to notify provider).

© 2011 Pearson Education, Inc.

GENERAL CHAPTER CONSIDERATIONS

1. Have students study and learn key terms listed at the beginning of the chapter.
2. Have students complete end-of-chapter exercises either in their book or on the MyNursingKit website.
3. Use the Classroom Response Questions provided in PowerPoint to assess students prior to lecture.

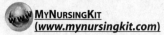

MyNursingKit (www.mynursingkit.com)

- Websites
- NCLEX® questions
- Critical Thinking Questions
- Case Studies
- Animations and Videos
- Drug Prototype Questions

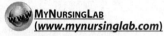

MyNursingLab (www.mynursinglab.com)

- Knowledge Quick Check
- Pre/Posttests
- Customized study plans
- *Separate purchase*

STUDENT WORKBOOK AND RESOURCE GUIDE

- Chapter 27 activities
- *Separate purchase*

PEARSON NURSE'S DRUG GUIDE

- *Separate purchase*

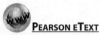

PEARSON eTEXT

- Students can search, highlight, take notes, and more all in electronic format.
- *Separate purchase*

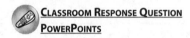

CLASSROOM RESPONSE QUESTION POWERPOINTS

TESTBANK

CHAPTER 28
DRUGS FOR HEMATOPOIETIC DISORDERS

LEARNING OUTCOME 1

Describe the process of hematopoiesis.

Concepts for Lecture

Hematopoiesis is the process of blood-cell production that begins with primitive stem cells that reside in bone marrow. Hematopoiesis is controlled homeostatically through hormones and growth factors. Demands of the body influence hematopoiesis; white blood cells (WBCs) can increase to ten times the normal concentration and red blood cells (RBCs) as much as five times when needed.

 POWERPOINT SLIDES

Figure 28.1 Hematopoiesis

 SUGGESTION FOR CLASSROOM ACTIVITIES

- Have students search reliable medical Internet sites for information on stem-cell research and share their findings with the class.

 SUGGESTION FOR CLINICAL ACTIVITIES

- Have students research bone-marrow disorders at *www.aamds.org/aplastic/*, and then during clinical have them observe the bone-marrow-donation process.

 REFERENCE

- Aplastic Anemia: *www.aamds.org/aplastic/*

 POWERPOINT SLIDES

Table 28.1 Hematopoietic Growth Factors

 SUGGESTION FOR CLASSROOM ACTIVITIES

- Have students draw diagrams illustrating erythropoietin metabolism in the body.

 SUGGESTION FOR CLINICAL ACTIVITIES

- Have students research the drug information describing various drugs used for bone-marrow disorders and clinical trials in progress. Provide time for the students to present their findings during postclinical.

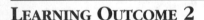

LEARNING OUTCOME 2

Explain how hematopoiesis is regulated.

Concepts for Lecture

1. Hematopoiesis is regulated through messages from hormones. This is important to pharmacology, as some of these hematopoietic growth factors are now available as medications through recombinant DNA technology. These growth factors are used pharmacologically to stimulate production of erythrocytes, leukocytes, and platelets. (See Table 28.1 for a list of hematopoietic growth factors.)
2. **Erythropoietin** is a hormone that stimulates the production of red blood cells when the kidneys sense a reduction in oxygen and the body experiences hemorrhage or hypoxia. Epoetin alpha and darbepoietin alpha are synthetic forms of erythropoietin.

© 2011 Pearson Education, Inc.

LEARNING OUTCOME 3

Explain why hematopoietic agents are often administered to patients following chemotherapy or organ transplant.

Concepts for Lecture

1. The goal of CSF pharmaotherapy is to produce a rapid increase in the number of neutrophils in patients who have suppressed immune systems. CSF therapy shortens the length of time patients are susceptible to life-threatening infections due to low numbers of neutrophils (neutropenia). Indications include patients undergoing chemotherapy or receiving bone marrow or stem cell transplants, or who have certain malignancies. By raising neutrophil counts, CSFs can assist in keeping antineoplastic dosing regimens on schedule (and more effective).

2. Filgrastim (Neupogen) is similar to natural G-CSF and is primarily used for chronic neutropenia or neutropenia secondary to chemotherapy. Pegfilgrastim (Neulasta) is a form of filgrastim bonded to a molecule of polyethylene glycol (PEG). The PEG decreases the renal excretion of the molecule, allowing it to remain in the body with a sustained duration of action. Sargramostim (Leukine) is similar to natural GM-CSF and is used to treat neutropenia in patients treated for acute myelogenous leukemia, and patients who are having autologous bone marrow transplantation.

3. The only hematopoietic growth factor available to enhance platelet production is oprelvekin (Neumega). (Produced through recombinant DNA technology, oprelvekin stimulates the production of megakaryocytes and thrombopoietin. Oprelvekin is functionally equivalent to interleukin-11 (IL-11), a substance secreted by monocytes and lymphocytes that signals cells in the immune system to respond to an infection. Oprelvekin is used to enhance the production of platelets in patients who are at risk for thrombocytopenia caused by cancer chemotherapy.

LEARNING OUTCOME 4

Explain the functions of colony-stimulating factors.

Concepts for Lecture

1. Regulation of white blood cell (WBC) production, or leukopoiesis, is more complicated than erythropoiesis because there are different types of leukocytes in the blood. Pharmacologically, the most important substances controlling production are colony-stimulating factors (CSFs). Also called leukopoietic growth factors, the CSFs comprise a small group of drugs that stimulate the growth and differentiation of one or more types of leukocytes. Doses for these medications are listed in Table 28.1.

2. When the body receives a bacterial challenge the production of CSFs increases rapidly. The CSFs are active at very low concentrations; each stem cell stimulated by these growth factors is capable of producing as many as 1,000 mature leukocytes. The CSFs not only increase the production of *new* leukocytes, but also activate *existing* white blood cells. Examples of enhanced functions include increased migration of leukocytes to the bacteria, increased antibody toxicity, and increased phagocytosis.

3. Colony-stimulating factors are named according to the types of blood cells they stimulate. Granulocytes CSF (G-CSF) increases production of neutrophils. Granulocyte/macrophage CSF (GM-CSF) stimulates production of both neutrophils and macrophages. Research into colony-stimulating factors is an emerging area of pharmacology.

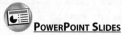

POWERPOINT SLIDES

SUGGESTION FOR CLASSROOM ACTIVITIES

- Invite an oncology nurse to talk to the class about reasons for administering hematopoietic agents to patients following chemotherapy.

SUGGESTION FOR CLINICAL ACTIVITIES

- Assign the student to care for a patient who is receiving a hematopoietic agent. Have the student create a medication card for that drug.

POWERPOINT SLIDES

SUGGESTION FOR CLASSROOM ACTIVITIES

- Assign students to develop concept maps of how blood cells are formed with a correlation to the colony-stimulating factor the blood cells are associated with.

SUGGESTION FOR CLINICAL ACTIVITIES

- Review the clients' charts with students, and look for white-blood-cell counts with differentials. Have them discuss what the results mean for the patients at postclinical conference.

Learning Outcome 5

Classify types of anemia based on their causes.

Concepts for Lecture

1. **Anemia** is a disorder in which blood has a reduced capacity to carry oxygen because of hemorrhage, excessive erythrocyte destruction, or insufficient erythrocyte synthesis. Anemia is a sign, not a distinct disease.

2. Classification of anemia is generally based on a description of the erythrocyte's size and color. Sizes are described as normal (normocytic), small (microcytic), or large (macrocytic). Color is based on the amount of hemoglobin present and is described as normal red (normochromic) or light red (hypochromic). This classification is shown in Table 28.2.

3. Although each type of anemia has specific characteristics, all have common signs and symptoms. If the anemia occurs gradually, the patient may remain asymptomatic, except during periods of physical exercise. As the condition progresses, the patient often exhibits pallor, a paleness of the skin and mucous membranes due to hemoglobin deficiency. Decreased exercise tolerance, fatigue, and lethargy occur because insufficient oxygen reaches muscles. Dizziness and fainting are common as the brain does not receive enough oxygen to function properly. The respiratory and cardiovascular systems compensate for the oxygen depletion by increasing respiration rate and heart rate. Chronic or severe disease can result in heart failure.

4. **Antianemic agents.** Depending on the type of anemia, several vitamins and minerals may be given to enhance the oxygen-carrying capacity of blood. The most common antianemic agents are cyanocobalamin (Crystamine, others), folic acid (Folvite, others), and ferrous sulfate (Feosol, others). These agents are listed in Table 28.3.

Learning Outcome 6

Identify the role of intrinsic factor in the absorption of vitamin B_{12}.

Concepts for Lecture

1. The **intrinsic factor** is a protein secreted by stomach cells. Intrinsic factor is required for vitamin B_{12} to be absorbed from the intestine. Figure 28.2 illustrates the metabolism of vitamin B_{12}. Inflammatory diseases of the stomach or surgical removal of the stomach may result in deficiency of intrinsic factor. Inflammatory diseases of the small intestine that affect food and nutrient absorption may also cause vitamin B_{12} deficiency. Because vitamin B_{12} is found primarily in foods of animal origin, strict vegetarians may require careful meal planning or a vitamin supplement to prevent deficiency.

2. The most profound consequence of vitamin B_{12} deficiency is a condition called **pernicious** or **megaloblastic anemia,** which affects both the hematologic and nervous systems. The hematopoietic stem cells produce abnormally large erythrocytes that do not fully mature. Red blood cells are most affected, though lack of maturation of all blood cell types may occur in severe disease.

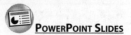

POWERPOINT SLIDES

Table 28.2 Classifications of Anemias
Table 28.3 Antianemic Agents

SUGGESTION FOR CLASSROOM ACTIVITIES

- Direct students to the website at *www.irondisorders.org/,* which is devoted to educating the public about the various iron-related diseases. Assign a paper with parameters based on this website.

SUGGESTION FOR CLINICAL ACTIVITIES

- Assign students to care for a patient with a type of anemia. Ask them to present a case study of that patient at postclinical.

REFERENCE

- Iron Disorders Institute: *www.irondisorders.org*

POWERPOINT SLIDES

Figure 28.2 Metabolism of Vitamin B_{12}
Table 28.3 Vitamins and Minerals

SUGGESTION FOR CLASSROOM ACTIVITIES

- Have the students develop a poster that illustrates the different etiologies of vitamin B_{12} deficiency.

SUGGESTION FOR CLINICAL ACTIVITIES

- Assign students to care for patients with vitamin B_{12} deficiency.

© 2011 Pearson Education, Inc.

3. The symptoms of pernicious anemia are often nonspecific and develop slowly, sometimes over decades. Nervous system symptoms may include memory loss, confusion, unsteadiness, tingling or numbness in the limbs, delusions, mood disturbances, and even hallucinations in severe deficiencies. Permanent nervous system damage may result if the disease remains untreated. Pharmacotherapy includes the administration of cyanocobalamin, a form of vitamin B_{12} (see the prototype drug feature in this chapter).

LEARNING OUTCOME 7

Describe the metabolism, storage, and transfer of iron in the body.

Concepts for Lecture

1. Iron is a mineral essential to the function of several mitochondrial enzymes involved in metabolism and energy production in the cell. Most iron in the body, 60 to 80% is associated with hemoglobin inside erythrocytes. Because free iron is toxic, the body binds the mineral to the protein complexes **ferritin, hemosiderin,** and **transferrin.** Ferritin and hemosiderin maintain iron stores *inside* cells, whereas transferrin *transports* iron to sites in the body where it is needed.
2. After erythrocytes die, nearly all the iron in their hemoglobin is incorporated into transferrin and recycled for later use. Because of this efficient recycling, only about 1 mg of iron is excreted from the body per day, making daily dietary iron requirements in most individuals quite small. Iron balance is maintained by the increased absorption of the mineral from the proximal small intestine during periods of deficiency. Because iron is found in greater quantities in meat products, vegetarians are at higher risk of iron-deficiency anemia.
3. Iron deficiency is the most common cause of anemia. More than 50% of patients diagnosed with iron deficiency anemia have GI bleeding, such as may occur from GI malignancies or chronic peptic ulcer disease. In the United States and Canada, iron deficiency most commonly occurs in women of childbearing age due to blood losses during menses and pregnancy. These conditions may require more than the recommended daily allowance (RDA) of iron (Chapter 42). The most significant effect of iron deficiency is a reduction in erythropoiesis, resulting in symptoms of anemia.

LEARNING OUTCOME 8

Describe the nurse's role in the pharmacologic management of hematopoietic disorders.

Concepts for Lecture

1. The role of the nurse in the pharmacological management of hematopoietic disorders involves careful monitoring of a patient's condition and providing education as it relates to the prescribed drug treatment. Assess the patient's medical, drug, dietary, and lifestyle history. Obtain baseline laboratory tests, especially a CBC, and vital signs. Hematocrit and hemoglobin levels provide a reference for evaluating drug effectiveness.
2. Hematopoietic growth factor therapy: Assess for food or drug allergies, contraindicated in individuals who are hypersensitive to many protein-based products. Assess for hypertension, because the drug can

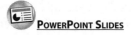
POWERPOINT SLIDES

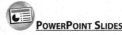
SUGGESTION FOR CLASSROOM ACTIVITIES

- Direct students to develop a concept map of how free iron, ferritin, hemosderin, and transferrin work in the body.

SUGGESTION FOR CLINICAL ACTIVITIES

- Assign the students to care for a patient being treated with iron supplements. Have them note adverse effects in these patients to present during postclinical conference.

POWERPOINT SLIDES

SUGGESTION FOR CLASSROOM ACTIVITIES

- Assign students to small groups, and have each group develop a client-education pamphlet for taking iron.

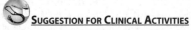
SUGGESTION FOR CLINICAL ACTIVITIES

- During clinical, have students provide patient education for those patients taking iron preparations.

raise blood pressure to dangerous levels. Risk of thromboembolic disease is increased with this drug, especially in those on dialysis, so monitor the patient for early signs of stroke or heart attack. Monitor for side effects such as nausea and vomiting, constipation, medication-site reaction, and headache. Premature infants are sensitive to benzyl alcohol, which may be present in epoetin alpha, so they must be given the preservative-free formulation to prevent "fetal gasping" syndrome. Epoetin alpha should be used with caution in pregnant and lactating patients (pregnancy category C). Patient teaching should include monitoring blood pressure, taking the drug as directed, using the appropriate injection technique, and reporting side effects.

3. Colony-stimulating factors: CSF is contraindicated in those with hypersensitivity to certain foreign proteins (e.g., *Escherichia coli*) or yeast products and a history of leukemia. Do not administer this drug simultaneously with chemotherapy. Obtain a baseline CBC with differential and platelet count to evaluate drug effectiveness. CSF may cause dysrhythmias and tachycardia; therefore, perform a thorough initial and ongoing cardiac assessment. Assess for hypertension and skeletal pain and abnormal ST-segment depression, which are side effects. Use with caution in patients with kidney and liver impairment. A serious side effect of sargramostim is respiratory distress that occurs during the IV infusion the first time the drug is administered. If this occurs, notify the physician and follow protocol related to continuing the infusion. Teach the patient to wash hands, avoid infectious people, and report symptoms of infection or respiratory problems.

4. Platelet Enhancers: Use with caution in patients with cardiac disease. Withhold oprelvekin for 12 hours before or after radiation therapy, because the breakdown of cells after radiation will decrease the effectiveness of the medication. Monitor patients with a history of edema because this drug aggravates fluid retention, and oprelvekin may cause pleural effusion or congestive heart failure. Teach patient to immediately report edema; change in urinary output or body weight; bleeding; and difficulty breathing. The patient should avoid activities that may produce injury.

5. **Antianemic agents**—Vitamin B$_{12}$ and folic acid: assess for causes of anemia, including GI dysfunction, GI surgery, tapeworm infestation, and gluten enteropathy. This drug is not an effective treatment for iron-deficiency anemias. Cyanocobalamin is contraindicated in patients with severe pulmonary disease and is used cautiously in patients with heart disease. Monitor potassium levels during pharmacotherapy because hypokalemia is a possible side effect of this drug. Assess patients for additional side effects, such as itching, rash, or flushing. Patients taking this drug may develop pulmonary edema and heart failure, so cardiovascular status should be monitored. Teaching should include importance of diet, rest, and reporting shortness of breath or edema.

6. Antianemic agents—iron: Iron dextran can be given as an intramuscular (IM) injection or as an IV infusion and is often used for patients who cannot tolerate oral iron preparations. Assess for allergies using a test dose; allergic reactions can be fatal. GI disturbances are common with iron, though they may diminish over time. Stools can become a harmless dark green or black color. Taking oral iron with food reduces GI distress but also greatly reduces absorption. Iron deficiency and iron-deficiency anemia have been identified as significant problems among children from 1 to 2 years of age; supplements should be administered. Accidental overdosing from the taking of products containing iron is one of the leading causes of fatal poisoning in children. It is extremely important that iron be kept out of the reach of children. Pregnant women and those with heavy menstrual flow have an increased demand for iron. Teach patients to take iron with food, use a straw to prevent staining teeth, and report signs of bleeding.

© 2011 Pearson Education, Inc.

LEARNING OUTCOME 9

For each of the drug classes listed in Drugs at a Glance, know representative drugs, and explain their mechanism of drug action, primary actions, and important adverse effects.

Concepts for Lecture

1. Hematopoietic growth factors: The prototype drug is erythropoietin, epoetin alpha (Epogen, Procrit). The mechanism of action involves the hormone (normally secreted by the kidneys), which travels to stem cells in the bone marrow with the message to increase erythrocyte production. The primary use is to treat anemia. Adverse effects include hypertension and seizures.
2. Colony-stimulating factor: The prototype drug is filgrastim (Neupogen). The mechanism of action is to increase neutrophil production and enhance phagocytosis and cytotoxic functions. The primary use is for chemotherapy, organ transplant, and AIDS complications. Adverse effects include bone pain, allergies, and thrombocytopenia.
3. Antianemic agents—vitamin supplement: The prototype drug is cyanocobalamin (Crystamine, vitamin B_{12}, others). The mechanism of action is replacement of vitamin B_{12}. The primary use is treatment of vitamin B_{12} deficiency. Adverse effects include diarrhea, hypokalemia, rash, and anaphylaxis.
4. Antianemic agents—iron supplement: The prototype drug is ferrous sulfate (Feosol, others). The mechanism of action is to supplement the iron needed by the body. Its primary use is treatment of iron deficiency. The adverse effects are nausea, heartburn, constipation, dark stools, cardiovascular collapse, aggravation of peptic ulcers or ulcerative colitis, hepatic necrosis, and anaphylaxis (iron dextran).

LEARNING OUTCOME 10

Use the nursing process to care for patients who are receiving drug therapy for hematopoietic disorders.

Concepts for Lecture

1. Patients receiving epoetin alpha—Assessment: Understand the reason the drug has been prescribed in order to assess for therapeutic effects (e.g., anemia secondary to chronic renal failure, cancer treatment). Obtain a complete health history including cardiovascular (including HTN, MI) and peripheral vascular disease, respiratory (including previous pulmonary embolism), neurologic (including CVA), hepatic, or renal disease. Obtain a drug history including allergies, current prescription and OTC drugs, herbal preparations, and alcohol use. Be alert to possible drug interactions. Obtain baseline. Obtain weight and vital signs, especially blood pressure. Evaluate appropriate laboratory findings (e.g., CBC, aPTT, INR, transferrin and serum ferritin levels, renal and liver function studies). Assess the patient's ability to receive and understand instruction. Assess for therapeutic effects (e.g., Hct, RBC count, significantly improved), patient's activity level and general sense of well-being has improved. Assess for adverse effects: HTN, headache, neurologic changes in level of consciousness or premonitory signs and symptoms of seizure activity (e.g., aura), angina, signs of thrombosis development in peripheral extremities (e.g., leg pain, pale extremity, diminished peripheral pulses).

POWERPOINT SLIDES

Prototype Drug
- erythropoietin, epoetin alpha (Epogen, Procrit)
- filgrastim (Neupogen)
- cyanocobalamin (Crystamine, vitamin B_{12}, others)
- ferrous sulfate (Feosol, others)

ANIMATIONS AND VIDEOS

- Mechanism in Action: Epoetin Alfa (Epogen, Procrit)

SUGGESTION FOR CLASSROOM ACTIVITIES

- Have each student make drug cards for each classification of drug used in hematopoietic therapy. Use two different drugs for each classification. The card should include mechanisms of action, primary actions, and important adverse effects.

SUGGESTION FOR CLINICAL ACTIVITIES

- Assign students to observe nurses taking care of patients receiving chemotherapy for a clinical day. Have the students report on any drugs for hematopoietic disorders the patients were receiving.

POWERPOINT SLIDES

NURSING PROCESS FOCUS

- Patients Receiving Epoetin Alpha
- Patients Receiving Filgrastim (Neupogen)
- Patients Receiving Ferrous Sulfate (Ferralyn)

SUGGESTION FOR CLASSROOM ACTIVITIES

- Divide students into small groups, and have each group develop a teaching plan for a patient receiving hematopoietic therapy.

SUGGESTION FOR CLINICAL ACTIVITIES

- Have students develop care plans for patients who are taking drugs for hematopoietic disorders in the clinical area.

2. Patients receiving epoetin alpha—Nursing diagnoses: *Ineffective Tissue Perfusion* related to underlying disorder, *Activity Intolerance* related to underlying disorder, *Fatigue* related to underlying disorder, *Deficient Knowledge* (drug therapy), *Risk for Injury* related to adverse drug effects.

3. Patients receiving epoetin alpha—Planning: The patient will experience therapeutic effects dependent on the reason the drug is being given (e.g., experience increase in activity level, less fatigue, and shortness of breath on exertion). Be free from or experience minimal adverse effects. Verbalize an understanding of the drug's use, adverse effects and required precautions. Demonstrate proper self-administration of the medication (e.g., dose, timing, when to notify provider).

4. Patients receiving epoetin alpha—Implementation: Monitor for therapeutic effects (RBC count CBC and platelet count). Encourage adequate rest periods and adequate fluid intake. Monitor for adverse effects, especially HTN, peripheral thrombosis, or seizure activity. Encourage adequate dietary intake of iron, folic acid, and vitamin B_{12}. Instruct patient and/or family in proper self-administration techniques followed by return demonstration.

5. Patients receiving epoetin alpha—Evaluation: The patient experiences increase in activity level, less fatigue and shortness of breath on exertion. Is free from or experiences minimal adverse effects. Verbalizes an understanding of the drug's use, adverse effects, and required precautions. Demonstrates proper self-administration of the medication (e.g., dose, timing, when to notify provider).

6. Patients receiving filgrastim (Neupogen)—Assessment: Understand the reason the drug has been prescribed in order to assess for therapeutic effects (e.g., neutropenia, leukopenia, secondary to cancer treatment, HIV, post-bone marrow transplant). Obtain a complete health history including recent or current infections, recent surgeries, injuries or wounds, yeast infections (e.g., thrush), vaccination history, cardiac conditions (e.g., dyrhythmias, CHF), respiratory, renal, and hepatic conditions. Obtain a drug history including allergies, current prescription and OTC drugs, herbal preparations, and alcohol use. Be alert to possible reactions. Obtain complete health history including allergies, drug history, reactions. Obtain baseline weight and vital signs. Assess level of fatigue. Evaluate appropriate findings (e.g., CBC, WBC, or ANC – absolute neutrophil count), renal and liver function studies, uric acid levels, and ECG. Assess patient's ability to receive and understand instruction. Include family and caregiver as needed. Assess for adverse effects: bone pain (especially lower back, posterior iliac crests, and sternum), fever, nausea, anorexia, hyperuricemia, anemia, ST depression on ECG, angina, respiratory distress, and allergic reaction. Continue to assess for infection and fatigue related to drug treatment (e.g., chemotherapy).

7. Patients receiving filgrastim (Neupogen)—Nursing Diagnoses: *Anxiety* related to concerns about seriousness of underlying disorder; insurance/financial concerns; *Fear* related to concerns about seriousness of underlying disorder; insurance/financial concerns; *Activity Intolerance* related to underlying disorder or drug treatment of disorder; *Fatigue* related to underlying disorder or drug treatment of disorder; *Deficient Knowledge* (drug therapy); *Risk for Infection* related to underlying disorder or drug treatment of disorder, *Risk for Impaired Oral Mucus Membranes* related to drug treatment or disorder, *Risk for Caregiver Role Strain* (family and caregivers).

8. Patients receiving filgrastim (Neupogen)—Planning: The patient will experience therapeutic effects dependent on the reason the drug is being given (e.g., experience increase WBC/ANC level, no signs or symptoms of infection). Be free from, or experience minimal adverse effects. Verbalize an understanding of the drug's use, adverse effects

© 2011 Pearson Education, Inc.

and required precautions. Demonstrate proper self-administration of the medication (e.g., dose, timing, when to notify provider).

9. Patients receiving filgrastim (Neupogen)—Implementation: Monitor for therapeutic effects. Encourage adequate rest periods and adequate fluid intake. Monitor for adverse effects: bone pain (especially lower back, posterior iliac crests, and sternum), fever, nausea, anorexia, hyperuricemia, anemia, S-T depression on ECG, angina, respiratory distress, and allergic reaction. Monitor for infection and fatigue related to drug treatment (e.g., chemotherapy). Monitor for hyperuricemia. Maintain meticulous infection control measures. Report any signs and symptoms of infections, especially viral or fungal, or fever immediately. Monitor ECG periodically for ST segment depression or dysrhythmias and report immediately. Monitor for signs of dyspnea or respiratory distress, especially when accompanied by tachycardia and hypotension, and report immediately. Monitor for signs and symptoms of allergic-type reactions. (Patient may be hypersensitive to proteins from *E. coli* used to develop the drug.) Monitor hepatic status during drug administration period. (Filgrastim may cause an elevation in liver enzymes.) Instruct patient and/or family in proper self-administration techniques.

10. Patients receiving filgrastim (Neupogen)—Evaluation: The patient experiences an increase WBC/ANC level, no signs or symptoms of infection). Is free from, or experiences minimal adverse effects. Verbalizes an understanding of the drug's use, adverse effects and required precautions. Demonstrates proper self-administration of the medication (e.g., dose, timing, when to notify provider).

11. Patients receiving ferrous sulfate (Ferralyn)—Assessment: Obtain complete health history, including allergies, drug history, possible drug reactions, history of peptic-ulcer disease, or recent blood loss. Obtain baseline weight and vital signs. Assess fatigue level. Evaluate appropriate laboratory findings (e.g., CBC, electrolytes, transferrin and serum ferritin levels, renal and liver function studies). Assess patient's ability to receive and understand instruction. Assess for adverse effects: itching, skin rash, hypokalemia, nausea, vomiting, heartburn, constipation, black stools (iron preparations), allergic reactions. Assess reason for drug administration, such as presence or history of anemia, or prophylaxis during infancy, childhood, and pregnancy. Assess CBC, specifically hematocrit and hemoglobin levels, to establish baseline values.

12. Patients receiving ferrous sulfate (Ferralyn)—Nursing diagnoses: *Risk for Imbalanced Nutrition* related to inadequate iron intake; *Risk for Impaired Gas Exchange* related to low RBC count, resulting in decreased oxygenation; *Risk for Injury* (weakness, dizziness, syncope) related to anemia; *Knowledge Deficit* related to drug therapy.

13. Patients receiving ferrous sulfate (Ferralyn)—Planning: The patient will experience increase in activity level, less fatigue, and shortness of breath on exertion. Be free from or experience minimal adverse effects. Verbalize an understanding of the drug's use, adverse effects, and required precautions. Demonstrate proper self-administration of the medication (e.g., dose, timing, when to notify provider).

14. Patients receiving ferrous sulfate (Ferralyn)—Implementation: Monitor CBC and changes in stool. Plan activities to allow for periods of rest to help patient conserve energy. Dilute oral liquid iron formulations and administer on an empty stomach through a straw held towards the back of the mouth to avoid staining of teeth. Monitor for adverse effects, including skin rash, hypokalemia, nausea, vomiting, constipation, heartburn, staining of teeth, black stools (iron preparations), and allergic reactions. Plan activities to allow for periods of rest to help patient conserve energy. Instruct patient and/or family in proper self-administration techniques. Keep all vitamins and iron preparations out of the reach of young children. (Iron poisoning may

be fatal in young children.) Monitor patient's dietary intake to ensure adequate fluid and fiber intake.

15. Patients receiving ferrous sulfate (Ferralyn)—Evaluation: The patient experiences increase in activity level, less fatigue and shortness of breath on exertion. Is free from or experiences minimal adverse effects. Verbalizes an understanding of the drug's use, adverse effects, and required precautions. Demonstrates proper self-administration of the medication (e.g., dose, timing, when to notify provider).

GENERAL CHAPTER CONSIDERATIONS

1. Have students study and learn key terms listed at the beginning of the chapter.
2. Have students complete end-of-chapter exercises either in their book or on the MyNursingKit website.
3. Use the Classroom Response Questions provided in PowerPoint to assess students prior to lecture.

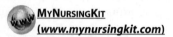 **MYNURSINGKIT**
(www.mynursingkit.com)
- Websites
- NCLEX® questions
- Critical Thinking Questions
- Case Studies
- Animations and Videos
- Drug Prototype Questions

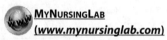 **MYNURSINGLAB**
(www.mynursinglab.com)
- Knowledge Quick Check
- Pre/Posttests
- Customized study plans
- *Separate purchase*

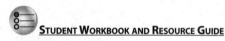 **STUDENT WORKBOOK AND RESOURCE GUIDE**
- Chapter 28 activities
- *Separate purchase*

PEARSON NURSE'S DRUG GUIDE
- *Separate purchase*

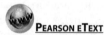 **PEARSON eTEXT**
- Students can search, highlight, take notes, and more all in electronic format.
- *Separate purchase*

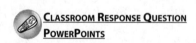 **CLASSROOM RESPONSE QUESTION POWERPOINTS**

 TESTBANK

© 2011 Pearson Education, Inc.

CHAPTER 29
DRUGS FOR SHOCK

LEARNING OUTCOME 1

Compare and contrast the different types of shock.

Concepts for Lecture

1. Shock is a collection of signs and symptoms in which vital tissues and organs are not receiving enough blood to function properly. Without adequate oxygen and other nutrients, cells cannot carry out normal metabolic processes. Shock is a medical emergency; failure to reverse the causes and symptoms of shock may lead to irreversible organ damage and death.
2. Shock is often classified by the underlying pathological process or by the organ system that is primarily affected. Types of shock include anaphylactic, cardiogenic, hypovolemic, neurogenic, and septic.
   a. Anaphylactic shock is an acute allergic reaction caused by a severe reaction to an allergen such as penicillin, nuts, shellfish, or animal proteins.
   b. Cardiogenic results from failure of the heart to pump sufficient blood to tissues caused by left heart failure, myocardial ischemia, MI, dysrhythmias, pulmonary embolism, myocardial or pericardial infection.
   c. Hypovolemic shock is due to loss of blood volume from hemorrhage, burns, excessive diuresis, severe vomiting or diarrhea.
   d. Neurogenic shock occurs when there is vasodilation due to overstimulation of the parasympathetic or understimulation of the sympathetic nervous systems due to trauma to spinal cord or medulla, severe emotional stress or pain, drugs that depress the central nervous system.
   e. Septic shock is a multiple organ dysfunction as a result of pathogenic organisms in the blood; it is often a precursor to acute respiratory distress syndrome and disseminated intravascular coagulation caused by widespread inflammatory response to bacterial, fungal, or parasitic infection. (See Table 29.1 for common of types of shock.)

POWERPOINT SLIDES

Table 29.1 Common Types of Shock

SUGGESTION FOR CLASSROOM ACTIVITIES

- Discuss the common types of shock listed in Table 29.1. Ask students to compare and contrast the types of shock.

SUGGESTION FOR CLINICAL ACTIVITIES

- Assign students to work in the ED, and have them report at postclinical on ED patients who were in a shock state.

LEARNING OUTCOME 2

Relate the general symptoms of shock to their physiologic causes.

Concepts for Lecture

1. Shock is a collection of nonspecific signs and symptoms. Key body systems affected by shock are the nervous, renal, and cardiovascular systems. Some symptoms are specific for certain types of shock, yet many similarities exist. Most types of shock have some symptoms in common: The patient has pale, cold, clammy skin; patient feels sick and weak; the patient exhibits behavioral changes, including restlessness, anxiety, confusion, depression, apathy, and unconsciousness. Thirst is a common complaint. Without immediate treatment, multiple body systems will be affected and respiratory or renal failure may result. (Figure 29.1 shows common symptoms of a patient in shock.)

POWERPOINT SLIDES

Figure 29.1 Symptoms of a Patient in Shock
Figure 29.2 Physiological Changes During Circulatory Shock: Pharmacological Intervention

SUGGESTION FOR CLASSROOM ACTIVITIES

- Have students draw a table of the symptoms of shock related to the physiological causes of shock.

2. The central problem in most types of shock is the inability of the cardiovascular system to send sufficient blood to the vital organs, with the heart and brain being affected early in the progression of the disease. Assessing the patient's cardiovascular status will provide important clues for a diagnosis of shock. Blood pressure is usually low and cardiac output diminished. Heart rate may be rapid with a weak, thready pulse. Breathing is usually rapid and shallow. Figure 29.2 illustrates the physiological changes that occur during circulatory shock.

LEARNING OUTCOME 3

Explain the initial treatment priorities for a patient who is in shock.

Concepts for Lecture

1. Shock is treated as a medical emergency, and the first goal is to provide basic life support. Rapid identification of the underlying cause, followed by aggressive treatment, is essential, because the patient's condition may deteriorate rapidly without specific emergency measures. The initial nursing interventions of maintaining the ABCs of life support—airway, breathing, and circulation—to sustain normal blood pressure are critical. The patient is immediately connected to a cardiac monitor, and a pulse oximeter is applied. More invasive monitoring (e.g., arterial line monitoring of blood pressure and pulse rate) is often required and should be started as soon as feasible. Unless contraindicated, oxygen is administered at 15 L/min via a nonrebreather mask. Neurological status and level of consciousness are carefully monitored. Additional nursing interventions consist of keeping the patient quiet and warm and offering psychological support and reassurance.
2. The remaining therapies for shock depend on the specific cause of the condition. The two primary pharmacotherapeutic goals are to restore normal fluid volume and composition and to maintain adequate blood pressure. For anaphylaxis, an additional goal is to prevent or stop the hypersensitive inflammatory response.

LEARNING OUTCOME 4

Compare and contrast the use of colloids and crystalloids in fluid replacement therapy.

Concepts for Lecture

1. Immediate fluid replacement is essential with significant fluid loss. Causes of fluid loss include hemorrhage, extensive burns, severe dehydration, persistent vomiting or diarrhea, and intensive diuretic therapy.
2. During hypovolemic shock, three categories of fluid-replacement agents are used: blood, colloids, and crystalloids.
3. Whole blood may be indicated in cases of massive hemorrhage when 30% or more of the total body blood volume is lost. The supply depends on donors; using it safely requires careful cross-matching; and infections such as hepatitis or HIV can be transmitted.
4. Colloids expand plasma volume and maintain blood pressure. These agents are administered to provide life-sustaining support following massive hemorrhage and to treat shock, as well as to treat burns, acute liver failure, and neonatal hemolytic disease. Colloids stay suspended

SUGGESTION FOR CLINICAL ACTIVITIES
• In the clinical area, have students access the standardized care plans for patients in shock. Discuss the care of a patient in shock at postclinical.

POWERPOINT SLIDES

SUGGESTION FOR CLASSROOM ACTIVITIES
• Invite an emergency-department nurse to speak to the students about shock and its treatment.

SUGGESTION FOR CLINICAL ACTIVITIES
• In the clinical area, create a mock drill for a patient that presents with shock. Have students role-play different responder roles. Use an empty room or ED area to stage the drill. Invite hospital personnel to participate.

POWERPOINT SLIDES

SUGGESTION FOR CLASSROOM ACTIVITIES
• Create a *Jeopardy*-type game using the types of IV solutions to identify as a crystalloid or colloid, types of shock, and physiology of shock. Divide students into teams, and play the game.

SUGGESTION FOR CLINICAL ACTIVITIES
• Visit areas of the hospital where IV solutions and blood products are stored. Have the students identify each as a colloid or crystalloid.

© 2011 Pearson Education, Inc.

in blood; they draw molecules from the body's cells and tissues into the blood vessels—this is called oncotic pressure. Examples of colloid fluids are normal human serum albumin, plasma protein fraction, dextran, and hetastarch (Hespan).

5. Crystalloids are IV solutions that contain electrolytes in concentrations resembling those of plasma. They are used to replace fluids that have been lost and to promote urine output. Examples of crystalloids are normal saline, lactated Ringer's, Plasmalyte, and hypertonic saline. Additional information on the role of crystalloids and colloids in correcting fluid balance disorders is included in Chapter 31.

LEARNING OUTCOME 5

List the drugs used in the pharmacotherapy of anaphylaxis, and discuss their indications.

Concepts for Lecture

1. Anaphylaxis is a potentially fatal condition in which body defenses produce a hyper-response to a foreign substance known as an *antigen* or *allergen.* During anaphylaxis, the body responds quickly, often just minutes after exposure to the allergen, by releasing massive amounts of histamine and other mediators of the inflammatory response. Antibiotics, especially penicillins, cephalosporins, and sulfonamides NSAIDs, such as aspirin, ibuprofen, and naproxen ACE inhibitors. Opioid analgesics and iodine-based contrast media used for radiographic exams may cause anaphylaxis.

2. The patient may experience itching, hives, and a tightness in the throat or chest. Swelling occurs around the larynx, causing a nonproductive cough and the voice to become hoarse. As anaphylaxis progresses, the patient experiences a rapid fall in blood pressure and difficulty breathing due to bronchoconstriction. The hypotension causes reflex tachycardia. Without medical intervention, anaphylaxis leads to a profound state of shock, which is often fatal. Figure 29.3 illustrates the symptoms of anaphylaxis.

3. Anaphylaxis is treated with a large number of different drugs, including sympathomimetics, antihistamines, and glucocorticoids. Therapy is symptomatic, in an effort to support the cardiovascular system and prevent further hyperreaction of the immune system. Drug therapy includes: giving oxygen immediately; administering antihistamines to prevent release of histamine; administering bronchodilators to relieve shortness of breath; and administering corticosteroids to suppress inflammation.

LEARNING OUTCOME 6

For each of the classes shown in Drugs at a Glance, know representative drug examples, and explain their mechanism of action, primary actions, and important adverse effects.

Concepts for Lecture

1. Fluid-replacement agent/colloid—prototype drug: normal serum albumin (Albuminar, Albutein). The mechanism of action for colloid agents is to maintain plasma osmotic pressure and transport substances through the blood. Its primary use is restoration of plasma volume and blood proteins. Adverse effects include allergies and protein overload.

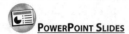 **POWERPOINT SLIDES**

Figure 29.3 Symptoms of Anaphylaxis

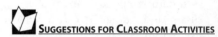 **SUGGESTIONS FOR CLASSROOM ACTIVITIES**

- Ask students to share experiences of observing a severe allergic response. Discuss the effects of histamine on the cardiovascular and respiratory systems.

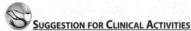 **SUGGESTION FOR CLINICAL ACTIVITIES**

- Have students prepare drug cards for the most commonly used antihistamine, corticosteroid, and bronchodilator used at the clinical facility to treat anaphylaxis. Ask them to bring the cards to postclinical, and discuss specific intravenous dosages.

 POWERPOINT SLIDES

Prototype Drug
- normal serum albumin (Albuminar, Albutein)
- norepinephrine (Levaterenol, Levophed)
- dopamine (Dopastat, Inotropin)
- epinephrine (Adrenalin)

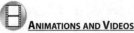 **ANIMATIONS AND VIDEOS**

- Mechanism in Action: Dopamine (Dopastat)
- Mechanism in Action: Epinephrine (Adrenalin)

2. Vasoconstrictors/sympathomimetics—prototype drug: norepinephrine (Levaterenol, Levophed). Vasoconstrictors/sympathomimetics are critical-care drugs sometimes needed during severe shock to maintain blood pressure. These drugs strongly activate alpha-adrenergic receptors in arterioles. The mechanism of action is to act directly on alpha-adrenergic receptors to raise blood pressure; they also have positive inotropic effects. The primary use is to treat acute shock and cardiac arrest. Adverse effects include tachycardia, bradycardia, and hypertension.

3. Inotropic agents—prototype drug: dopamine (Dopastat, Inotropin). Inotropic agents are useful in reversing the decreased cardiac output resulting from shock by increasing the strength of myocardial contraction. Their mechanism of action is dose dependent: Low doses have a dopaminergic effect; high doses have a beta-adrenergic effect. Their primary use is in the treatment of hypervolemic and cardiogenic shock. Adverse effects include dysrhythmias, hypertension, and gangrene.

4. Sympathomimetic/anaphylaxis—prototype drug: epinephrine (Adrenalin). The mechanism of action is as a nonselective adrenergic agonist (sympathomimetic). The primary use is treatment of anaphylaxis, shock, and cardiac arrest. Adverse effects include hypertension and dysrhythmias.

LEARNING OUTCOME 7

Use the steps of the nursing process to care for patients who are receiving drug therapy for shock.

Concepts for Lecture

1. **Patients receiving IV replacement therapy for shock— Assessment:** Prior to administration, obtain a complete health history, including allergies, drug history, and possible drug interactions. Obtain baseline weight and vital signs, level of consciousness, breath sounds, urinary and cardiac output. Evaluate appropriate laboratory findings (e.g., Hgb and Hct, WBC count, electrolytes, arterial blood gases, total protein and albumin levels, aPTT, aPT or INR, blood cultures, renal and liver function studies). Assess the patient's ability to receive and understand instruction. Assess for and promptly report adverse effects: tachycardia, hypertension, dysrhythmias, decreasing level of consciousness, increasing dyspnea, lung congestion, pink-tinged frothy sputum, decreased urinary output, allergic reactions.

2. **Patients receiving IV replacement therapy for shock—Nursing diagnoses:** *Decreased Cardiac Output* (cardiovascular); *Ineffective Tissue Perfusion* (cardiopulmonary, septic shock); *Impaired Gas Exchange* (cardiopulmonary); *Ineffective Airway Clearance* (anaphylaxis); *Deficient Fluid Volume* (volume loss, third-spacing); *Anxiety* or *Fear* related to concerns about severity of condition; *Deficient Knowledge* (drug therapy); *Risk for Injury* related to adverse effects of drug therapy or administration; *Risk for Excessive Fluid Volume* related to drug therapy.

3. **Patients receiving IV replacement therapy for shock—Planning:** The patient will experience therapeutic effects dependent on the reason the drug is being given (e.g., improved blood pressure, cardiac and urine output within normal limits). Be free from or experience minimal adverse effects. Verbalize an understanding of the drug's use, adverse effects, and required precautions.

4. **Patients receiving IV replacement therapy for shock— Implementation:** Continue frequent assessments as above for therapeutic effects dependent on the reason the drug therapy is given. Pulse, blood pressure, and respiratory rate should be within normal limits or

SUGGESTION FOR CLASSROOM ACTIVITIES

- Have each student make drug cards for each classification of drug used in treatment of shock. Use two different drugs for each classification. The card should include mechanisms of action, primary actions, and important adverse effects.

SUGGESTION FOR CLINICAL ACTIVITIES

- During a clinical rotation, assign the students to an intensive care unit with directions to observe the care of a patient with septic shock.

POWERPOINT SLIDES

SUGGESTION FOR CLASSROOM ACTIVITIES

- Divide students into small groups, and have each group develop a teaching plan for a patient receiving fluid-replacement therapy.

© 2011 Pearson Education, Inc.

within parameters set by health care provider, ABGs, and/or pulse oximetry. Provide supportive nursing measures (e.g., moistening lips if patient is intubated, explanations for all procedures, frequent orientation). Monitor for signs of fluid volume excess (e.g., increasing BP, hypertension, tachycardia, bounding pulse, confusion, decreasing level of consciousness), and notify health care provider if blood pressure or pulse is abnormal. Continue frequent cardiac monitoring (e.g., ECG, cardiac output, and urine output). Frequently monitor CBC, electrolyte, aPTT, aPT, or INR levels. Monitor respiratory status. Weigh patient daily and report weight gain or loss of 1 kg (approximately 2 lbs) or more in a 24 hour period. Closely monitor for signs and symptoms of allergy if colloids are used.

5. **Patients receiving IV replacement therapy for shock—Evaluation:** The patient experiences therapeutic effects dependent on the reason the drug is being given (e.g., improved blood pressure, cardiac and urine output within normal limits). The patient is free from or experiences minimal adverse effects and verbalizes an understanding of the drug's use, adverse effects, and required precautions.

GENERAL CHAPTER CONSIDERATIONS

1. Have students study and learn key terms listed at the beginning of the chapter.
2. Have students complete end-of-chapter exercises either in their book or on the MyNursingKit website.
3. Use the Classroom Response Questions provided in PowerPoint to assess students prior to lecture.

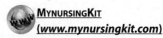
MyNursingKit
(www.mynursingkit.com)
- Websites
- NCLEX® questions
- Critical Thinking Questions
- Case Studies
- Animations and Videos
- Drug Prototype Questions

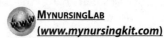
MyNursingLab
(www.mynursingkit.com)
- Knowledge Quick Check
- Pre/Posttests
- Customized study plans
- *Separate purchase*

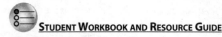
STUDENT WORKBOOK AND RESOURCE GUIDE
- Chapter 29 activities
- *Separate purchase*

PEARSON NURSE'S DRUG GUIDE
- *Separate purchase*

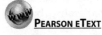
PEARSON eTEXT
- Students can search, highlight, take notes, and more all in electronic format.
- *Separate purchase*

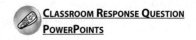
CLASSROOM RESPONSE QUESTION POWERPOINTS

TESTBANK

© 2011 Pearson Education, Inc.

CHAPTER 30
DIURETIC THERAPY AND DRUGS FOR RENAL FAILURE

LEARNING OUTCOME 1

Explain the role of the kidneys in maintaining fluid, electrolyte, and acid–base balance.

Concepts for Lecture

1. The kidneys are the primary organs for regulating fluid balance, electrolyte composition, and acid–base balance of body fluids. They also secrete the enzyme renin, which helps regulate blood pressure and erythropoietin, a hormone that stimulates red blood cell production. In addition, the kidneys are responsible for the production of calcitriol, the active form of vitamin D, which helps maintain bone homeostasis.
2. The urinary system consists of two kidneys, two ureters, one bladder, and a urethra. The functional unit of the kidney is the nephron.

LEARNING OUTCOME 2

Explain the processes that change the composition of filtrate as it travels through the nephron.

Concepts for Lecture

1. The nephron is the functional unit of the kidney. Blood enters a nephron and is filtered through Bowman's capsule. The fluid is called filtrate. Water and small molecules pass into the proximal tubule. Filtrate passes through the loop of Henle, then the distal tubule. Filtrate empties into collecting ducts and leaves the nephron as urine. The three major processes of urine formation are filtration, reabsorption, and secretion. As filtrate travels through the nephron, its composition changes dramatically as a result of the processes of reabsorption and secretion.
2. Reabsorption: Filtrate in Bowman's capsule is the same composition as plasma minus large proteins. Some substances in the filtrate cross the wall of the nephron and reenter the blood. Most of the water in the filtrate is reabsorbed. Glucose, amino acids, sodium, chloride, calcium, and bicarbonate are reabsorbed.
3. Secretion: Some substances pass from the blood through the walls of the nephron and become part of the filtrate. Potassium, phosphate, hydrogen, ammonium ion, and some acid drugs are secreted into the filtrate. Reabsorption and secretion are critical to the pharmacokinetics of many drugs.
4. Nephron structure and function: see Figure 30.1.

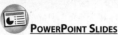

POWERPOINT SLIDES

SUGGESTION FOR CLASSROOM ACTIVITIES

- Direct students to draw a concept map of the functions of the kidney.

SUGGESTION FOR CLINICAL ACTIVITIES

- In the clinical area the students will complete an assessment of the urinary system and include an analysis of intake and output for the past 24 hours.

POWERPOINT SLIDES

Figure 30.1 The Nephron

SUGGESTION FOR CLASSROOM ACTIVITIES

- Direct students to draw a diagram of the renal system illustrating the processes of filtration, reabsorption, and secretion as they occur in the nephron.

SUGGESTION FOR CLINICAL ACTIVITIES

- In the clinical area the student will review the urinalysis, blood urea nitrogen, and creatinine levels for the patients assigned. Each student will present an analysis of those results including normal levels, possible reasons for abnormalities, and implications for nursing care.

© 2011 Pearson Education, Inc.

LEARNING OUTCOME 3

Describe the adjustments in pharmacotherapy that must be considered for patients with renal failure.

Concepts for Lecture

1. Renal failure is a decrease in the ability of the kidneys to function. Drugs can accumulate to high levels in the body. The dosage levels for most medication dosages need to be adjusted. Administering the average dose to a person in renal failure can be fatal.
2. The diagnosis of renal failure is made by analyzing the following diagnostic studies: urinalysis, serum creatinine, diagnostic imaging, renal biopsy, and glomerular filtration rate (GFR). Glomerular filtration rate is the best marker for estimating renal function; it measures the volume of water filtered per minute.
3. Renal failure is classified as acute or chronic, depending on its onset. Acute renal failure requires immediate treatment. The accumulation of waste products can be fatal. The most common cause of acute renal failure is hypoperfusion. The cause must be rapidly identified; some of the usual causes are heart failure, dysrhythmias, hemorrhage, and dehydration.
4. Chronic renal failure occurs over months or years. The patient usually has a history of diabetes mellitus or hypertension. Chronic renal failure may be undiagnosed for a long time. Nephrotoxic drugs can cause acute or chronic renal failure. (See Table 30.1 for a list of nephrotoxic drugs.)
5. Pharmacotherapy for renal failure attempts to cure the cause of the dysfunction. Diuretics are used to increase urine output. Cardiovascular drugs treat hypertension or heart failure associated with renal failure. (See Table 30.2 for the pharmacologic treatment of renal failure.) Dietary management includes restriction of protein and reduction of sodium, potassium, phosphorous, and magnesium.

LEARNING OUTCOME 4

Identify indications for diuretics.

Concepts for Lecture

1. Diuretics are drugs that alter the volume and/or composition of body fluids. They are indicated for the treatment of HTN, heart failure, and disorders characterized by accumulation of edema fluid.
2. Diuretics increase the rate of urine flow. Excretion of excess fluid is used to treat hypertension, heart failure, kidney failure, liver failure or cirrhosis, and pulmonary edema.

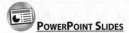
POWERPOINT SLIDES

Table 30.1 Nephrotoxic Drugs
Table 30.2 Pharmacological Management of Renal Failure

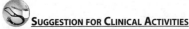
SUGGESTION FOR CLASSROOM ACTIVITIES

- Have students compare and contrast the etiology and treatment of acute and chronic renal failure.

SUGGESTION FOR CLINICAL ACTIVITIES

- In the clinical area, direct students to the standardized care plans for renal failure. Are there separate care plans for acute and chronic renal failure? Discuss the care plans in postclinical.

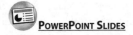
POWERPOINT SLIDES

SUGGESTION FOR CLASSROOM ACTIVITIES

- Have students make concept maps that show the relationship between diuretics and the physiological reasons they are administered.

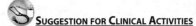
SUGGESTION FOR CLINICAL ACTIVITIES

- Assign students to care for patients who are taking diuretics.

LEARNING OUTCOME 5

Describe the general adverse effects of diuretic pharmacotherapy.

Concepts for Lecture

Pharmacotherapy with diuretics can cause fluid and electrolyte disturbances. Some of the side effects are dehydration, orthostatic hypotension, and imbalances of sodium and potassium.

LEARNING OUTCOME 6

Compare and contrast the loop, thiazide, and potassium-sparing diuretics.

Concepts for Lecture

1. Loop diuretics:The most effective diuretics are called *loop* or *high-ceiling* diuretics. Drugs in this class act by blocking the reabsorption of sodium and chloride in the loop of Henle. When given intravenously, they have the ability to cause large amounts of fluid to be excreted by the kidney in a very short time. Loop diuretics are used to reduce the edema associated with heart failure, hepatic cirrhosis, and chronic renal failure. Furosemide and torsemide are also approved for hypertension. (The loop diuretics are shown in Table 30.3.)
2. Thiazide diuretics:The thiazides comprise the largest, most commonly prescribed class of diuretics. These drugs act on the distal tubule to block Na^+ reabsorption and to increase potassium and water excretion. Their primary use is for the treatment of mild to moderate hypertension; however, they are also indicated for edema due to mild to moderate heart failure, liver failure, and renal failure. They are less efficacious than the loop diuretics and are not effective in patients with severe renal failure. (The thiazide diuretics are shown in Table 30.4.)
3. Potassium-sparing diuretics:Hypokalemia is one of the most serious adverse effects of the thiazide and loop diuretics. The therapeutic advantage of the potassium-sparing diuretics is that increased diuresis can be obtained without affecting blood potassium levels. This group of diuretics works in one of two ways, either by blocking sodium or by blocking aldosterone. (The potassium-sparing diuretics are shown in Table 30.5.)
4. Miscellaneous diuretics:A few diuretics (shown in Table 30.6) cannot be classified as loop, thiazide, or potassium-sparing agents. These diuretics have limited and specific indications. Three of these drugs inhibit carbonic anhydrase, an enzyme that affects acid–base balance by its ability to form carbonic acid from water and carbon dioxide. The osmotic diuretics include the drug mannitol. It is used to maintain urine flow in patients with acute renal failure or during prolonged surgery.

POWERPOINT SLIDES

SUGGESTION FOR CLASSROOM ACTIVITIES

- Direct students to the American Dietetics Association website at *www.eatright.org*. Have them list foods high in sodium and potassium.

SUGGESTION FOR CLINICAL ACTIVITIES

- Have students view charts of patients who have sodium and potassium laboratory results. What are the normals? What do abnormals indicate? What nursing implications arise with the abnormal laboratory results?

POWERPOINT SLIDES

SUGGESTION FOR CLASSROOM ACTIVITIES

- Divide the students into small groups, and have them prepare questions and answers for different categories of drugs used to treat renal failure. Include questions on each drug's classification and mechanisms of action for each type of disease.

SUGGESTION FOR CLINICAL ACTIVITIES

- Assign students to care for patients receiving diuretic therapy.

POWERPOINT SLIDES

Figure 30.1 The Nephron
Table 30.3 Loop Diuretics
Table 30.4 Thiazide and Thiazide-like Diuretics
Table 30.5 Potassium-sparing Diuretics
Table 30.6 Miscellaneous Diuretics

SUGGESTION FOR CLASSROOM ACTIVITIES

- Direct students to diagram the sites of diuretic action along the nephron.

SUGGESTION FOR CLINICAL ACTIVITIES

- Direct each student to present information on the diuretics their patients received during the clinical. Include an assessment of any possible or any actual side effects noted.

© 2011 Pearson Education, Inc.

LEARNING OUTCOME 7

Describe the nurse's role in the pharmacologic management of renal failure and in diuretic therapy.

Concepts for Lecture

1. The role of the nurse in the pharmacological management of renal failure and in diuretic therapy involves careful monitoring of a patient's condition and providing education as it relates to the prescribed drug treatment. The nurse obtains a medical, drug, dietary, and lifestyle history from each patient. Assessment of weight, intake and output, skin turgor and moisture, vital signs (check blood pressure lying, sitting, and standing), breath sounds, and the presence of edema will indicate the effectiveness of the diuretic.

2. **Loop (high-ceiling) diuretics:** Obtain baseline, and monitor periodically during drug therapy the patient's lab values, weight, and current level of urine output. It is critical to measure the patient's electrolytes, especially potassium, sodium, and chloride, prior to loop diuretic therapy. Monitor the patient's blood urea nitrogen (BUN), serum creatinine, uric acid, and blood-glucose levels. Assess for adverse effects such as circulatory collapse (due to loss of fluid), dysrhythmias, hearing loss, renal failure, and anemia. Orthostatic hypotension, hypokalemia, hyponatremia, and polyuria are additional common side effects. Observe for a rash or pruritis, which can indicate hypersensitivity to loop diuretics. Teach patients to take diuretics in the morning, change positions slowly, and to monitor weight. Patients should take potassium supplements, if ordered, and consume potassium-rich foods.

3. **Thiazide and thiazide-like diuretics:** Obtain baseline, and monitor periodically during drug therapy the patient's lab values, weight, and current level of urine output. It is critical to measure the patient's electrolytes, especially potassium, sodium, and chloride, prior to loop-diuretic therapy. Monitor the patient's blood urea nitrogen (BUN), serum creatinine, uric acid, and blood-glucose levels. Increased potassium loss may occur when used with digoxin. Patients taking lithium have an increased risk of toxicity when taking thiazide diuretics. Hypersensitivity reactions may occur more frequently in patients who are allergic to sulfa-based medications. These reactions often present as rashes. Use with caution in pregnant women. Do not administer thiazide diuretics to lactating women. Teach patients to use sunscreen to decrease photosensitivity. Patients should take potassium supplements, if ordered, and consume potassium-rich foods, report any tenderness or pain in joints, which may indicate gout.

4. **Potassium-sparing diuretics:** The advantage of these medications is that the patient will not experience hypokalemia. It is critical to assess electrolytes, especially potassium and sodium levels, prior to administering potassium-sparing diuretics. Monitor the patient's BUN and serum creatinine. Be alert for adverse effects that may include hyperkalemia and GI bleeding, confusion, dizziness, muscle weakness, blurred vision, impotence, amenorrhea, or gynecomastia. Spironolactone may also decrease the effectiveness of anticoagulants. Patients taking digoxin or lithium may be at increased risk for toxicity when taking potassium-sparing diuretics. Do not use triamterene in lactating women. Teach patients to immediately report signs and symptoms of hyperkalemia, such as irritability, anxiety, abdominal cramping, or irregular heartbeat. Avoid use of potassium-based salt substitutes. When in direct sunlight, use sunscreen to decrease photosensitivity. Avoid performing tasks that require mental alertness until the effects of the medication are known. Do not eat excess amounts of foods high in potassium.

POWERPOINT SLIDES

SUGGESTION FOR CLASSROOM ACTIVITIES

- Invite a nurse from the dialysis unit to talk to the students about renal failure, pharmacological therapies with the patient in renal failure, and the dialysis process. Direct students to search the following website to prepare for the guest lecture: *www.nephrologychannel.com*.

SUGGESTION FOR CLINICAL ACTIVITIES

- Assign students to observe in the renal dialysis unit. Have them interview the patients and ask about the types of diuretics they have used.

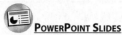
REFERENCE

- *www.nephrologychannel.com*

LEARNING OUTCOME 8

For each of the classes shown in Drugs at a Glance, know representative drugs, and explain the mechanism of drug action, primary actions, and important adverse effects.

Concepts for Lecture

1. The most efficacious diuretics are the loop or high-ceiling agents. The mechanism of action is to block the reabsorption of sodium in the loop of Henle. Prototype drug: furesomide (Lasix); increases urine output even when blood flow to kidney is diminished. Mechanism of action: to block reabsorption of sodium in loop of Henle. Primary use: to treat hypertension and reduce edema associated with heart failure, hepatic cirrhosis, and renal failure. Adverse effects are rapid excretion of large amounts of water dehydration, electrolyte imbalances, and ototoxicity. Other examples: Torsemide, which has a longer half-life than furosemide and offers the advantage of once-a-day dosing; and bumetanide (Bumex), which is 40 times more potent than furosemide but has a shorter duration of action. Loop diuretics are shown in Table 30.3.

2. The thiazides act by blocking sodium absorption in the distal tubule of the nephron and are the most widely prescribed class of diuretics. The prototype drug in this class is chlorothiazide (Diuril). The most common indication for chlorothiazide is mild to moderate hypertension or in combination with other antihypertensives for severe hypertension. It is also used to treat fluid retention due to heart failure, liver disease, and corticosteroid or estrogen therapy. When given orally, it may take as long as four weeks to obtain the *optimum* therapeutic effect. Adverse effects are dehydration, orthostatic hypotension, and hypokalemia.

3. Though less effective than the loop diuretics, potassium-sparing diuretics are used in combination with other agents; they help prevent hypokalemia. The prototype drug is spironolactone (Aldactone). The mechanism of action is to block the action of aldosterone. The primary use is to significantly reduce mortality in heart failure. The major adverse effect is hyperkalemia.

4. Several less commonly prescribed classes, such as the osmotic diuretics and the carbonic anhydrase inhibitors, have specific indications. Carbonic anhydrase inhibitors such as acetazolamide (Diamox) inhibit formation of carbonic acid. The primary use is to decrease intraocular fluid pressure in patients with glaucoma. Adverse effects can be allergic reactions, as these drugs contain sulfa, and fluid and electrolyte imbalances.

5. Osmotic diuretics such as mannitol quickly reduce plasma volume. They are used to reduce intracranial pressure due to cerebral edema and to maintain urine flow in prolonged surgery, acute renal failure, or severe renal hypoperfusion. Adverse effects include headache, dizziness, tremors, dry mouth, fluid and electrolyte imbalances, and thrombophlebitis.

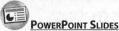

POWERPOINT SLIDES

Prototype Drug
- furosemide (Lasix)
- chlorothiazide (Diuril)
- spironolactone (Aldactone)

ANIMATIONS AND VIDEOS

- Mechanism in Action: Spironolactone (Aldactone)

SUGGESTION FOR CLASSROOM ACTIVITIES

- Divide students into four small groups to represent the four classes of diuretics. Have each group develop a game to use with their classmates to assist in memorizing, comparing, and contrasting the different classifications and side effects.

SUGGESTION FOR CLINICAL ACTIVITIES

- Direct students to access the National Kidney and Urologic Diseases Information Clearinghouse (NKUDIC) at *kidney.niddk .nih.gov/ index.htm* and search for client-education pamphlets. Ask them to use these pamphlets as needed when they are doing patient education.

REFERENCE

- National Kidney and Urologic Diseases Information Clearinghouse (NKUDIC): *kidney.niddk.nih.gov/index.htm*

© 2011 Pearson Education, Inc.

LEARNING OUTCOME 9

Use the nursing process to care for patiients who are receiving drug therapy for renal failure and diuretic therapy.

Concepts for Lecture

1. **Patients receiving drug therapy for renal failure and diuretic therapy—Assessment:** Obtain a complete health history (cardiovascular disease, diabetes, pregnancy, or breast-feeding), including data on recent surgeries or trauma. Obtain patient's medication history, including nicotine and alcohol consumption and use of herbal supplements or alternative therapies to determine possible drug allergies and/or interactions. Obtain dietary and lifestyle history. Evaluate appropriate laboratory findings such as electrolytes, glucose, CBC, hepatic or renal function studies, uric acid levels, and lipid profiles. Obtain baseline weight, vital signs (especially BP and pulse), breath sounds, and cardiac monitoring (e.g., ECG, cardiac output). Assess for location and character/amount of edema. Assess baseline hearing and balance. Assess patient's ability to receive and understand instruction. Assess for and promptly report adverse effects: hypotension, palpitations, dizziness or lightheadedness, musculoskeletal weakness or cramping, nausea, vomiting, abdominal cramping, diarrhea, headache.

2. **Patients receiving drug therapy for renal failure and diuretic therapy—Nursing diagnoses:** *Deficient Fluid Volume* related to adverse effects of diuretics; *Fatigue; Decreased Cardiac Output* related to adverse effects of diuretics; *Deficient Knowledge* (drug therapy); *Risk for Falls; Risk for Injury* related to hypotension, dizziness associated with adverse effects; *Risk for Functional Incontinence* related to diuretic use; *Risk for Noncompliance* related to adverse effects of drug therapy.

3. **Patients receiving drug therapy for renal failure and diuretic therapy—Planning:** The patient will experience a decrease in blood pressure. Be free from or experience minimal adverse effects. Verbalize an understanding of the drug's use, adverse effects and required precautions. Demonstrate proper self-administration of the medication (e.g., dose, timing, when to notify provider).

4. **Patients receiving drug therapy for renal failure and diuretic therapy—Implementation:** Continue frequent assessments above for therapeutic effects blood pressure and pulse. Continue to monitor vital signs. Take blood pressure lying, sitting, and standing to detect orthostatic hypotension. Continue to monitor electrolytes, glucose, CBC, lipid profiles, liver function studies, creatinine, and uric acid levels. Continue to monitor hearing and balance, reporting persistent tinnitus or vertigo promptly. Ensure patient safety, especially in the elderly. Observe for lightheadedness or dizziness. Weigh patient daily and report weight gain or loss of 1 kg or more in a 24 hour period. Measure intake and output. Monitor nutritional status and encourage appropriate intake to prevent electrolyte imbalances. Observe for signs of hypokalemia or hyperkalemia. Use with caution in patients taking corticosteroids, ACE inhibitors, angiotensin-receptor blockers (ARBs), digoxin, or lithium. Observe for signs of hyperglycemia. Use with caution in patients with diabetes. Observe for symptoms of gout. Observe for sunburning if prolonged sun exposure. Observe for signs of infection. Instruct patient and/or family in proper self-administration of drug.

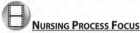

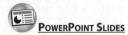

POWERPOINT SLIDES

NURSING PROCESS FOCUS
- Care for patients who are receiving drug therapy for renal failure

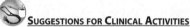

SUGGESTION FOR CLASSROOM ACTIVITIES
- Divide students into small groups and have each group develop a teaching plan for a patient receiving diuretic therapy.

SUGGESTIONS FOR CLINICAL ACTIVITIES
- Assign students to present a diuretic teaching session to a patient receiving diuretic therapy during clinical.
- Have the student report on the teaching session during postclinical conference.

5. Patients receiving drug therapy for renal failure and diuretic therapy—Evaluation: The patient experiences a decrease in blood pressure. Is free from or experiences minimal adverse effects. Verbalizes an understanding of the drug's use, adverse effects, and required precautions. Demonstrates proper self-administration of the medication (e.g., dose, timing, when to notify provider).

GENERAL CHAPTER CONSIDERATIONS

1. Have students study and learn key terms listed at the beginning of the chapter.
2. Have students complete end-of-chapter exercises either in their book or on the MyNursingKit website.
3. Use the Classroom Response Questions provided in PowerPoint to assess students prior to lecture.

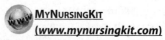

MYNURSINGKIT (*www.mynursingkit.com*)

- Websites
- NCLEX® questions
- Critical Thinking Questions
- Case Studies
- Animations and Videos
- Drug Prototype Questions

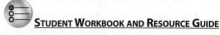

MYNURSINGLAB (*www.mynursingkit.com*)

- Knowledge Quick Check
- Pre/Posttests
- Customized study plans
- *Separate purchase*

STUDENT WORKBOOK AND RESOURCE GUIDE

- Chapter 30 activities
- *Separate purchase*

PEARSON NURSE'S DRUG GUIDE

- *Separate purchase*

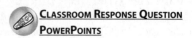

PEARSON eTEXT

- Students can search, highlight, take notes, and more all in electronic format.
- *Separate purchase*

CLASSROOM RESPONSE QUESTION POWERPOINTS

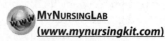

TESTBANK

© 2011 Pearson Education, Inc.

CHAPTER 31
DRUGS FOR FLUID BALANCE, ELECTROLYTE, AND ACID–BASE DISORDERS

LEARNING OUTCOME 1

Describe conditions for which IV fluid therapy may be indicated.

Concepts for Lecture

1. There is a continuous exchange of fluids across membranes separating the intracellular and extracellular fluid compartments. Large molecules and those that are ionized are less able to cross membranes.
2. The volume and composition of fluids in the body must be maintained within narrow limits. Excess fluid volume can lead to hypertension, congestive heart failure, or peripheral edema, whereas depletion results in dehydration and perhaps shock. Body fluids must also contain specific amounts of essential ions or electrolytes, and be maintained at particular pH values. Accumulation of excess acids or bases can change the pH of body fluids and rapidly result in death if left untreated. Control of water balance in the compartments is essential to homeostasis. Imbalances of body fluid, electrolytes, and acid–base are frequent indications for IV therapy.

LEARNING OUTCOME 2

Explain how changes in the osmolality or tonicity of a fluid can cause water to move to a different compartment.

Concepts for Lecture

1. Osmolality is the concentration of an osmotic solution and is dependent on the number of dissolved solutes (usually sodium, glucose, or urea) in a body fluid. Normal osmolality is 275–295 mOsm/kg. Changes in the osmolality of body fluids can cause water to move to different compartments. The greatest contributor to osmolality is sodium, which is controlled by the hormone aldosterone. Tonicity describes the ability of a solution to cause a change in water movement across a membrane due to osmotic forces. It is a general term, not a precise measurement.
2. Osmosis means water moves from areas of low osmolality to areas of high osmolality. When a patient is given hypertonic intravenous fluid, the water moves from the interstitial space to plasma. Hypotonic intravenous fluid causes water to move from plasma to the interstitial space. Isotonic intravenous fluid does not cause a fluid shift.
3. Overall fluid balance is achieved through complex mechanisms that regulate fluid intake and output. The most important regulator of fluid intake is thirst. The primary regulators of fluid output are the kidneys, renin-angiotensin mechanism, aldosterone, and antidiuretic hormone (ADH).

POWERPOINT SLIDES

SUGGESTIONS FOR CLASSROOM ACTIVITIES

- Discuss the specific locations of intracellular fluid and extracellular fluids.
- Discuss the indications of water imbalances in an infant, an adult, and an elderly person.

SUGGESTION FOR CLINICAL ACTIVITIES

- Assign students to care for a patient with an intravenous infusion

POWERPOINT SLIDES

Figure 31.2 Movement of Fluids and Solution Tonicity

ANIMATIONS AND VIDEOS

- Fluid Balance

SUGGESTION FOR CLASSROOM ACTIVITIES

- Direct students to diagram the movement of fluids through osmosis in the interstitial compartment and the plasma compartment when either hypotonic or hypertonic IV fluids are given.

SUGGESTION FOR CLINICAL ACTIVITIES

- Assign students to care for a patient with dehydration or a patient at risk for dehydration.

4. Deficit-fluid-balance disorders can cause dehydration or shock. A deficit fluid balance is treated with oral or intravenous fluids. Excess-fluid-balance disorders are treated with diuretics.

LEARNING OUTCOME 3

Compare and contrast the use of colloids and crystalloids in IV therapy.

Concepts for Lecture

1. Intravenous fluid therapy using crystalloids and colloids replaces lost fluids. Causes of water and electrolyte loss are gastrointestinal fluid loss, vomiting, diarrhea, laxatives, suctioning, perspiration, burns, hemorrhage, excessive diuresis, and ketoacidosis.
2. Crystalloids contain electrolytes and are distributed primarily to the interstitial spaces. They are used to replace fluids and promote urine output and can expand the circulating *intravascular* fluid volume without causing major fluid shifts between compartments. Crystalloids are capable of leaving the plasma and moving to the interstitial spaces and intracellular fluid. The compartment entered depends on tonicity of intravenous fluid.
3. Colloids are large molecules that are too large to easily cross the capillary membrane. They stay in the intravascular space to rapidly expand plasma volume. Colloids also draw water from the intracellular fluid and interstitial spaces into the plasma, thereby increasing osmotic pressure. They are important in treating hypovolemic shock due to burns, hemorrhage, or surgery.

LEARNING OUTCOME 4

Explain the importance of electrolyte balance in the body.

Concepts for Lecture

Electrolytes are positively or negatively charged inorganic molecules that are essential to nerve conduction, membrane permeability, water balance, and other critical body functions. Imbalances may lead to serious abnormalities. (See Table 31.3 for important electrolytes and Table 31.4 for electrolyte imbalances.)

 POWERPOINT SLIDES

Table 31.1 Selected Crystalloid Intravenous Solutions
Table 31.2 Selected Colloid Intravenous Solutions

 SUGGESTION FOR CLASSROOM ACTIVITIES

- Discuss situations in which crystalloids (isotonic, hypotonic, and hypertonic) and colloids would be used for treatment.

 SUGGESTION FOR CLINICAL ACTIVITIES

- Assign students to use the information on "heat and water" from the SportsMed website at *www.rice.edu/~jenky/mednav.html* to do a concept map that illustrates the care of a patient with dehydration; present the concept map at postclinical after students care for a patient with dehydration.

 POWERPOINT SLIDES

Table 31.3 Important Electrolytes
Table 31.4 Electrolyte Imbalances

 SUGGESTION FOR CLASSROOM ACTIVITIES

- Review the types of electrolyte imbalances.

 SUGGESTION FOR CLINICAL ACTIVITIES

- Assign students to care for a patient with an electrolyte imbalance.

© 2011 Pearson Education, Inc.

LEARNING OUTCOME 5

Explain the pharmacotherapy of sodium and potassium imbalances.

Concepts for Lecture

1. Sodium is the major electrolyte in extracellular fluid. It is essential for maintaining osmolality, water balance, and acid–base balance. Water travels with or toward sodium. Sodium movement is the link between water retention, blood volume, and blood pressure. It is regulated by the kidneys and aldosterone. (See Figure 31.3.)

2. Hypernatremia occurs when the sodium level rises above 145 mEq/L. The most common cause is kidney disease. Sodium accumulates due to decreased excretion or because of high, net-water loss such as watery diarrhea, fever, or burns. High doses of glucocorticoids or estrogens also promote sodium retention. Hypernatremia increases the osmolality of the plasma, drawing fluid from interstitial spaces and cells, thus causing cellular dehydration. Patients may exhibit thirst, fatigue, weakness, muscle twitching, convulsions, altered mental status, and a decreased level of consciousness. Mild hypernatremia can be treated with a low-salt diet. Acute hypernatremia may be corrected with hypotonic intravenous fluids or diuretics.

3. Hyponatremia occurs when the sodium level falls below 135 mEq/L. It is caused by excessive dilution of plasma, as occurs with excessive antidiuretic hormone (ADH) secretion or excess administration of hypotonic intravenous solutions. Patients may suffer a significant loss of sodium due to vomiting, diarrhea, gastrointestinal suctioning, or diuretic use. Early symptoms of hyponatremia include nausea, vomiting, anorexia, and abdominal cramping. Later signs include altered neurologic function such as confusion, lethargy, convulsions, coma, and muscle twitching or tremors. Treatment of hyponatremia caused by excessive dilution is to administer loop diuretics to cause an isotonic diuresis. For hyponatremia caused by sodium loss, treat with oral sodium chloride or intravenous fluids containing salt such as normal saline or lactated Ringers.

4. Potassium is essential for proper nerve and muscle function and maintaining acid–base balance. It is influenced by aldosterone; for each sodium ion that is reabsorbed, one potassium ion is secreted into the renal tubules. Potassium imbalances can be serious, even fatal.

5. Hyperkalemia occurs when the potassium level rises above 5 mEq/L. It is caused by high consumption of potassium-rich foods or dietary supplements or administration of potassium-sparing diuretics and accumulates when renal disease causes decreased excretion. Symptoms of hyperkalemia include dysrhythmias and heart block, which are the most serious. Other symptoms are muscle twitching, fatigue, paresthesias, dyspnea, cramping, and diarrhea. Treatment of hyperkalemia is to restrict dietary sources, decrease the dose of potassium-sparing diuretics, administer glucose and insulin, administer calcium to counteract potassium toxicity on the heart, and administer polystyrene sulfonate (Kayexalate) and sorbitol to decrease the potassium in the body.

6. Hypokalemia occurs when the potassium level falls below 3.5 mEq/L. It may be caused by high doses of loop diuretics, strenuous muscle activity, and severe vomiting or diarrhea. Neurons and muscle fibers are most sensitive to potassium loss, so symptoms include muscle weakness, lethargy, anorexia, dysrhythmias, and cardiac arrest. Treatment of mild hypokalemia is to increase dietary intake. Oral or parenteral potassium supplements are given for more serious cases of hypokalemia.

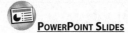

POWERPOINT SLIDES

Table 31.3 Important Electrolytes
Table 31.4 Electrolyte Imbalances

SUGGESTION FOR CLASSROOM ACTIVITIES

- Ask students to make a table illustrating causes, signs and symptoms, and pharmacotherapies for hypernatremia, hyponatremia, hyperkalemia, and hypokalemia.

SUGGESTION FOR CLINICAL ACTIVITIES

- Assign students to care for a patient with an electrolyte disturbance.

© 2011 Pearson Education, Inc.

LEARNING OUTCOME 6

Discuss common causes of alkalosis and acidosis and the medications used to treat these disorders.

Concepts for Lecture

1. Acidosis is excess acid (pH below 7.35), and alkalosis is excess base (pH above 7.45). Both are symptoms of an underlying disorder. They may be fatal if not treated rapidly. The body uses buffers to maintain overall pH within narrow limits. The kidneys and lungs collaborate to remove excess metabolic acid. (See Figure 31.4 for an illustration of acid–base imbalance.) (Common causes of acidosis and alkalosis are shown in Table 31.5.)

2. Acidosis may be respiratory (caused by hypoventilation) or metabolic (caused by diarrhea, kidney failure, diabetes, excess alcohol, or starvation). Symptoms of acidosis affect the central nervous system and include lethargy, confusion, coma, and deep, rapid respirations in an attempt to blow off excess acid. The goal is to quickly reverse the effects of excess acid in the blood. Administration of sodium bicarbonate is the appropriate pharmacologic therapy.

3. Alkalosis may also be respiratory (in this case caused by hyperventilation due to asthma, anxiety, or high altitude) or metabolic (caused by prolonged constipation, excess sodium bicarbonate, diuretics that cause potassium depletion, or severe vomiting). Symptoms are due to central-nervous-system stimulation, including nervousness, hyperactive reflexes, and convulsions, and slow, shallow respirations in an attempt to retain acid. Treatment of alkalosis is administration of ammonium chloride in severe cases and administration of sodium chloride with potassium chloride in mild cases.

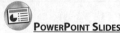
POWERPOINT SLIDES

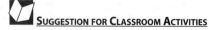
Figure 31.4 Illustration of Acid–Base Imbalance
Table 31.5 Common Causes of Acidosis and Alkalosis

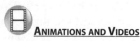
ANIMATIONS AND VIDEOS

- Acids

SUGGESTION FOR CLASSROOM ACTIVITIES

- Direct the students to create concept maps illustrating the causes, signs, and symptoms of acid–base disorders and the pharmacotherapies used to treat alkalosis and acidosis.

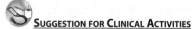
SUGGESTION FOR CLINICAL ACTIVITIES

- Assign students to care for a patient with an acid–base imbalance.

LEARNING OUTCOME 7

Describe the nurse's role in the pharmacologic management of fluid balance, electrolyte, and acid–base disorders.

Concepts for Lecture

1. The role of the nurse in the pharmacological management of fluid balance, electrolyte, and acid–base disorders involves careful monitoring of a patient's condition and providing education as it relates to the prescribed drug treatment. Obtain baseline medical, surgical, and drug history; lifestyle and dietary habits, including use of herbal or alternative therapies; and a detailed description of symptomology and current therapies. Obtain baseline weight and vital signs, level of consciousness, breath sounds, and urinary output as appropriate. Evaluate appropriate laboratory findings (e.g., electrolytes, CBC, urine specific gravity and urinalysis, BUN and creatinine, total protein and albumin levels, aPTT, aPT, or INR, renal and liver function studies).

2. **Colloidal solutions:** The primary nursing responsibility when caring for the patient receiving plasma volume expanders is monitoring fluid-volume status. Monitor closely for both fluid-volume deficit and fluid-volume excess. Closely assess neurologic status and urinary output. Report a hematocrit below 30% to the physician immediately. Teach the patient to report any signs of bleeding, hypersensitivity, or fluid-volume overload.

3. **Sodium replacement therapy:** Assess sodium and electrolyte balance. Be alert for signs of hyponatremia and hypernatremia. Monitor

POWERPOINT SLIDES

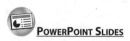

SUGGESTION FOR CLASSROOM ACTIVITIES

- Invite a nurse from an intensive care unit or an emergency room nurse to speak about pharmacological management of fluid balance, electrolyte, and acid–base disorders.

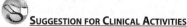
SUGGESTION FOR CLINICAL ACTIVITIES

- Direct students to develop a teaching plan for the pharmacological management of their assigned patients with a fluid balance, electrolyte, or acid–base disorder.

© 2011 Pearson Education, Inc.

serum sodium levels, urine specific gravity, and serum and urine osmolarity closely when administering hypertonic solutions. Teach the patient to report any symptoms that may relate to fluid overload during infusion of hypertonic saline solutions. Also teach the patient to drink adequate amounts of water or balanced sports drinks to replenish lost fluids and electrolytes.

4. **Potassium-replacement therapy:** Monitor for cardiac abnormalities; do not use in patients with severe renal impairment and those who use potassium-sparing diuretics. Potassium supplements are also contraindicated with acute dehydration or heat cramps and in patients with digoxin intoxication with AV-node disturbance. Instruct patients to take oral potassium with meals to avoid irritating the GI tract.

5. **Sodium bicarbonate therapy:** Monitor arterial blood-gas reports; use cautiously in patients with cardiac disease or renal impairment. Teach patients to use alternative OTC antacids to prevent excess sodium or bicarbonate from being absorbed into systemic circulation.

6. **Ammonium chloride therapy:** Assess the pH in arterial blood-gas levels prior to administration. This drug is contraindicated in the presence of liver disease because its acidifying action depends on proper liver functioning to convert ammonium ions to urea. Infuse slowly to avoid ammonium toxicity and to decrease irritation to the veins.

LEARNING OUTCOME 8

For each of the classes listed in Drugs at a Glance, know representative drugs, and explain the mechanism of drug action, primary actions, and important adverse effects.

Concepts for Lecture

1. **Colloids** are fluid-replacement agents. Prototype drug: dextran 40 (Gentran 40, Hyskon, 10% LMD, Rheomacrodex). Mechanism of action: to raise the oncotic pressure of the blood, thereby causing fluid to move from the interstitial spaces of the tissues to the intravascular space (blood). Primary use: Because it has the capability of expanding plasma volume within minutes after administration, it is used as fluid replacement for patients experiencing hypovolemic shock due to hemorrhage, surgery, or severe burns. Adverse effects: hypersensitivity reactions, fluid overload, and hypertension.

2. **Electrolytes.** Prototype drug: sodium chloride. Mechanism of action: as an electrolyte/sodium supplement. Primary use: administered for hyponatremia when serum levels fall below 130 mEq/L. Adverse effects: hypernatremia and pulmonary edema.

3. **Electrolytes.** Prototype drug: potassium chloride. Mechanism of action: as an electrolyte/potassium supplement. Primary use: to prevent or treat hypokalemia. Adverse effects: gastrointestinal irritation and hyperkalemia; it is contraindicated in patients with chronic renal failure or those taking a potassium-sparing diuretic.

4. **Acid–base agents.** Prototype drug: sodium bicarbonate. Mechanism of action: to raise the pH of body fluids. Primary use: to treat metabolic acidosis. Adverse effects: metabolic alkalosis caused by receiving too much bicarbonate ion and hypokalemia.

 POWERPOINT SLIDES

Prototype Drug
- dextran 40 (Gentran 40, Hyskon, 10% LMD, Rheomacrodex).
- sodium chloride
- potassium chloride
- sodium bicarbonate

 SUGGESTION FOR CLASSROOM ACTIVITIES

- Divide students into five groups. Assign each group a class of drugs from this chapter to create a game that teaches other students the mechanism of action and adverse effects of that classification.

SUGGESTION FOR CLINICAL ACTIVITIES

- Assign students to care for patients who are receiving drugs for fluid balance, electrolyte, and acid–base disorders. Have each student make a drug card for the medications and present at postclinical.

LEARNING OUTCOME 9

Use the nursing process to care for patients who are receiving drug therapy for fluid balance, electrolyte, and acid–base disorders.

Concepts for Lecture

1. **Patients who are receiving drug therapy for fluid balance, electrolyte, and acid–base disorders. Assessment:** Prior to administration, obtain a complete health history, including allergies, drug history, and possible drug interactions. Assess for the presence of fluid-volume deficit. Obtain the following laboratory studies: CBC, serum electrolytes, renal function (BUN and serum creatinine), total protein and albumin levels, aPTT, aPT, or INR, and liver function studies.

2. **Patients who are receiving drug therapy for fluid balance, electrolyte, and acid–base disorders. Nursing diagnoses:** *Deficient Fluid Volume; Decreased Cardiac Output; Fatigue; Activity Intolerance; Deficient Knowledge* (drug therapy); *Risk for Falls, Risk for Injury* related to hypotension, dizziness associated with adverse effects; Risk for Excessive Fluid Volume related to drug therapy; Risk for Ineffective Health Maintenance regarding drug effects and dietary needs.

3. **Patients who are receiving drug therapy for fluid balance, electrolyte, and acid–base disorders. Planning:** The patient will experience therapeutic effects dependent on the reason the drug is being given (e.g., increased urinary output and relief of dehydration, electrolyte values within normal limits). Be free from or experience minimal adverse effects; verbalize an understanding of the drug's use, adverse effects, and required precautions; demonstrate proper self-administration of the medication (e.g., dose, timing, when to notify provider).

4. **Patients who are receiving drug therapy for fluid balance, electrolyte, and acid–base disorders. Implementation:** Monitor hemodynamic status every 15 to 60 minutes, including blood pressure, urinary output, weight, and invasive pressure-monitoring devices. Monitor for signs of fluid-volume excess or deficit. Monitor for hypersensitivity reactions; signs of circulatory overload; and changes in complete blood count results. Closely monitor for signs and symptoms of allergy (colloids). Monitor IV sites closely when infusing potassium or ammonium. Instruct patients to consume foods high in potassium (hypokalemia) and avoid salt substitues (hyperkalemia). Instruct patient to report dyspnea, itching, feelings of throat tightness, palpitations, chest pain or tightening, or headache immediately. Ensure patient safety (ambulation). Monitor CBC, electrolytes, aPTT, aPT, or INR levels.

5. **Patients who are receiving drug therapy for fluid balance, electrolyte, and acid–base disorders. Evaluation:** The patient experiences therapeutic effects dependent on the reason the drug is being given (e.g., increased urinary output and relief of dehydration, electrolyte values within normal limits). Is free from or experiences minimal adverse effects; verbalizes an understanding of the drug's use, adverse effects and required precautions; demonstrates proper self-administration of the medication (e.g., dose, timing, when to notify provider).

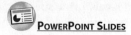

POWERPOINT SLIDES

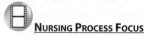

NURSING PROCESS FOCUS

- Care for patients who are receiving drug therapy for fluid balance, electrolyte, and acid–base disorders.

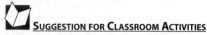

SUGGESTION FOR CLASSROOM ACTIVITIES

- Divide students into small groups, and have each group develop a teaching plan for a patient receiving therapy for a fluid balance, an electrolyte, and an acid–base disorder.

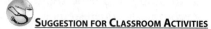

SUGGESTION FOR CLASSROOM ACTIVITIES

- Have the students implement teaching plans for patients receiving therapy for a fluid balance, electrolyte, or acid–base disorder in the clinical area.

© 2011 Pearson Education, Inc.

GENERAL CHAPTER CONSIDERATIONS

1. Have students study and learn key terms listed at the beginning of the chapter.
2. Have students complete end-of-chapter exercises either in their book or on the MyNursingKit website.
3. Use the Classroom Response Questions provided in PowerPoint to assess students prior to lecture.

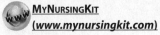

MyNursingKit (*www.mynursingkit.com*)

- Websites
- NCLEX® questions
- Critical Thinking Questions
- Case Studies
- Animations and Videos
- Drug Prototype Questions

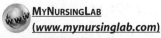

MyNursingLab (*www.mynursinglab.com*)

- Knowledge Quick Check
- Pre/Posttests
- Customized study plans
- *Separate purchase*

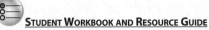

STUDENT WORKBOOK AND RESOURCE GUIDE

- Chapter 31 activities
- *Separate purchase*

PEARSON NURSE'S DRUG GUIDE

- *Separate purchase*

PEARSON eTEXT

- Students can search, highlight, take notes, and more all in electronic format.
- *Separate purchase*

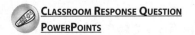

CLASSROOM RESPONSE QUESTION POWERPOINTS

TESTBANK

© 2011 Pearson Education, Inc.

CHAPTER 32
DRUGS FOR IMMUNE SYSTEM MODULATION

LEARNING OUTCOME 1

Compare and contrast specific and nonspecific body defenses.

Concepts for Lecture

1. **Nonspecific body defenses** are the first line of defense, a barrier to microbes or environmental hazards. They deny entrance of pathogens to the body by providing general responses that are not specific to a particular threat. Examples of nonspecific body defenses are the skin, phagocytes, natural killer cells, complement system, fever, interferons, and inflammation.

2. **Specific body defenses** are the second line of defense, activated by specific antigens, and each is effective against one particular microbe species. For example, a specific defense may act against only a single species of bacteria and be ineffective against all others. This type of defense is known as the immune response. Foreign agents that elicit an immune response are called antigens. The primary cell of the immune response that interacts with antigens is the lymphocyte. Two major divisions of the immune system are antibody-mediated (humoral) or cell-mediated immunity.

LEARNING OUTCOME 2

Compare and contrast the humoral and cell-mediated immune responses.

Concepts for Lecture

1. **Humoral immunity** is initiated when an antigen encounters a B cell. The activated B cell divides rapidly to form clones of itself. Most cells in this clone are called plasma cells; their primary function is to secrete antibodies that are specific to the antigen that initiated the challenge. Circulating through the body, antibodies, also known as immunoglobulins, physically interact with the antigen to neutralize it or mark the foreign agent for destruction by other cells of the immune response. Peak production of antibodies occurs about 10 days after an antigen challenge. Memory B cells can speed a future defense against a specific antigen. (The important functions of antibodies are illustrated in Figure 32.2.)

2. **Cell-mediated immunity** involves lymphocytes called T cells. Two major types of T cells are called helper T cells (CD_4 receptor) and cytotoxic T cells (CD_8 receptor). The helper T cells are responsible for activating most other immune cells, including B cells. Cytotoxic T cells travel throughout the body, directly killing certain bacteria, parasites, virus-infected cells, and cancer cells. Activated T cells form clones and produce huge amounts of cytokines—hormonelike proteins that regulate the intensity and duration of the immune response and mediate cell-to-cell communication. Specific cytokines include interleukins, gamma interferon, and perforin.

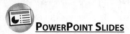 **POWERPOINT SLIDES**

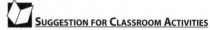 **SUGGESTION FOR CLASSROOM ACTIVITIES**

- Ask students to give examples of how pathogens can gain entry to a body through the nonspecific body defenses.

SUGGESTION FOR CLINICAL ACTIVITIES

- Direct the students to assess their patients' nonspecific body defenses and give a summary of that assessment during postclinical.

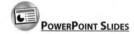 **POWERPOINT SLIDES**

Figure 32.2 Functions of Antibodies

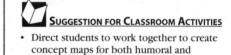 **SUGGESTION FOR CLASSROOM ACTIVITIES**

- Direct students to work together to create concept maps for both humoral and cell-mediated immunity steps.

SUGGESTION FOR CLINICAL ACTIVITIES

- Compare and contrast the humoral and cell-mediated immune responses that students may observe in their clinical patients.

© 2011 Pearson Education, Inc.

LEARNING OUTCOME 3

For each of the major vaccines, give the recommended dosage schedule.

Concepts for Lecture

The nurse plays a key role in encouraging patients to be vaccinated according to established guidelines. The recommended dosage schedule for vaccines: Diphtheria, tetanus, and pertussis (DPT, Tri-Immunol, Tripedia, Acel-Imune, Infanrix, Certiva)—given IM; 0.5 mL at ages 2 months, 4 months, 6 months, and 18 months. Haemophilus type B conjugate (HibTITER, ActHIB, PedvaxHIB)—given IM; 0.5 mL at ages 2 months, 4 months, 6 months, and 15 months. Children ages 12–14 months who have not been vaccinated receive a single dose. Hepatitis B (Recombivax HB, Engerix-B)—given to children: 2.5-5 mcg at birth; then 0.5 mL at 1–4 months and 6–18 months. Adults: 0.5 mL in three doses, with the second dose 30 days after the first, and the final dose six months after the first. Influenza vaccine (Fluzone, FluShield, Fluvirin)—given to children: IM, two doses, one month apart; then annual dose. Adults: IM, single annual dose. Measles, mumps, and rubella (MMR II)—given subcutaneously; 0.5 mL single dose at age 15 months to puberty. Pneumococcal, polyvalent (Pneumovax 23, Pnu-Immune 23) or 7-valent (Prenvar)—given to children (Prenvar): IM, four doses at ages 2 months, 4 months, 6 months, and 12–15 months. Adults (Pneumovax 23 or Pnu-Immune 23): subcutaneously or IM; 0.5 mL as a single dose. Poliovirus, inactivated (IPOL)—given subcutaneously; 0.5 mL at ages 4–8 weeks, 2–4 months, and 6–12 months. Varicella zoster/chickenpox (Varivax)—for children younger than 12 months: given as a single dose; for patients 12 months and older: given subcutaneously; 0.5 mL, two doses given 4–8 weeks apart. (See Table 32.2 for the recommended dosage schedule in table form.)

LEARNING OUTCOME 4

Distinguish between active immunity and passive immunity.

Concepts for Lecture

1. **Activity immunity** occurs when the immune system is stimulated to produce antibodies. Exposure to the antigen through surviving the illness produces active immunity. Vaccines are biological agents used to prevent illness by boosting antibody production and producing active immunity.
2. **Passive immunity** is obtained when preformed antibodies are transferred from one person to another. Examples are maternal antibodies crossing the placenta; administration of immune globulin and antivenom; and treatment for botulism, tetanus, and rabies. This therapy is for people who are exposed or have a high risk of exposure and immunosuppressed people. (See Table 32.1.)

POWERPOINT SLIDES

Table 32.2 Selected Vaccines and Their Schedules

SUGGESTION FOR CLASSROOM ACTIVITIES

- Direct the students to access the state health website or the CDC website to find vaccination schedules.

SUGGESTION FOR CLINICAL ACTIVITIES

- Assign students to observe administration of vaccines in a clinical or public health setting.

POWERPOINT LECTURE SLIDES

Table 32.1 Immune Globulin Preparations

ANIMATIONS AND VIDEOS

- **Pharmacotherapy Illustrated 32.1** Mechanism of Active and Passive Immunity

SUGGESTIONS FOR CLASSROOM ACTIVITIES

- Direct the students to draw a concept map for both active and passive immunity.
- Direct students to work in small groups to create concept maps that compare and contrast the four types of immunosuppressants.

SUGGESTIONS FOR CLINICAL ACTIVITIES

- Assign students to observe the administration of immune globulin in the clinical area.
- Assign students to care for patients taking immunosuppressant drugs.

LEARNING OUTCOME 5

Identify indications for pharmacotherapy with biologic response modifiers.

Concepts for Lecture

1. **Immunostimulants** are biologic response modifiers, including interferons and interleukins that boost the patient's immune system. They are used to treat certain viral infections, immunodeficiencies, and specific cancers. Biologic response modifiers are cytokines produced through recombinant DNA technology that boost specific functions of the immune system.

2. **Interferons** are secreted by lymphocytes and macrophages that have been infected with a virus; they slow the spread of viral infections and enhance the activity of leukocytes. These drugs have antiviral, anticancer, and anti-inflammatory properties. The actions of interferons include modulation of immune functions such as increasing phagocytosis and enhancing the cytotoxic activity of T cells. There are two major classes. Interferon alpha is used to treat leukemia, AIDS, and hepatitis B or C. Interferon beta is used to treat multiple sclerosis, granulomatous disease, and severe osteoporosis.

3. **Interleukins** are used to treat metastatic renal carcinoma and to stimulate platelet production in immunosuppressed patients. They enhance capabilities of the immune system, stimulate cytotoxic T cells, increase B-cell and plasma-cell production, and promote inflammation. (See Table 32.3 for a list of immunostimulants.)

LEARNING OUTCOME 6

Explain the need for immunosuppressant medications following organ and tissue transplants.

Concepts for Lecture

1. Transplanted organs have antigens that trigger the immune response. This response, called transplant rejection, is often a humoral response (acute response). The antibodies destroy transplanted tissue within days. The cell-mediated response is slower, occurring about two weeks after surgery. Chronic rejection can occur months to years later.

2. **Immunosuppressants** inhibit the patient's immune system. They are used to treat severe autoimmune disease and prevent tissue rejection following organ transplantation, which would be impossible without immunosuppressants. Unfortunately, they are toxic to bone marrow and increase the risk of infections and lymphoma.

LEARNING OUTCOME 7

Identify the classes of medications used as immunosuppressants.

Concepts for Lecture

Immunosuppressants include glucocorticoids, antimetabolites, antibodies, and calcineurin inhibitors. Glucocorticoids inhibit inflammation and are often drugs of choice in the short-term therapy of severe inflammation. Antimetabolites such as sirolimus (Rapamune) and azathioprine (Imuran) inhibit aspects of lymphocyte replication. By

 POWERPOINT SLIDES

Table 32.3 Immunostimulants

 SUGGESTION FOR CLASSROOM ACTIVITIES
- Direct students to create a concept map of biologic modifiers.

 SUGGESTION FOR CLINICAL ACTIVITIES
- Assign students to care for patients taking biologic modifiers.

 POWERPOINT SLIDES

 SUGGESTION FOR CLASSROOM ACTIVITIES
- Invite a nurse who works in organ donation to speak to the class.

 SUGGESTION FOR CLINICAL ACTIVITIES
- Assign students to care for patients who have had organ transplants.

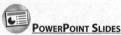 **POWERPOINT SLIDES**

Table 32.4 Immunosuppressants

© 2011 Pearson Education, Inc.

binding to the intracellular messenger calcineurin, cyclosporine (Sandimmune, Neoral) and tacrolimus (Prograf) disrupt T-cell function. The calcineurin inhibitors are of value in treating psoriasis, an inflammatory disorder of the skin. Antibodies to human T cells are produced by animal immune systems that recognize injected human cells as foreign. When purified and injected into humans, these mouse antibodies will attack T cells (or T-cell receptors). Muromonab-CD3 (Orthoclone OKT3) is administered to prevent rejection of kidney, heart, and liver transplants and to deplete the bone marrow of T-cells prior to marrow transplant. Basiliximab (Simulect) and daclizumab (Zenapax) are given to prevent acute rejection of kidney transplants. Infliximab (Remicade) is used to suppress the severe inflammation that often accompanies autoimmune disorders such as Crohn's disease and rheumatoid arthritis. Note that the suffix "ab" in the generic name refers to antibody. (For immunosuppressants, see Table 32.4.)

LEARNING OUTCOME 8

Describe the nurse's role in the pharmacologic management of immune disorders.

Concepts for Lecture

1. The role of the nurse in the pharmacologic management of immune disorders involves careful monitoring of a patient's condition and providing education as it relates to the prescribed drug treatment. Obtain baseline medical, surgical, and drug history; lifestyle and dietary habits, including use of herbal or alternative therapies; and a detailed description of symptomology and current therapies. Obtain baseline vital signs, especially blood pressure and temperature, height and weight. Assess oral and dental health. Evaluate appropriate laboratory findings (e.g., CBC, platelets, electrolytes, glucose, hepatic and renal labs, lipid levels). Assess patient's ability to receive and understand instruction.

2. **Immunization agents:** Assess for any risk-based precautions, such as pregnancy, diabetes, heart disease, renal failure, and various other serious and debilitating conditions, and provide education on the importance of receiving vaccinations. Answer all questions and concerns patients and family members may have regarding the risks and benefits of vaccines. Instruct patients and family on the recommended immunization schedule and the importance of any recommended follow-up vaccines.

3. **Immunostimulants:** Assessment of infections and cancer verifies the need for these drugs. Immunostimulants are contraindicated for patients with renal or liver disease and those who are pregnant. Before starting therapy, obtain the results of lab tests, including a complete blood count, electrolytes, renal function, and liver enzymes to provide baseline data. Keep the patient well hydrated during pharmacotherapy. Use of immunostimulants can lead to the development of encephalopathy; therefore, assess for changes in mental status, including suicidal ideation.

4. **Immunosuppressants:** These are contraindicated in patients with leukemia, metastatic cancer, active infection, or renal or liver disease or those who are pregnant. Obtain vital signs and results of lab testing, including a complete blood count, electrolytes, and liver profile, to provide baseline data and reveal any abnormalities. Monitor vital signs, especially temperature, and blood tests for indications of infection. Carefully monitor the degree of bone-marrow suppression (thrombocytopenia and leukopenia). Monitor patients who are taking azathioprine (Imuran) for the development of secondary malignancies.

SUGGESTION FOR CLASSROOM ACTIVITIES

- Direct students to work in small groups to create concept maps that compare and contrast the four types of immunosuppressants.

SUGGESTION FOR CLINICAL ACTIVITIES

- Assign students to care for patients taking immunosuppressant drugs.

POWERPOINT LECTURE SLIDES

SUGGESTION FOR CLASSROOM ACTIVITIES

- Invite a nurse from a clinic or public-health unit to speak about the vaccination process.

SUGGESTION FOR CLINICAL ACTIVITIES

- Direct the students to develop a teaching plan to encourage the community to vaccinate children. Direct them to include a schedule of vaccination.

LEARNING OUTCOME 9

For each of the drug classes listed in Drugs at a Glance, know representative drugs, and explain their mechanism of drug action, primary actions related to the immune system, and important adverse effects.

Concepts for Lecture

1. **Immunization agent—vaccine.** Prototype drug: hepatitis B vaccine (Engerix-B, Recombivax HB). Mechanism of action: by vaccine, the provision of active immunity. Primary use: to treat individuals who are at risk of exposure to hepatitis B virus (HBV). Adverse effects: pain and inflammation at the injection site. Some patients experience transient fever or fatigue.

2. **Immunostimulant—interferon.** Prototype drug: interferon alpha-2a (Roferon-A). Mechanism of action: This biologic response modifier enhances or stimulates the immune system to remove antigens. It also suppresses the growth of cancer cells. Primary use: cancers (hairy cell leukemia, malignant melanoma, non-Hodgkin's lymphoma, AIDS-related Kaposi's sarcoma), as well as viral infections (human papilloma virus, chronic hepatitis virus B and C). Off-label indications may include chronic myelogenous leukemia, bladder cancer, herpes simplex virus, renal cell cancer, varicella-zoster virus, and West Nile virus. Adverse effects: flulike syndrome of fever, chills, dizziness, and fatigue occurs in 50% of patients, although this usually diminishes as therapy progresses. Headache, nausea, vomiting, diarrhea, and anorexia are relatively common. Depression and suicidal ideation have been reported. With prolonged therapy, serious toxicity such as immunosuppression, hepatotoxicity, and neurotoxicity may be observed.

3. **Immunosuppressant—calineurin inhibitor.** Prototype drug: cyclosporine (Neoral, Sandimmune). Mechanism of action: to inhibit helper T cells. Primary use: for prophylaxis of kidney, heart and liver transplant rejection, psoriasis and xerophthalmia, an eye condition. Adverse effects: 75% of patients experience reduction in urine flow and over 50% will experience hypertension. Other common side effects are headache, gingival hyperplasia, and elevated hepatic enzymes. Long-term therapy increases the risk of malignancy, especially lymphomas and skin cancers.

LEARNING OUTCOME 10

Use the nursing process to care for patients receiving drug therapy for immune conditions.

Concepts for Lecture

1. **Immunostimulant Therapy—Assessment:** Obtain a complete health history including previous history of hepatic, renal, cardiovascular, neurologic, or autoimmune disease, HIV infection, fever or active infections, pregnancy or breast-feeding; previous allergic response to immunizations or to products contained within immunization (e.g., yeast sensitivity, sensitivity to eggs or albumin products). Obtain a drug history, especially the use of immunosuppressants or corticosteroids. Obtain an immunization history and any unusual reactions or responses that occurred. Obtain baseline vital signs, especially temperature. Evaluate appropriate laboratory findings (e.g., CBC, platelets, electrolytes, titres, hepatic and renal labs). Assess patient's ability to receive and understand instruction. Assess for and immediately report

POWERPOINT SLIDES

Prototype Drug
- hepatitis B vaccine (Engerix-B, Recombivax HB)
- interferon alpha-2a (Roferon-A)
- cyclosporine (Neoral, Sandimmune)

ANIMATIONS AND VIDEOS

- Mechanism in Action: Interferon alfa-2A (Roferon-A)

SUGGESTION FOR CLASSROOM ACTIVITIES

- Direct students to create exam questions and answers from the prototype drugs, and encourage them to use the mechanism of action, indications, and adverse effects in the questions. Use several of the questions in the exam for this unit.

SUGGESTION FOR CLINICAL ACTIVITIES

- Direct students to observe the care plans for their patients who are taking drugs for immune disorders. Discuss the care plans during post-clinical.

POWERPOINT SLIDES

NURSING PROCESS FOCUS

- Care for patients receiving drug therapy for immune disorders

SUGGESTION FOR CLASSROOM ACTIVITIES

- Direct the students to access the CDC website to find current traveler's health information on immunizations.

SUGGESTION FOR CLINICAL ACTIVITIES

- Have each student present a teaching plan for a drug used for immune disorders to the patient as applicable.

© 2011 Pearson Education, Inc.

adverse effects: fever, dizziness, confusion, muscle weakness, tachycardia, hypotension, syncope, dyspnea, pulmonary congestion, skin rashes, bruising or bleeding, anaphylactic reactions.

2. **Patients Receiving Immunostimulant Therapy—Nursing Diagnoses:** *Health Seeking Behaviors* (expressed desire to obtain vaccinations); *Ineffective Health Maintenance* related to failure to complete immunization schedule; *Deficient Knowledge* (vaccination schedule, recommendations); *Risk for Injury* related to drug adverse effects.

3. **Patients Receiving Immunostimulant Therapy—Planning:** The patient will experience therapeutic effects dependent on the reason the drug is being given (e.g., active immunity); be free from or experience minimal adverse effects. Verbalize an understanding of the drug's use, adverse effects, and required precautions. Demonstrate proper self-administration of the medication (e.g., dose, timing, when to notify provider for immunostimulants).

4. **Patients Receiving Immunostimulant Therapy—Implementation:** Monitor vital signs, especially temperature, and neurologic status. Report all significant adverse effects to health care provider for reporting to VAERS—Vaccine Adverse Event Reporting System (*vaers.hhs.gov*). Treat minor adverse (side) effects symptomatically. Assess for possibility of pregnancy, previous history of organ transplantation, and home environment. Avoid or defer immunizations in any patient with a fever, autoimmune disease, or those taking corticosteroids. Assess patients for previous use of BCG vaccine and consult with health care provider before giving PPD ("Mantoux"). Monitor for signs of opportunistic and superinfections, or an increase in bruising or bleeding in patients receiving interferon therapy. Monitor neurologic and mental status in patients receiving interferon therapy. (Psychosis, depression, and suicidal ideations are potential adverse effects of interferon use.)

5. **Patients Receiving Immunostimulant Therapy—Evaluation:** The patient will experience therapeutic effects dependent on the reason the drug is being given (e.g., active immunity); Is free from, or experiences minimal adverse effects. Verbalizes an understanding of the drug's use, adverse effects, and required precautions. Demonstrates proper self-administration of the medication (e.g., dose, timing, when to notify provider).

6. **Patients Receiving Immunosuppressant Therapy—Assessment:** Obtain a complete health history including previous history or current case of cancer, fever or active infections (especially herpes, varicella, and CMV), hepatic, renal, cardiovascular, neurologic, or autoimmune disease, dermatologic conditions, HIV infection, pregnancy or breastfeeding. Obtain vital signs, especially blood pressure, temperature, height, and weight. Assess mental alertness and dental health. Obtain a dietary history, especially the intake of grapefruit or grapefruit juice. Evaluate appropriate laboratory findings (e.g., CBC, platelets, electrolytes, glucose, hepatic and renal labs, lipid levels). Assess for and immediately report adverse effects: fever, chills, visible signs of infection, nausea, vomiting, dizziness, confusion, muscle weakness, tremors, tachycardia, hypertension, angina, syncope, dyspnea, pulmonary congestion, skin rashes, bruising or bleeding, decreased urine output.

REFERENCE

- **Current recommendations may be found on the CDC Traveler's Health website:** *wwwn.cdc.gov/travel*
- Vaccine Adverse Event Reporting System: *vaers.hhs.gov*

7. **Patients Receiving Immunosuppressant Therapy—Nursing Diagnoses:** *Anxiety or Fear* related to concerns about condition, treatment; *Ineffective Therapeutic Regimen Management* related to complexity of disease, treatment; *Social Isolation; Deficient Knowledge* (drug therapy); *Risk for Infection; Risk for Injury; Risk for Impaired Oral Mucus Membranes* related to drug treatment.

8. **Patients Receiving Immunosuppressant Drug Therapy—Planning:** The patient will experience therapeutic effects dependent on the reason the drug is being given (e.g., free from signs of transplant rejection, excessive/auto-immune response limited and decreasing) and be free from or experience minimal adverse effects. Verbalizes an understanding of the drug's use, adverse effects and required precautions. Demonstrates proper self-administration of the medication (e.g., dose, timing, when to report to provider).

9. **Patients Receiving Immunosuppressant Therapy—Implementation:** Monitor vital signs, especially blood pressure and temperature. Observe for signs and symptoms of infection. Assess for changes in level of consciousness, disorientation or confusion, or tremors. Monitor CBC, platelets, electrolytes, glucose, liver and renal function studies, lipid levels (leukopenia, anemia, thrombocytopenia, hyperglycemia, and hyperkalemia). Inspect oral mucus membranes and dental health (oral candidiasis and gingivitis). Assess for pregnancy. Assess diet and consumption of grapefruit or grapefruit juice. Assess for development of hirsutism or alopecia. Assess for and immediately report adverse effects: fever, chills, visible signs of infection, nausea, vomiting, dizziness, confusion, muscle weakness, tremors, tachycardia, hypertension, angina, syncope, dyspnea, pulmonary congestion, skin rashes, bruising or bleeding, decreased urine output.

10. **Patients Receiving Immunosuppressant Therapy—Evaluation:** The patient experiences therapeutic effects (free from signs of transplant rejection; excessive/auto-immune response limited and decreasing) and is free from or experiences minimal adverse effects. Verbalizes an understanding of the drug's use, adverse effects and required precautions. Demonstrates proper self-administration of the medication (e.g., dose, timing, when to report to provider).

© 2011 Pearson Education, Inc.

General Chapter Considerations

1. Have students study and learn key terms listed at the beginning of the chapter.
2. Have students complete end-of-chapter exercises either in their book or on the MyNursingKit website.
3. Use the Classroom Response Questions provided in PowerPoint to assess students prior to lecture.

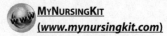

MyNursingKit (www.mynursingkit.com)

- Websites
- NCLEX® questions
- Critical Thinking Questions
- Case Studies
- Animations and Videos
- Drug Prototype Questions

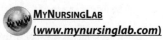

MyNursingLab (www.mynursinglab.com)

- Knowledge Quick Check
- Pre/Posttests
- Customized study plans
- *Separate purchase*

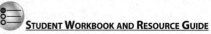

Student Workbook and Resource Guide

- Chapter 32 activities
- *Separate purchase*

Pearson Nurse's Drug Guide

- *Separate purchase*

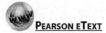

Pearson eText

- Students can search, highlight, take notes, and more all in electronic format.
- *Separate purchase*

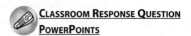

Classroom Response Question PowerPoints

Testbank

CHAPTER 33
DRUGS FOR INFLAMMATION AND FEVER

LEARNING OUTCOME 1

Explain the pathophysiology of inflammation and fever.

Concepts for Lecture

1. Inflammation is a natural, nonspecific body defense that limits the spread of invading microorganisms or injury. Occurs in response to an injury or antigen. The central purpose of inflammation is to contain the injury or destroy the microorganism. Inflammation is not a disease, but a symptom of an underlying disorder. By neutralizing the foreign agent and removing cellular debris and dead cells, repair of the injured area can proceed at a faster pace. Inflammation limits the spread of injury or antigens by containing the injury or destroying the microorganism. Acute inflammation occurs over several days, whereas chronic inflammation may continue for months or years.
2. Signs and symptoms of inflammation include swelling, pain, warmth, and redness.

LEARNING OUTCOME 2

Outline the basic steps in the acute inflammatory response.

Concepts for Lecture

1. Damaged tissue releases chemical mediators that alert the surrounding area of injury. The chemical mediators are histamine, leukotrienes, bradykinin, complement, and prostaglandins. (See Table 33.1 to see the sources and actions of these mediators.)
2. There are five basic steps in acute inflammation. They occur after cellular injury causes release of chemical mediators. The steps are vasodilation, vascular permeability (edema), cellular infiltration (pus), thrombosis (clots), and stimulation of nerve endings (pain). (See Figure 33.1 for an illustration of the steps of inflammation.)

LEARNING OUTCOME 3

Explain the role of chemical mediators in the inflammatory response.

Concepts for Lecture

1. Histamine is a key chemical mediator in inflammation. It is stored in mast cells and initiates the inflammatory response. It directly stimulates pain receptors. Release of histamine produces vasodilation, allowing

POWERPOINT SLIDES

SUGGESTION FOR CLASSROOM ACTIVITIES

- Direct students to break into small groups and share signs and symptoms of inflammation they have experienced personally or observed in others.

SUGGESTION FOR CLINICAL ACTIVITIES

- Document signs of inflammation as appropriate in the clinical area.

POWERPOINT SLIDES

Table 33.1 Chemical Mediators of Inflammation
Figure 33.1 Steps in Acute Inflammation

SUGGESTION FOR CLASSROOM ACTIVITIES

- Direct students to create and discuss concept maps of acute inflammation.

SUGGESTION FOR CLINICAL ACTIVITIES

- Assign students to care for patients with infections. Direct them to describe the steps of acute inflammation that they observed in those patients.

POWERPOINT SLIDES

SUGGESTION FOR CLASSROOM ACTIVITIES

- Contrast symptoms of H_1 and H_2 receptor stimulation.

© 2011 Pearson Education, Inc.

capillaries to become leaky, causing tissue swelling. Histamine is responsible for the symptoms of anaphylaxis.

2. There are two different receptors with which histamine interacts to elicit a response. H_1 receptors are present in the smooth muscle of the vascular system, the bronchial tree, and the digestive tract. Stimulation of these receptors results in itching, pain, edema, vasodilation, bronchoconstriction, and the characteristic symptoms of inflammation and allergy. In contrast, H_2 receptors are primarily present in the stomach, and their stimulation results in the secretion of large amounts of hydrochloric acid.

LEARNING OUTCOME 4

Outline the general strategies for treating inflammation.

Concepts for Lecture

1. Identify and treat the underlying cause. Inflammation is usually self-limiting and nonpharmacologic treatments such as ice packs and rest should be used for mild symptoms. Anti-inflammatory creams, ointments, patches, suppositories, and intranasal sprays are used for inflammation of the skin and mucous membranes of the mouth, nose, rectum and vagina. Many of these are available over the counter (OTC).

2. The goal is to prevent or decrease the intensity of the inflammatory response and reduce fever. Common diseases that benefit from anti-inflammatory agents include allergic rhinitis, anaphylaxis, ankylosing spondylitis, contact dermatitis, Crohn's disease, glomerulonephritis, Hashimoto's thyroiditis, peptic ulcer disease, rheumatoid arthritis, systemic lupus erythematosus, and ulcerative colitis.

LEARNING OUTCOME 5

Compare and contrast the actions and adverse effects of the different nonsteroidal anti-inflammatory drugs (NSAIDs).

Concepts for Lecture

1. Nonsteroidal anti-inflammatory drugs (NSAIDs) are the primary drugs for the treatment of simple inflammation. This drug class includes aspirin, ibuprofen, and COX-2 inhibitors (see Table 33.2). All have about the same efficacy, but the side effects vary. All are also analgesics and antipyretics. Acetaminophen has no anti-inflammatory action and *is not an NSAID*.

2. There are two forms of the enzyme cyclooxygenase (COX) (see Table 33.3). Cyclooxygenase-1 (COX-1) is present in all tissues. It reduces gastric-acid secretion, promotes renal blood flow, and promotes platelet aggregation. Inhibition of COX-1 results in bleeding, gastric upset, and reduced renal function. Cyclooxygenase-2 (COX-2) is present at sites of injury. It promotes inflammation, sensitizes pain receptors, and mediates fever in the brain. Inhibition of COX-2 results in suppression of inflammation.

3. Aspirin treats inflammation by inhibiting both COX-1 and COX-2. It is readily available, inexpensive, and effective. Large doses are needed to relieve severe inflammation. Adverse effects include irritation to the digestive system, bleeding, and salicylism (tinnitus, dizziness, headache, excessive perspiration).

SUGGESTION FOR CLINICAL ACTIVITIES

- Assign several students to care for patients with inflammatory disorders and several to care for patients with gastrointestinal disorders who are taking histamine 2 receptor blockers. Discuss how the two types of histamine receptors affect the body.

POWERPOINT SLIDES

SUGGESTION FOR CLASSROOM ACTIVITIES

- Direct students to identify other conditions for which anti-inflammatory agents are used.

SUGGESTION FOR CLINICAL ACTIVITIES

- Assign students to care for patients being treated with anti-inflammatory agents.

POWERPOINT SLIDES

Table 33.2 Selected Nonsteroidal Anti-inflammatory Drugs
Table 33.3 Forms of Cyclooxygenase

SUGGESTION FOR CLASSROOM ACTIVITIES

- Direct students to make posters that compare and contrast actions and side effects of the NSAIDs.

SUGGESTION FOR CLINICAL ACTIVITIES

- Assign students to observe the medication-administration records for their assigned patients. Note the frequency and indications for nonsteroidal anti-inflammatory drugs. How are these drugs used in your medical facilities? Is acetaminophen used as frequently?

4. Ibuprofen is an alternative to aspirin. It inhibits COX-1 and COX-2. A common side effect is nausea and vomiting. Ibuprofen causes less gastric irritation and bleeding than aspirin.

5. COX-2 inhibitors are the newest and most controversial class. They do not inhibit COX-1; thus, they do not affect blood coagulation and do not irritate the digestive system. They were the treatment of choice for moderate to severe inflammation until 2004 when rofecoxib (Vioxx) was found to double the risk of heart attack and stroke and was subsequently removed from the market. Valdecoxib (Bextra) was also removed in 2005. Celecoxib (Celebrex) is the only remaining COX-2 inhibitor.

LEARNING OUTCOME 6

Explain the role of glucocorticoids in the pharmacologic management of inflammation.

Concepts for Lecture

Systemic glucocorticoids are effective in treating acute or severe inflammation. They are naturally released from the adrenal cortex, suppress histamine and prostaglandins, and can inhibit the immune system to reduce inflammation. (See Table 33.4 for a list of glucocorticoids.) Serious adverse effects may include suppression of adrenal-gland function, hyperglycemia, mood changes, cataracts, peptic ulcers, electrolyte imbalances, and osteoporosis. Glucocorticoids can also mask infections; this creates the potential for existing infections to grow rapidly and undetected. For this reason, glucocorticoids are contraindicated in active infections. Glucocorticoids are used for short-term treatment of acute inflammation. If they are absolutely necessary for long-term treatment, the dose is kept as low as possible, and use of alternate-day dosing is established. Cushing's syndrome may result when glucocorticoids are used long term. They must be gradually discontinued.

LEARNING OUTCOME 7

For each of the classes listed in Drugs at a Glance, know representative drugs, and explain their mechanisms of drug action, primary actions related to inflammation and fever, and important adverse effects.

Concepts for Lecture

1. **Anti-inflammatory Drugs—NSAIDs.** Prototype drug: ibuprofen (Advil, Motrin, others). Mechanism of action: to inhibit prostaglandin synthesis. Primary use: for musculoskeletal disorders such as rheumatoid arthritis and osteoarthritis, mild to moderate pain, reduction of fever, and primary dysmenorrheal pain. Adverse effects: nausea, heartburn, epigastric pain, and dizziness.

2. **Anti-inflammatory Drugs—Systemic Glucocorticoids.** Prototype drug: prednisone (Meticorten). Mechanism of action: being metabolized to an active form of glucocorticoids. Primary use: to treat inflammation. Adverse effects: Cushing's syndrome if used for long-term therapy.

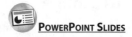 **POWERPOINT SLIDES**

 SUGGESTION FOR CLASSROOM ACTIVITIES

- Discuss the actions and side effects of glucocorticoids with a case study. Have students create concept maps of the case study.

 SUGGESTION FOR CLINICAL ACTIVITIES

- Assign students to care for patients taking glucocorticoids.

 POWERPOINT SLIDES

Table 33.2 Selected Nonsteroidal Anti-inflammatory Drugs
Table 33.4 Selected Glucocorticoids for Severe Inflammation

Prototype Drug
- ibuprofen (Advil, Motrin, others)
- prednisone (Meticorten)
- acetaminophen (Tylenol)

 ANIMATION AND VIDEOS

- Mechanism in Action: Acetaminophen (*Tylenol*)

© 2011 Pearson Education, Inc.

3. **Antipyretics.** Prototype drug: acetaminophen (Tylenol). Mechanism of action: to reduce fever by direct action at the level of the hypothalamus and dilation of peripheral blood vessels, which enables sweating and dissipation of heat. Primary use: to relieve pain and reduce fever. It has no anti-inflammatory properties. Adverse effects: possible liver damage. It has less gastric irritation than aspirin and does not affect blood coagulation.

LEARNING OUTCOME 8

Use the nursing process to care for patients receiving drug therapy for inflammation and fever.

Concepts for Lecture

1. **Assessment:** Obtain a complete health history (hepatic, renal, respiratory, cardiovascular or neurologic disease, pregnancy or breast-feeding), including data on origin of fever, recent surgeries, or trauma. Obtain baseline vital signs and weight. Obtain patient's complete medication history, including nicotine and alcohol consumption, herbal-supplement use, and use of alternative therapies, to determine possible drug allergies and/or interactions. Evaluate appropriate laboratory findings (e.g., CBC, coagulation panels, bleeding time, electrolytes, glucose, lipid profile, hepatic or renal function studies). Assess patient's ability to receive and understand instruction. Assess for and promptly report adverse effects: symptoms of GI bleeding (dark or "tarry" stools, hematemesis or coffee-ground emesis, blood in the stool), abdominal pain, severe tinnitus, dizziness, drowsiness, lightheadedness, confusion, agitation, euphoria or depression, palpitations, tachycardia, hypertension, increased respiratory rate and depth, pulmonary congestion, edema.
2. **Nursing Diagnoses:** *Pain; Hyperthermia; Risk for Injury* (hepatic toxicity); *Fluid Volume Deficit* related to fever; *Risk for Injury* related to adverse drug effects; *Risk for Infections* related to adverse drug effects of glucocorticoids; *Risk for Impaired Skin Integrity* related to adverse drug effects of glucocorticoids.
3. **Planning:** The patient will experience diminished fever, decreased or absent pain, decreased signs and symptoms of inflammation; be free from or experience minimal adverse effects. Verbalize an understanding of the drug's use, adverse effects, and required precautions. Demonstrate proper self-administration of the medication (e.g., dose, timing, when to notify provider).
4. **Implementation:** Assess for intolerance to ASA for possible cross-hypersensitivity to other NSAIDs or acetaminophen. Monitor hepatic and renal function. Monitor for abdominal pain and change in color of stool (gastrointestinal bleeding), hearing and balance (ototoxicity), and vision. Monitor electrolytes, blood-glucose and lipid levels periodically (hyperglycemia from corticosteroids). Monitor for signs and symptoms of infection in patients on corticosteroids. Monitor for osteoporosis and unusual changes in mood or affect in patients on corticosteroids. Weigh the patient on corticosteroids. Weigh the patient daily and report weight gain of 1 kg or more in a 24-hour period or more than 2 kg per week or increasing peripheral edema. Avoid use of aspirin or salicylates in children under 18. Do not stop corticosteroids abruptly. Use with caution in patients with a history of excessive alcohol consumption. Use with caution in patients with diabetes.

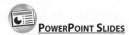
SUGGESTION FOR CLASSROOM ACTIVITIES

- Create a *Jeopardy*-like game for students to play based on the prototype drugs.

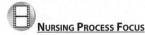
SUGGESTION FOR CLINICAL ACTIVITIES

- Direct students to create drug cards for each of the anti-inflammatory and antipyretic drugs given to their patients in clinical this week.

POWERPOINT SLIDES

NURSING PROCESS FOCUS

- Care for patients receiving drug therapy for inflammation and fever

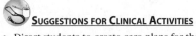
SUGGESTION FOR CLASSROOM ACTIVITIES

- Divide students into small groups, and have each group develop a teaching plan for a patient receiving drug therapy for fever.

SUGGESTIONS FOR CLINICAL ACTIVITIES

- Direct students to create care plans for their patients who are exhibiting fevers.

5. **Evaluation:** The patient experiences diminished fever, decreased or absent pain, decreased signs and symptoms of inflammation; is free from or experiences minimal adverse effects. Verbalizes an understanding of the drug's use, adverse effects, and required precautions. Demonstrates proper self-administration of the medication (e.g., dose, timing, when to notify provider).

GENERAL CHAPTER CONSIDERATIONS

1. Have students study and learn key terms listed at the beginning of the chapter.
2. Have students complete end-of-chapter exercises either in their book or on the MyNursingKit website.
3. Use the Classroom Response Questions provided in PowerPoint to assess students prior to lecture.

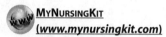

MyNursingKit
(*www.mynursingkit.com*)
- Websites
- NCLEX® questions
- Critical Thinking Questions
- Case Studies
- Animations and Videos
- Drug Prototype Questions

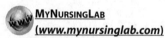

MyNursingLab
(*www.mynursinglab.com*)
- Knowledge Quick Check
- Pre/Posttests
- Customized study plans
- *Separate purchase*

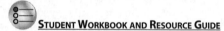

STUDENT WORKBOOK AND RESOURCE GUIDE
- Chapter 33 activities
- *Separate purchase*

PEARSON NURSE'S DRUG GUIDE
- *Separate purchase*

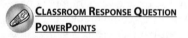

PEARSON eTEXT
- Students can search, highlight, take notes, and more all in electronic format.
- *Separate purchase*

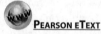

CLASSROOM RESPONSE QUESTION POWERPOINTS

TESTBANK

© 2011 Pearson Education, Inc.

CHAPTER 34
DRUGS FOR BACTERIAL INFECTIONS

LEARNING OUTCOME 1

Distinguish between the terms pathogenicity and virulence.

Concepts for Lecture

1. Pathogens are organisms that can cause disease by bypassing the body's defenses. Examples of some pathogens are bacteria, viruses, fungi, intracellular organisms, and multicellular animals. Pathogens generally cause disease by one of two basic mechanisms: invasiveness or toxin production. **Invasiveness** is the ability of a pathogen to grow extremely rapidly and cause direct damage to surrounding tissues by their sheer numbers. The second mechanism is the production of toxins. Even very small amounts of some bacterial toxins may disrupt normal cellular activity and, in extreme cases, result in death.
2. Pathogenicity is the ability of an organism to cause infection. Virulence is the ability of a microbe to produce disease when present in minute numbers.

LEARNING OUTCOME 2

Explain how bacteria are described and classified.

Concepts for Lecture

Bacteria are described by their shape—bacilli (rod shape), cocci (spherical), or spirilla (spiral); their ability to utilize oxygen—aerobic (with oxygen) or anaerobic (without), and by their staining characteristics—gram positive or gram negative.

LEARNING OUTCOME 3

Compare and contrast the terms bacteriostatic and bacteriocidal.

Concepts for Lecture

1. Anti-infective drugs are known as antibacterial, antimicrobial, or antibiotic. They are classified by their chemical structures (e.g., aminoglycoside, fluoroquinolone) or by their mechanism of action (e.g., cell-wall

POWERPOINT SLIDES

SUGGESTION FOR CLASSROOM ACTIVITIES
- Discuss how pathogens can cause disease.

SUGGESTION FOR CLINICAL ACTIVITIES
- During clinical, direct students to interview a patient with an infection to present at post-clinical.

POWERPOINT SLIDES

Table 34.1 Common Bacterial Pathogens and Disorders

SUGGESTION FOR CLASSROOM ACTIVITIES
- Bring models, pictures, or diagrams of bacteria in a microscopic view. Discuss gram stain and shape of the bacteria.

SUGGESTION FOR CLINICAL ACTIVITIES
- Assign students to spend time in the pathology department or laboratory department at the clinical facility. Direct the student to report on how bacteria are identified in the laboratory.

POWERPOINT SLIDES

Table 34.1 Bacterial Pathogens and Disorders.
Figure 34.1 Mechanisms of Action of Antimicrobial Drugs

inhibitor, folic-acid inhibitor). (See Table 34.1 for a look at bacterial pathogens and disorders.)

2. Anti-infective drugs act by affecting the target organism's unique structure, metabolism, or life cycle. The goal is to eliminate the pathogen by bactericidal properties (to kill bacteria) or bacteriostatic properties (to slow the growth of bacteria). (See Figure 34.1 for Mechanisms of action of antimicrobial drugs.)

SUGGESTION FOR CLASSROOM ACTIVITIES

- Discuss how antibiotics work by targeting the differences in bacterial cells from human cells.

SUGGESTION FOR CLINICAL ACTIVITIES

- Assign students to spend time in the pharmacy to observe all the different types of anti-infectives. Direct the student to report on a particular aspect of an anti-infective at post-clinical.

LEARNING OUTCOME 4

Using a specific example, explain how resistance can develop to an anti-infective drug.

Concepts for Lecture

1. Acquired resistance occurs when a pathogen acquires a gene for bacterial resistance, either through mutation or from another microbe. Through mutation, the antibiotics destroy sensitive bacteria, and insensitive (mutated) bacteria remain. Mutations are random and occur during cell division; mutated bacteria multiply. It is important to remember that antibiotics do not create mutations. Acquired resistance can also be caused by another microbe when resistant bacteria are passed to others.

2. The widespread use of antibiotics has not caused resistance, but over-prescribing of antibiotics has worsened the problem because it results in loss of antibiotic effectiveness. Practitioners should only prescribe when necessary. Long-time use increases resistant strains. Nosocomial infections are often resistant. Prophylactic use is sometimes appropriate. The nurse should instruct the patient to take the full dose. (See Figure 34.2 for an illustration of acquired resistance.)

POWERPOINT SLIDES

Figure 34.2 An Illustration of Acquired Resistance

SUGGESTION FOR CLASSROOM ACTIVITIES

- Direct students to concept map bacterial resistance.

SUGGESTION FOR CLINICAL ACTIVITIES

- Direct students to research the most common type of nosocomial infection at their clinical site. Research this topic on the CDC website; are the findings the same?

LEARNING OUTCOME 5

Describe the nurse's role in the pharmacologic management of bacterial infections.

Concepts for Lecture

1. The role of the nurse in the pharmacologic management of bacterial infections involves careful monitoring of a patient's condition and providing education as it relates to the prescribed drug treatment. Obtain baseline medical, surgical, and drug history; lifestyle and dietary habits, including use of herbal or alternative therapies; and a detailed description of symptomology and current therapies. Obtain specimens for culture and sensitivity prior to the start of antibiotic therapy. Monitor for indications of response to therapy, including reduced fever, normal WBC count, improved appetite, and absence of symptoms such as cough. After parenteral administration, observe the patient for possible allergic reactions for 30 minutes, especially with the first dose. Monitor for superinfections. Replacement of natural colon flora with probiotic supplements or cultured dairy products such as yogurt or buttermilk may help to alleviate symptoms. Teach patients to wear medic alert bracelets if allergic to antibiotics, to report any symptoms

POWERPOINT SLIDES

SUGGESTION FOR CLASSROOM ACTIVITIES

- Discuss the role of the nurse in monitoring patients who are taking drugs for bacterial infections.

SUGGESTION FOR CLINICAL ACTIVITIES

- Direct students to create a teaching plan for the patient taking drugs for bacterial infections.

© 2011 Pearson Education, Inc.

of an allergic reaction, and to not stop taking the drug until the complete prescription has been taken.

2. **Drug therapy with penicillins:** Assess previous drug reactions to penicillin. If the patient has a history of a severe penicillin allergic reaction, also avoid cephalosporins. Monitor for hyperkalemia and hypernatremia. Monitor cardiac status, including ECG changes.

3. **Cephalosporin therapy:** Assess for the presence or history of bleeding disorders because cephalosporins may reduce prothrombin levels through interference with vitamin K metabolism. Assess renal and hepatic function. Avoid alcohol; some cephalosporins cause a disulfiram (Antabuse)–like reaction when alcoholic beverages are consumed.

4. **Tetracycline therapy:** This is contraindicated for use with patients who are pregnant and lactating because of the drug's effect on linear skeletal growth of the fetus and child. Tetracycline therapy is also contraindicated in children less than 8 years of age because of the drug's ability to cause permanent mottling and discoloration of the teeth. Tetracyclines decrease the effectiveness of oral contraceptives, so advise female patients to use an alternate method of birth control while taking the medication. Use with caution in patients with impaired kidney or liver function. Tetracyclines cause photosensitivity. Do not take these medications with milk products, iron supplements, magnesium-containing laxatives, or antacids.

5. **Macrolide therapy:** Assess for the presence of respiratory infection. Examine the patient for history of cardiac disorders, because macrolides may exacerbate existing heart disease. Monitor hepatic enzymes with certain macrolides, such as erythromycin estolate. Multiple drug–drug interactions occur with macrolides.

6. **Aminoglycoside therapy:** Monitor for ototoxicity and nephrotoxicity during the course of therapy. Hearing loss may occur after therapy has been completed. Neuromuscular function may also be impaired. Increase fluid intake, unless otherwise contraindicated, to promote excretion.

7. **Fluoroquinolone therapy:** Because these agents may decrease leukocytes, monitor the WBC count. Carefully monitor patients with liver and renal dysfunction, because the drug is metabolized by the liver and excreted by the kidneys. Inform the patient that these drugs may cause dizziness and lightheadedness and advise against driving or performing hazardous tasks during drug therapy. Inform patients receiving norfloxacin (Noroxin) that photophobia is possible. Some fluoroquinolones, such as ciprofloxacin (Cipro), may affect tendons, especially in children.

8. **Sulfonamide therapy:** Assess for anemia or other hematological disorders, because sulfonamides may cause hemolytic anemia and blood dyscrasias. Assess renal function, because sulfonamides may increase the risk for crystalluria. Avoid administering these agents in patients with a history of hypersensitivity to sulfonamides, because this can induce a skin abnormality called Stevens–Johnson syndrome. Avoid exposure to direct sunlight; use sunscreen and protective clothing to decrease the effects of photosensitivity.

9. **Antituberculosis therapy:** Assess the patient for a history of alcohol abuse, AIDS, liver disease, or kidney disease, because many antituberculosis drugs are contraindicated in those conditions. Use caution in patients with renal dysfunction, those who are pregnant or lactating, or those with a history of convulsive disorders. Assess for gouty arthritis. Because some antituberculosis drugs interact with oral contraceptives and decrease their effectiveness, female patients with childbearing potential should use an alternate form of birth control while using these medications. If taking isoniazid, avoid foods containing tyramine, such as aged cheese, smoked and pickled fish, beer and red wine, bananas, and chocolate.

© 2011 Pearson Education, Inc.

LEARNING OUTCOME 6

Explain the importance of culture and sensitivity testing to anti-infective chemotherapy.

Concepts for Lecture

1. Careful selection of the correct antibiotic, through the use of culture and sensitivity testing, is essential for effective pharmacotherapy and to limit adverse effects. Broad-spectrum antibiotics are effective for a wide variety of bacteria. Narrow-spectrum antibiotics are effective for a narrow group of bacteria.
2. Culture and sensitivity testing is examination of a specimen for microorganisms. The specimen is grown in the lab and identified. It is tested for sensitivity to different antibiotics. Bacteria may take several days to identify. Viruses may take several weeks to identify. Broad-spectrum antibiotics may be started before the lab culture is completed.

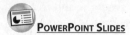 **POWERPOINT SLIDES**

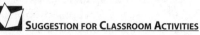 **SUGGESTION FOR CLASSROOM ACTIVITIES**

- Discuss the process of culture and sensitivity testing.

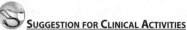 **SUGGESTION FOR CLINICAL ACTIVITIES**

- Assign students to spend part of a clinical day in the medical laboratory to observe the process of culture and sensitivity testing.

LEARNING OUTCOME 7

Identify the mechanism of development and symptoms of superinfections caused by anti-infective therapy.

Concepts for Lecture

1. **Multidrug therapy** may be affected by antagonism, which occurs when combining two drugs decreases the efficacy of each of the drugs. Use of multiple antibiotics increases the risk of resistance. Multidrug therapy can be used when multiorganisms cause the infection, for the treatment of tuberculosis, for the treatment of HIV.
2. **Superinfections** are secondary infections that may occur during antibiotic therapy if too many host flora are killed by an antibiotic. Host flora prevent the growth of pathogenic organisms. Pathogenic microorganisms have a chance to multiply when they can opportunistically take advantage of a suppressed immune system. Signs and symptoms include diarrhea, bladder pain, painful urination, or abnormal vaginal discharge.
3. Host factors such as immune-system status, local conditions at the infection site, allergic reactions, age, pregnancy status, and genetics influence the choice of antibiotic.

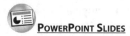 **POWERPOINT SLIDES**

 SUGGESTION FOR CLASSROOM ACTIVITIES

- Discuss the etiology and manifestations of superinfections.

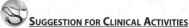 **SUGGESTION FOR CLINICAL ACTIVITIES**

- Assign students to care for a patient with a superinfection.

LEARNING OUTCOME 8

For each of the drug classes listed in Drugs at a Glance, know representative drug examples, and explain their mechanism of action, primary actions, and important adverse effects.

Concepts for Lecture

1. **Penicillin.** Prototype drug: penicillin G (Pentids). Mechanism of action: to kill bacteria by disrupting their cell walls. Primary use: as the drug of choice against streptococci, pneumococci, and staphylococci organisms that do not produce penicillinase; also a medication of choice for gonorrhea and syphilis. Adverse effects: diarrhea, nausea, and vomiting; superinfections; and anaphylaxis. (See Table 34.2.)

POWERPOINT SLIDES

Table 34.2 Penicillins
Table 34.3 Cephalosporins
Table 34.4 Tetracyclines
Table 34.5 Macrolides
Table 34.6 Aminoglycosides
Table 34.7 Fluoroquinolones
Table 34.8 Sulfonamides
Table 34.9 Selected Miscellaneous Antibacterials

© 2011 Pearson Education, Inc.

2. **Cephalosporin.** Prototype drug: cefotaxime (Claforan). Mechanism of action: to act as a third-generation cephalosporin with a broad spectrum of activity against gram-negative organisms. Primary use: to be effective against many bacterial species that have developed resistance to earlier-generation cephalosporins—serious infections of the lower respiratory tract, central nervous system, genitourinary system, bones, blood, and joints. Adverse effects: hypersensitivity, anaphylaxis, diarrhea, vomiting, nausea, and pain at the injection site. (See Table 34.3.)

3. **Tetracycline.** Prototype drug: tetracycline HCL (Achromycin, others). Mechanism of action: to be effective against a broad range of gram-positive and gram-negative organisms. Primary use: for chlamydiae, rickettsiae, and mycoplasma. Adverse effects: superinfections. Tetracycline irritates the GI mucosa and may cause nausea, vomiting, epigastric burning, diarrhea, discoloration of the teeth, and photosensitivity. (See Table 34.4.)

4. **Macrolide.** Prototype drug: erythromycin (E-Mycin, Erythrocin). Mechanism of action: to act as a spectrum similar to that of the penicillins and to be effective against most gram-positive bacteria. Primary use: as the preferred drug for infections of *Bordetella pertussis* (whooping cough), *Corynebacterium diphtheriae*, and most gram-positive bacteria. Adverse effects: nausea, abdominal cramping, and vomiting. The most severe adverse effect is hepatotoxicity. (See Table 34.5.)

5. **Aminoglycoside.** Prototype drug: gentamicin (Garamycin). Mechanism of action: to act as a broad-spectrum, bacteriocidal antibiotic. Primary use: for serious urinary, respiratory, nervous, or GI infections when less-toxic antibiotics are contraindicated. It is often used in combination with other antibiotics or when drugs from other classes have proven ineffective. It is used parenterally, or as drops (Genoptic), for eye infections. Adverse effects: ototoxicity and nephrotoxicity. (See Table 34.6.)

6. **Fluoroquinolone.** Prototype drug: ciprofloxacin (Cipro). Mechanism of action: to inhibit bacterial DNA gyrase, thus affecting bacterial replication and DNA repair. Primary use: to be more effective against gram-negative than gram-positive organisms. It is prescribed for respiratory infections, bone and joint infections, GI infections, ophthalmic infections, sinusitis, and prostatitis. Adverse effects: nausea, vomiting, diarrhea, phototoxicity, headache, and dizziness. (See Table 34.7.)

7. **Sulfonamide.** Prototype drug: trimethoprim-sulfamethoxazole (Bactrim, Septra). Mechanism of action: to kill bacteria by inhibiting bacterial metabolism of folic acid, or folate. Primary use: for urinary tract infections. It is also approved for the treatment of *Pneumocystis carinii* pneumonia, for shigella infections of the small bowel, and for acute episodes of chronic bronchitis. Adverse effects: skin rashes, nausea, vomiting, agranulocytosis, or thrombocytopenia. (See Table 34.8.).

8. **Miscellaneous.** Examples of miscellaneous antibiotics are clindamycin (Cleocin)—used for oral infections caused by bacteriocides. An adverse effect associated with clindamycin is pseudomembranous colitis. Metronidazole (Flagyl) is used to treat *H. pylori* infections of the stomach; vancomycin (Vancocin)—effective for MRSA infections; adverse effects include ototoxicity, nephrotoxicity, and red man syndrome. **Some of the new miscellaneous antibiotics are:** *Oxazolidinones*—linezolid (Zyvox) is as effective as vancomycin against MRSA; *Cyclic lipopeptides*—daptomycin (Cubicin) is used to treat serious skin infections; *Carbapenems*—imipenem (Primaxin) has some of the broadest spectrums; *Ketolides*—telithromycin (Ketek) is used for respiratory infections; *Glycylcyclines*—tigecycline (Tygacil) is used for drug-resistant abdominal infections and complicated skin infections. (See Table 34.9.)

Prototype Drug
- penicillin G (Pentids)
- cefotaxime (Claforan)
- tetracycline HCL (Achromycin, others)
- erythromycin (E-Mycin, Erythrocin)
- gentamicin (Garamycin)
- ciprofloxacin (Cipro)
- trimethoprim-sulfamethoxazole (Bactrim, Septra)

ANIMATIONS AND VIDEOS
- Mechanism in Action: Penicillin (Pentids)
- Mechanism in Action: Ciprofloxacin (Cipro)

SUGGESTION FOR CLASSROOM ACTIVITIES
- Have each student make drug cards for each classification of drug used to treat bacterial infections. Use two different drugs for each classification. The card should include actions, uses, routes of administration, dosages, and adverse effects.

SUGGESTION FOR CLINICAL ACTIVITIES
- Divide students into small groups, and have each group develop a teaching plan for a patient receiving medications for a bacterial infection.

© 2011 Pearson Education, Inc.

LEARNING OUTCOME 9

Explain how the pharmacotherapy of tuberculosis differs from that of other infections.

Concepts for Lecture

1. Tuberculosis is caused by *Mycobacterium tuberculosis*. Its cell wall is resistant to anti-infectives, so the body's immune response attempts to isolate the pathogen by walling it off. Tuberculosis may remain dormant in walled-off areas called tubercles, but a decreased immune system can give tuberculosis the opportunity to become active.

2. Therapy is long term. Six to twelve months of drug therapy is needed to reach isolated pathogens in the tubercles, and the therapy must be continued for the full course even if there are no symptoms. Patients with multidrug-resistant infections require therapy for 24 months. Multidrug therapy consists of two to four antibiotics that are administered concurrently. Multiple-drug therapies are needed in the treatment of tuberculosis because the complex microbes are slow growing and commonly develop drug resistance. Therapy is initiated with first-choice drugs, and then when resistance develops, second-choice drugs are used. The second-choice drugs are more toxic and less effective than first-choice drugs.

3. Chemoprophylaxis means that antituberculosis drugs are used prophylactically in high-risk populations. Close contacts and family members of recently infected tuberculosis patients begin therapy immediately after a patient has a positive tuberculin test. Patients with AIDS, those who are HIV-positive, or those who are receiving immunosuppressant drugs also receive therapy.

LEARNING OUTCOME 10

Use the nursing process to care for patients who are receiving drug therapy for bacterial infections.

Concepts for Lecture

1. **Patients Receiving Antibacterial Therapy—Assessment:** Obtain a complete health history including allergies, drug history, and possible drug interactions. Assess signs and symptoms of current infection noting location, characteristics, presence or absence of drainage and character of drainage, duration, presence or absence of fever or pain. Evaluate appropriate laboratory findings (e.g., CBC, culture and sensitivity, hepatic and renal function studies). Report immediately severe diarrhea, especially containing mucus, blood, or pus, yellowing of sclera or skin decreased urine output or darkened urine. Assess for possibility of pregnancy or breast-feeding in patients prescribed tetracycline antibiotics.

2. **Patients Receiving Antibacterial Therapy—Nursing diagnoses:** *Infection; Pain*, related to infection; *Hyperthermia; Deficient Knowledge* (drug therapy); *Risk for Injury*, related to adverse drug effects; *Risk for Deficient Fluid Volume*, related to fever, diarrhea caused by adverse drug effects; *Risk for Noncompliance*, related to adverse drug effects, deficient knowledge, or cost of medication.

3. **Patients Receiving Antibacterial Therapy—Planning:** The patient will report diminished signs and symptoms of infection, decreased fever; be free from or experience minimal adverse effects. Verbalize an understanding of the drug's use, adverse effects, and required precautions. Demonstrate proper self-administration of the medication (e.g., dose, timing, when to notify provider).

 POWERPOINT SLIDES

 SUGGESTION FOR CLASSROOM ACTIVITIES

- Discuss reasons why patients with tuberculosis are often noncompliant with the prescribed drug therapy.

SUGGESTION FOR CLINICAL ACTIVITIES

- Assign students to spend clinical time at the local public health agency. Have them research the policies and plan for a tuberculosis outbreak at the local university. What are the admission policies at a university regarding tuberculosis screening? How does this affect students from foreign countries?

 POWERPOINT SLIDES

 NURSING PROCESS FOCUS

- Patients Receiving Antibacterial Therapy
- Patients Receiving Antituberculosis Agents

 SUGGESTION FOR CLASSROOM ACTIVITIES

- Divide students into small groups, and have each group develop a teaching plan for a patient receiving drug therapy for bacterial infections.

 SUGGESTION FOR CLINICAL ACTIVITIES

- Assign students to review the care plans on their patients who are receiving drug therapy for bacterial infections. Have each student suggest one way in which he or she can contribute.

© 2011 Pearson Education, Inc.

4. **Patients Receiving Antibacterial Therapy—Implementation:** Monitor vital signs and symptoms of infection to determine antibacterial effectiveness. Monitor for hypersensitivity and allergic reaction. Monitor for severe diarrhea. Monitor periodic lab work: hepatic and renal function tests, CBC, urinalysis, culture and sensitivity, peak and trough drug levels. Administer drug around the clock. Monitor for superinfection. Monitor intake of OTC products such as antacids, calcium supplements, iron products, and laxatives containing magnesium. Monitor for photosensitivity. Monitor for hepatic, renal, and/or ototoxicity (e.g., jaundice, RUQ pain, darkened urine, diminished urine output, tinnitus, vertigo). Determine the interactions of the prescribed antibiotics with various foods and beverages. Monitor IV site for signs and symptoms of tissue irritation, severe pain, and extravasation. Monitor for side effects, renal function, symptoms of ototoxicity, and compliance with antibiotic therapy. Monitor for development of "Red Man" syndrome in patients receiving vancomycin.

5. **Patients Receiving Antibacterial Therapy—Evaluation: Planning:** The patient will report diminished signs and symptoms of infection, decreased fever; be free from or experience minimal adverse effects. Verbalize an understanding of the drug's use, adverse effects, and required precautions. Demonstrate proper self-administration of the medication (e.g., dose, timing, when to notify provider).

6. **Patients Receiving Antituberculosis Agents—Assessment:** Obtain a complete health history including allergies, drug history, and possible drug interactions. Assess signs and symptoms of current infection noting symptoms, duration, or any recent changes. Assess for concurrent infections, particularly HIV. Assess for presence or history of tuberculosis, immunosuppressant status, and kidney or liver disease. Assess cognitive ability to comply with long-term therapy. Evaluate appropriate laboratory findings (e.g., CBC, AFB culture and sensitivity, hepatic and renal function studies).

7. **Patients Receiving Antituberculosis Agents—Nursing diagnoses:** *Infection; Fatigue; Imbalanced Nutrition, Less than Body Requirements,* related to fatigue, adverse drug effects; *Deficient Knowledge* (drug therapy, infection control measures); *Risk for Noncompliance,* related to adverse drug effects, deficient knowledge, length of treatment required, or cost of medication; *Risk for Social Isolation,* related to disease, length of treatment.

8. **Patients Receiving Antituberculosis Agents—Planning:** The patient will report diminished signs and symptoms of infection, decreased fever and fatigue, increased appetite). Be free from or experience minimal adverse effects. Verbalize an understanding of the drug's use, adverse effects and required precautions. Demonstrate proper self-administration of the medication (e.g., dose, timing, when to notify provider).

9. **Patients Receiving Antituberculosis Agents—Implementation:** Monitor for hepatic side effects. Monitor for neurologic side effects. Collect sputum specimens. Monitor for dietary compliance when patient is taking isoniazid. Monitor for side effects specific to various antituberculosis drugs. Monitor for hepatic, renal, and/or ototoxicity (e.g., jaundice, RUQ pain, darkened urine, diminished urine output, tinnitus, vertigo). Establish infection-control measures. Establish therapeutic environment to ensure adequate rest, nutrition, hydration, and relaxation. Monitor patient's ability and motivation to comply with therapeutic regimen.

10. **Patients Receiving Antituberculosis Agents—Evaluation:** The patient reports diminished signs and symptoms of infection, decreased fever and fatigue, increased appetite). Is free from or experiences minimal adverse effects. Verbalizes an understanding of the drug's use, adverse effects, and required precautions. Demonstrates proper self-administration of the medication (e.g., dose, timing, when to notify provider).

© 2011 Pearson Education, Inc.

GENERAL CHAPTER CONSIDERATIONS

1. Have students study and learn key terms listed at the beginning of the chapter.
2. Have students complete end-of-chapter exercises either in their book or on the MyNursingKit website.
3. Use the Classroom Response Questions provided in PowerPoint to assess students prior to lecture.

MYNURSINGKIT
(www.mynursingkit.com)

- Websites
- NCLEX® questions
- Critical Thinking Questions
- Case Studies
- Animations and Videos
- Drug Prototype Questions

MYNURSINGLAB
(www.mynursinglab.com)

- Knowledge Quick Check
- Pre/Posttests
- Customized study plans
- *Separate purchase*

STUDENT WORKBOOK AND RESOURCE GUIDE

- Chapter 34 activities
- *Separate purchase*

PEARSON NURSE'S DRUG GUIDE

- *Separate purchase*

PEARSON ETEXT

- Students can search, highlight, take notes, and more all in electronic format.
- *Separate purchase*

CLASSROOM RESPONSE QUESTION
POWERPOINTS

TESTBANK

© 2011 Pearson Education, Inc.

CHAPTER 35
DRUGS FOR FUNGAL, PROTOZOAL, AND HELMINTHIC INFECTIONS

LEARNING OUTCOME 1

Compare and contrast the pharmacotherapy of superficial and systemic fungal infections.

Concepts for Lecture

Fungi are single-celled or multicellular organisms. They are more complex than bacteria and include mushrooms, yeasts, and molds; their purpose is to decompose dead organisms. (See Table 35.1 for a list of fungi.) Humans are exposed to fungi when they handle contaminated soil or inhale spores. Fungal infections are classified as superficial or systemic. The superficial infections affect hair, skin, nails, and mucous membranes and are treated with topical agents. The systemic infections affect internal organs, are less common, and can be fatal in immunosuppressed patients; systemic infections are treated with oral or parenteral agents. Fungi are unaffected by most antibiotics.

LEARNING OUTCOME 2

Identify the types of patients who are at greatest risk for acquiring serious fungal infections.

Concepts for Lecture

The human body is quite resistant to fungi. Most serious fungal infections occur in patients with suppressed immune defenses; for example, a patient with HIV. Community-acquired infections can affect those with intact immune systems. Opportunistic infections are those nosocomial infections that occur in the immunosuppressed patient. (See Table 35.1.)

LEARNING OUTCOME 3

Identify protozoan and helminthic infections that may benefit from pharmacotherapy.

Concepts for Lecture

1. **Protozoans** are single-celled animals that cause disease in Africa, South America, and Asia. They thrive in areas of poor sanitation, and travelers may transmit the organisms. Drugs used to treat bacterial and fungal infections are ineffective.
2. **Malaria** is the most common protozoal disease and the second most fatal infectious disease in the world. It is caused by the protozoan *Plasmodium* and transmitted by the bite of a female *Anopheles* mosquito. Malaria requires multidrug therapy due to the complicated life

POWERPOINT SLIDES

Table 35.1 Fungal Pathogens

SUGGESTION FOR CLASSROOM ACTIVITIES

• Compare and contrast superficial and systemic fungal infections.

SUGGESTION FOR CLINICAL ACTIVITIES

• Assign students to locate the infection-control manual at clinical and research the policies on fungal infections.

POWERPOINT SLIDES

Table 35.1 Fungal Pathogens

SUGGESTION FOR CLASSROOM ACTIVITIES

• Discuss how fungal infections develop in patients with suppressed immune systems.

SUGGESTION FOR CLINICAL ACTIVITIES

• Assign students to care for patients with fungal infections.

POWERPOINT SLIDES

Figure 35.1 Life Cycle of *Plasmodium*
Table 35.6 Nonmalarial Protozoal Infections

SUGGESTION FOR CLASSROOM ACTIVITIES

• Discuss the different types of protozoal and helminthic infections. Note the most common geographical locations.

cycle of the parasite. Drugs may be administered for prophylaxis, as therapy for acute attacks, and for prevention of relapses. (See Figure 35.1 for the life cycle of *Plasmodium*.)

3. **Goals of antimalarial therapy** include prevention, treatment, and prevention of relapse. Prevention includes the Centers for Disease Control recommendations for prophylactic antimalarials prior to, during, and for one week after visits to infested areas. The treatment interrupts the erythrocytic stage and eliminates the merozoites from red blood cells. Prevention of relapse involves elimination of the latent forms of *Plasmodium* residing in the liver.

4. **Nonmalarial protozoan infections** also thrive in unsanitary conditions. These other protozoal diseases include amebiasis, toxoplasmosis, giardiasis, cryptosporidiosis, trichomoniasis, trypanosomiasis, and leishmaniasis. (See Table 35.6 for a list of these infections.) Treatment of non-*Plasmodium* protozoan disease requires a different set of medications from those used for malaria.

5. **Helminths** are parasitic worms that cause significant disease in certain regions of the world. The group includes roundworms (nematodes), flukes (trematodes), tapeworms (cestodes), and enterobiasis (pinworms). Enterobiasis is the most common helminth infection in the United States. Most helminths enter the body through the skin or gastrointestinal tract. Pharmacotherapy for helminths is to kill the parasites locally and disrupt their life cycles. Resistance has not yet become a problem.

LEARNING OUTCOME 4

Explain how an understanding of the *Plasmodium* life cycle is important to the effective pharmacotherapy of malaria.

Concepts for Lecture

Pharmacotherapy of malaria attempts to interrupt the complex life cycle of *Plasmodium* (see Figure 35.1). The pharmacotherapy is aimed at prevention, treatment, and prevention of relapse. Prevention involves administering prophylactic antimalarials prior to, during, and for one week after visits to infested areas. Treatment involves interrupting the erythrocytic stage and eliminating the merozoites from red blood cells. Prevention of relapse means attempting to eliminate the latent forms of *Plasmodium* residing in the liver.

LEARNING OUTCOME 5

Describe the nurse's role in the pharmacologic management of fungal, protozoan, and helminth infections.

Concepts for Lecture

1. The role of the nurse in the pharmacologic management of fungal, protozoal, and helminth infections involves careful monitoring of a patient's condition and providing education as it relates to the prescribed drug treatment. Obtain baseline medical, surgical, and drug history; lifestyle and dietary habits, including use of herbal or alternative therapies; and a detailed description of symptomology and current therapies. Obtain baseline culture and sensitivity tests prior to the beginning of therapy. Contraindicated in patients with known hypersensitivity to the drugs.

 SUGGESTION FOR CLINICAL ACTIVITIES
- Assign students to small groups and have them design a patient-education pamphlet on pinworms.

 POWERPOINT SLIDES

Figure 35.1 Life cycle of *Plasmodium*

 SUGGESTION FOR CLASSROOM ACTIVITIES
- Direct students to draw a concept map of the life cycle of *Plasmodium*.

 SUGGESTION FOR CLINICAL ACTIVITIES
- Have students prepare a teaching plan that would be used to teach to patients on prevention of malaria.

 POWERPOINT SLIDES

 SUGGESTION FOR CLASSROOM ACTIVITIES
- Discuss the role of the nurse in monitoring patients who are taking drugs for fungal, protozoal, and helminth infections.

 SUGGESTION FOR CLINICAL ACTIVITIES
- Direct students to create a teaching plan for the patient taking drugs for fungal, protozoal, and helminth infections.

© 2011 Pearson Education, Inc.

2. **Systemic antifungal therapy:** This class of antifungal drugs should be used cautiously in those with renal impairment, patients with severe bone-marrow suppression, and patients who are pregnant. Amphotericin B (Fungizone) causes some degree of kidney damage in 80% of the patients who take it, so closely monitor fluid and electrolyte status. Amphotericin B can cause ototoxicity: assess for hearing loss, vertigo, unsteady gait, or tinnitus.

3. **Azole therapy:** Do not give ketoconazole (Nizoral) to patients with chronic alcoholism because this drug can be toxic to the liver. Assess for nausea, vomiting, abdominal pain, or diarrhea. Also monitor for signs and symptoms of hepatotoxicity, such as pruritus, jaundice, dark urine, and skin rash. Azoles may affect glycemic control in diabetic patients, so monitor blood-sugar levels carefully in these patients. Monitor for alcohol use because it increases the risk of side effects, such as nausea and vomiting, and increases blood pressure.

4. **Superficial antifungal therapy:** Assess for signs of contact dermatitis; if this is present, withhold the drug and notify the primary health care provider. Do not use superficial antifungals, such as nystatin (Mycostatin), intravaginally during pregnancy to treat infections caused by *Gardnerella vaginalis* or *Trichomonas* species; use cautiously in patients who are lactating. The medications may be "swished and swallowed" or "swished and spit" when used to treat oral candidiasis. Monitor for side effects such as nausea, vomiting, and diarrhea when the patient is taking high doses.

5. **Antiprotozoal drugs:** Contraindicated in patients with hematological disorders or severe skin disorders such as psoriasis or with patients who are pregnant. Use cautiously in patients with preexisting cardiovascular disease and those who are lactating. Test for G6PD deficiency. Chloroquine (Aralen) may precipitate anemia in those with G6PD deficiency and may cause bone-marrow depression. Obtain a baseline ECG because of potential cardiac complications associated with some antimalarial drugs. Monitor for GI side effects such as vomiting, diarrhea, and abdominal pain; oral antimalarials can be given with food to reduce GI distress. Monitor for signs of toxicity.

6. **Nonmalarial, antiprotozoal drug therapy:** Antiprotozoal therapy is contraindicated in patients with blood dyscrasias or active organic disease of the CNS and during the first month of pregnancy. These drugs are contraindicated in alcoholics; the medication is not administered until more than 24 hours after the patient's last drink of alcohol. Closely monitor vital signs and thyroid function during therapy, because serum iodine may increase and cause thyroid enlargement with iodoquinol (Yodoxin). Monitor for GI distress; oral medications can be given with food to decrease unpleasant effects. Patients taking metronidazole (Flagyl) may complain of dryness of the mouth and a metallic taste. Monitor for signs of CNS toxicity, such as seizures, paresthesia, nausea, and vomiting, and for allergic responses, such as urticaria and pruritus.

7. **Antihelminthic drugs:** Antihelminthic therapy should be used cautiously in patients who are pregnant or lactating, have preexisiting liver disease, or are younger than age 2. Identification of the specific worm must be done before treatment is initiated by analyzing samples of feces, urine, blood, sputum, or tissue. Monitor lab results; cases of leukopenia, thrombocytopenia, and agranulocytosis have been associated with the use of albendazole (Albenza). The patient needs to be educated on the nature of the worm infestation. Inform the patient that some types of worms will be expelled in stool as they are eradicated. Instruct the patient to take showers rather than baths and to change undergarment, linens, and towels daily.

© 2011 Pearson Education, Inc.

LEARNING OUTCOME 6

For each of the classes shown in Drugs at a Glance, know representative examples, and explain their mechanism of drug action, primary actions, and important adverse effects.

Concepts for Lecture

1. **Antifungal Drugs—Agents for Systemic Infections.** Prototype drug: amphotericin B (Fungizone). Mechanism of action: binds to ergosterol in fungal-cell membranes, causing them to become permeable or leaky. Primary use: has a wide spectrum of activity that includes most of the fungi pathogenic to humans. Adverse effects: fever and chills, vomiting, and headache at the beginning of therapy, which subside as treatment continues. Phlebitis is common during IV therapy. Some degree of nephrotoxicity is observed in most patients. Electrolyte imbalances frequently occur. Cardiac arrest, hypotension, and dysrhythmias are possible. (See Table 35.2.)

2. **Antifungal Drugs—Agents for Systemic Infections.** Prototype drug: fluconazole (Diflucan). Mechanism of action: to interfere with the synthesis of ergosterol. Primary use: to penetrate most body membranes to reach fungal infections in the CNS, bone, eyes, urinary tract, and respiratory tract. May not be effective against nonalbicans *Candida* species. Adverse effects: nausea, vomiting, and diarrhea with high doses. (See Table 35.3.)

3. **Antifungal Drugs—Superficial Infections.** Prototype drug: nystatin (Mycostatin). Mechanism of action: binds to sterols in the fungal-cell membrane, allowing leakage of intracellular contents. Primary use: topically used for *Candida* infections of the vagina, skin, and mouth. It may also be used orally to treat candidiasis of the intestine. Adverse effects: few, other than minor skin irritation; when given orally, it may cause nausea, vomiting, and diarrhea. (See Table 35.4.)

4. **Antiprotozoal Drugs—Antimalarial Agents.** Prototype drug: chloroquine (Aralen). Mechanism of action: concentrates in the food vacuoles of *Plasmodium* residing in red blood cells. Once in the vacuole, it is believed to prevent the metabolism of heme, which then builds to toxic levels within the parasite. Primary use: it has been the prototype medication for treating malaria for over 60 years. Adverse effects: nausea and diarrhea. At higher doses, CNS and cardiovascular toxicity may be observed. (See Table 35.5.)

5. **Antiprotozoal Drugs—Nonmalarial Antiprotozoal Agents.** Prototype drug: metronidazole (Flagyl). Mechanism of action: to act as an antiprotozoal drug that also has antibiotic activity against anaerobic bacteria. Primary use: to treat most forms of amebiasis. Adverse effects: anorexia, nausea, diarrhea, dizziness, and headache. Dryness of the mouth and an unpleasant metallic taste may be experienced. (Table 35.7.)

6. **Antihelminthic Drugs.** Prototype drug: mebendazole (Vermox). Mechanism of action: to act as a broad-spectrum antihelminthic drug. Primary use: in the treatment of a wide range of helminth infections. Adverse effects: few, but as the worms die, some abdominal pain, distension, and diarrhea may be experienced. (See Table 35.8.)

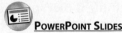

POWERPOINT SLIDES

Table 35.2 Drugs for Systemic Mycoses
Table 35.3 Azole Antifungals
Table 35.4 Selected Drugs for Superficial Mycoses
Table 35.5 Selected Drugs for Malaria
Table 35.7 Selected Drugs for Nonmalarial Protozoal Infections
Table 35.8 Selected Drugs for Helminthic Infections

Prototype Drug
- amphotericin B (Fungizone)
- fluconazole (Diflucan)
- nystatin (Mycostatin)
- chloroquine (Aralen)
- metronidazole (Flagyl)
- mebendazole (Vermox)

ANIMATIONS AND VIDEOS

- Mechanism in Action: Fluconazole (Diflucan)

SUGGESTIONS FOR CLASSROOM ACTIVITIES

- Have each student make drug cards for each classification of drug used to treat fungal, protozoal, and helminth infections. Use two different drugs for each classification. The card should include actions, uses, routes of administration, dosages, and adverse effects.
- Divide students into small groups and have each group develop a teaching plan for a patient receiving medications for fungal, protozoal, and helminth infections.

SUGGESTION FOR CLINICAL ACTIVITIES

- Assign students to care for patients receiving drugs for fungal, protozoal, and helminth infections during the clinical rotation. Use medication cards to explain drug class, action, adverse effects, and the usual dose to the clinical instructor.

© 2011 Pearson Education, Inc.

LEARNING OUTCOME 7

Use the nursing process to care for patients receiving drug therapy for fungal, protozoan, and helminth infections.

Concepts for Lecture

1. **Patients Receiving Amphotericin B—Assessment:** Obtain a complete health history, including allergies, drug history, allergies, and possible drug interactions. Assess signs and symptoms of current infection noting location, characteristics, presence or absence of drainage and character of drainage, duration, presence or absence of fever or pain. Obtain a culture and sensitivity of suspected area of infection to determine need for therapy. Obtain baseline vital signs, especially pulse and blood pressure. Obtain renal function including blood tests (CBC, chemistry panel, BUN, and creatinine).

2. **Patients Receiving Amphotericin B—Nursing Diagnoses:** *Infection* (current or risk for concurrent bacterial infection); *Pain,* related to infection; *Hyperthermia; Deficient Knowledge* (drug therapy); *Risk for Injury,* related to adverse drug effects; *Risk for Deficient Fluid Volume,* related to fever, diarrhea caused by adverse drug effects; *Risk for Decreased Cardiac Output, Ineffective Tissue Perfusion,* related to adverse effects of IV antifungals; *Risk for Noncompliance,* related to adverse drug effects, deficient knowledge, or length of therapy.

3. **Patients Receiving Amphotericin B—Planning:** Patient will experience therapeutic effects (e.g., diminished signs and symptoms of infection, decreased fever); be free from or experience minimal adverse effects. Verbalize an understanding of the drug's use, adverse effects, and required precautions. Demonstrate proper self-administration of the medication (e.g., dose, timing, when to notify provider).

4. **Patients Receiving Amphotericin B—Implementation:** Monitor vital signs frequently, especially pulse and blood pressure, during and after infusion. Monitor kidney function. Monitor for GI distress. Monitor for fluid overload and electrolyte imbalance, especially hypokalemia. Monitor for signs and symptoms of toxicity and hypersensitivity. Monitor IV site frequently for any signs of extravasation or thrombophlebitis.

5. **Patients Receiving Amphotericin B—Evaluation:** The patient experiences therapeutic effects (e.g., diminished signs and symptoms of infection, decreased fever); is free from or experiences minimal adverse effects. Verbalizes an understanding of the drug's use, adverse effects and required precautions. Demonstrates proper self-administration of the medication (e.g., dose, timing, when to notify provider).

6. **Patients Receiving Pharmacotherapy for Superficial Fungal Infections—Assessment:** Obtain a complete health history including allergies, drug history, and possible drug interactions. Obtain a culture and sensitivity of suspected area of infection to determine need for therapy. Obtain baseline liver-function tests.

7. **Patients Receiving Pharmacotherapy for Superficial Fungal Infections—Nursing diagnoses:** *Infection* (current or risk for concurrent bacterial infection); *Pain,* related to infection; *Hyperthermia; Deficient Knowledge* (drug therapy); *Risk for Injury,* related to adverse drug effects; *Ineffective Tissue Perfusion,* related to adverse effects of IV antifungals; *Risk for Noncompliance,* related to adverse drug effects, deficient knowledge, or length of therapy.

8. **Patients Receiving Pharmacotherapy for Superficial Fungal Infections—Planning:** The patient will experience therapeutic effects (e.g., diminished signs and symptoms of infection, decreased fever); be free from or experience minimal adverse effects. Verbalize an understanding of the drug's use, adverse effects, and required precautions.

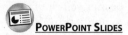

POWERPOINT SLIDES

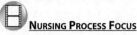

NURSING PROCESS FOCUS

- Patients Receiving Amphotericin B
- Patients Receiving Pharmacotherapy for Superficial Fungal Infections

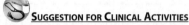

SUGGESTION FOR CLASSROOM ACTIVITIES

- Divide students into small groups, and have each group develop a teaching plan for a patient receiving drug therapy for fungal, protozoal, and helminth infections.

SUGGESTION FOR CLINICAL ACTIVITIES

- Instruct students to analyze their patients' care plans and make contributions to those care plans related to drug therapy for fungal, protozoal, and helminth infections.

Demonstrate proper self-administration of the medication (e.g., dose, timing, when to notify provider).

9. **Patients Receiving Pharmacotherapy for Superficial Fungal Infections—Implementation:** Monitor for possible side effects or hypersensitivity. Encourage compliance with instructions when taking oral antifungals. Monitor topical application. Avoid occlusive dressings. Monitor for contact dermatitis with topical formulations. Encourage infection-control practices.

10. **Patients Receiving Pharmacotherapy for Superficial Fungal Infections—Evaluation:** The patient experiences therapeutic effects (e.g., diminished signs and symptoms of infection, decreased fever); is free from or experiences minimal adverse effects. Verbalizes an understanding of the drug's use, adverse effects, and required precautions. Demonstrates sproper self-administration of the medication (e.g., dose, timing, when to notify provider).

GENERAL CHAPTER CONSIDERATIONS

1. Have students study and learn key terms listed at the beginning of the chapter.
2. Have students complete end-of-chapter exercises either in their book or on the MyNursingKit website.
3. Use the Classroom Response Questions provided in PowerPoint to assess students prior to lecture.

 MYNURSINGKIT
(*www.mynursingkit.com*)

- Websites
- NCLEX® questions
- Critical Thinking Questions
- Case Studies
- Animations and Videos
- Drug Prototype Questions

 MYNURSINGLAB
(*www.mynursinglab.com*)

- Knowledge Quick Check
- Pre/Posttests
- Customized study plans
- *Separate purchase*

 STUDENT WORKBOOK AND RESOURCE GUIDE

- Chapter 35 activities
- *Separate purchase*

PEARSON NURSE'S DRUG GUIDE

- *Separate purchase*

 PEARSON ETEXT

- Students can search, highlight, take notes, and more all in electronic format
- *Separate purchase*

 CLASSROOM RESPONSE QUESTION POWERPOINTS

 TESTBANK

© 2011 Pearson Education, Inc.

CHAPTER 36
DRUGS FOR VIRAL INFECTIONS

LEARNING OUTCOME 1

Describe the major structures of viruses.

Concepts for Lecture

Viruses are nonliving agents that infect bacteria, plants, and animals. A virus is an intracellular parasite and must be in a host cell to replicate and cause infection. A mature infective particle is called a virion. Viruses are intracellular parasites that must be inside a host to cause infection. Viruses are primitive structures, surrounded by a capsid (protein coat) and containing a few dozen genes. These genes are either ribonucleic acid (RNA) or deoxyribonucleic acid (DNA). DNA contains information needed for replication. (Figure 36.1 illustrates the structure of HIV.)

 POWERPOINT SLIDES

Figure 36.1 Structure of HIV

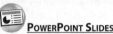 **SUGGESTION FOR CLASSROOM ACTIVITIES**

- Direct students to draw a concept map of how a virus infects a host cell.

 SUGGESTION FOR CLINICAL ACTIVITIES

- Direct students to research information in the infection-control manual at the clinical site on types of diseases caused by viruses.

LEARNING OUTCOME 2

Identify viral infections that benefit from pharmacotherapy.

Concepts for Lecture

Most viral infections are self-limiting and require no pharmacotherapy; for example, the rhinovirus that causes the common cold. Some viruses cause serious disease and require aggressive therapy. For example, HIV is fatal if left untreated. Another example, herpesviruses can cause significant pain and disability if left untreated. Antiviral therapy is challenging for several reasons. Viruses mutate rapidly, and the drug becomes ineffective. It is difficult for the drug to find the virus without injuring normal cells. Also, each antiviral drug is specific to one particular virus.

 POWERPOINT SLIDES

Figure 36.2 Replication of HIV

 SUGGESTION FOR CLINICAL ACTIVITIES

- Assign students to spend time in the laboratory observing how viruses are identified in that setting.

LEARNING OUTCOME 3

Explain the purpose and expected outcomes of HIV pharmacotherapy.

Concepts for Lecture

1. HIV targets the CD4 receptor on the T4 lymphocyte, using reverse transcriptase to make viral DNA from RNA. Virions bud from the host cell, and the enzyme protease enables the virion to infect other T4 lymphocytes. The result is gradual destruction of the immune system. HIV is called a "retrovirus" because of this reverse synthesis. (Figure 36.2 illustrates the replication cycle.)
2. Antiretroviral drugs used in the treatment of HIV-AIDS do not cure the disease, but they do help many patients to live symptom-free longer. New drugs for this disease have been developed, and rates of transmission from mother to newborn have been reduced. There has been

 POWERPOINT SLIDES

Figure 36.2 Replication Cycle

 SUGGESTION FOR CLASSROOM ACTIVITIES

- The National Institutes of Health (NIH) provides a comprehensive site called "AIDS info" at *aidsinfo.nih.gov/*. This site is treatment oriented and supplies the latest recommendations for the pharmacotherapy of HIV-AIDS. Direct students to access this site and research one of the topics.

a 70% decline in the death rate in the United States, but in African nations the incidence of HIV infections is still very high.

3. The latent phases of HIV occur when the virus lies dormant, and people are often unaware they have HIV. Once the diagnosis is confirmed, a decision about starting or delaying treatment must be made. The current protocol is to defer treatment in asymptomatic adults who have CD4 counts above 350 cells/mcL. Therapy is initiated when CD4 is under 200 cells/mcL or when symptoms appear. Therapeutic goals are to reduce HIV RNA load in the blood to an undetectable level or less than 50 copies/mL; an increased lifespan; a higher quality of life; and decreased risk of transmission from mother to child. Pharmacotherapy may be initiated in the acute (symptomatic) or chronic (asymptomatic) phase of HIV infection.

SUGGESTION FOR CLINICAL ACTIVITIES
- Assign students to care for a patient who has HIV infection.

REFERENCE
- The National Institutes of Health (NIH) "AIDS info": *aidsinfo.nih.gov/*

LEARNING OUTCOME 4

Explain the advantages of HAART in the pharmacotherapy of HIV infection.

Concepts for Lecture

Highly Active Antiretroviral Therapy (HAART) is the process of using drugs from five drug classes in various combinations in the pharmacotherapy of HIV-AIDS. The five drug classes are nucleoside reverse transcriptase inhibitor (NRTI), nonnucleoside reverse transcriptase inhibitor (NNRTI), protease inhibitor (PI), nucleotide reverse transcriptase inhibitor (NtRTI), and fusion (entry) inhibitor. The nucleotide reverse transcriptase inhibitors and the fusion inhibitors have been recently developed. Treatment failures are common with antiretroviral therapy. Patients have nontolerance of adverse effects, they do not adhere to the complex regimen, resistant strains can emerge, and genetic variability is a factor. Drug companies are responding to make treatment simpler. Therapy is always changing, and health care practitioners need to stay current with the latest treatments.

POWERPOINT SLIDES

SUGGESTION FOR CLASSROOM ACTIVITIES
- Discuss HAART combinations.

SUGGESTION FOR CLINICAL ACTIVITIES
- Review blood and body precautions in the clinical area.

LEARNING OUTCOME 5

Describe the nurse's role in the pharmacologic management of patients receiving antiretroviral and antiviral drugs.

Concepts for Lecture

1. The role of the nurse in the pharmacologic management of patients receiving antiretroviral and antiviral drugs involves careful monitoring of a patient's condition and providing education as it relates to the prescribed drug treatment. Obtain baseline medical, surgical, and drug history; lifestyle and dietary habits, including use of herbal or alternative therapies; and a detailed description of symptomology and current therapies.

2. **NRTI, NNRTI, and PI therapy:** Although NRTIs, NNRTIs, and PIs act by different mechanisms, the associated nursing care is similar. It is vital that the nurse establish a trusting, nonjudgmental relationship with the patient and his or her lifestyle. Assess the patient's understanding of the HIV disease process. Assess for symptoms of HIV and any opportunistic infections. Monitor plasma HIV RNA (viral load) assays, CD4 counts, complete blood count, liver and renal profiles, and blood-glucose levels throughout antiretroviral therapy. Assess for bone-marrow

POWERPOINT SLIDES

SUGGESTION FOR CLASSROOM ACTIVITIES
- Discuss the role of the nurse in monitoring patients who are taking drugs for viral infections.

SUGGESTION FOR CLINICAL ACTIVITIES
- Direct students to create a teaching plan for the patient taking drugs for viral infections.

© 2011 Pearson Education, Inc.

suppression, liver toxicity, and Stevens–Johnson syndrome. Advise the patient not to drive or perform hazardous activities until reactions to the medications are known. Be aware of the many conditions and drugs that are problematic with antiretroviral therapy. Teach patients how to practice blood and body-fluid precautions.

3. **Antiviral Therapy:** For patients with preexisting renal or hepatic disease, use the drugs with extreme caution. Although many antiviral medications are listed as pregnancy categories B or C, judicious use is still warranted during pregnancy. Emphasize compliance with antiviral therapy, such as taking the exact amount around the clock even if sleep is interrupted. Although most antiviral drugs are well tolerated, some cause GI distress and should be taken with food.

Learning Outcome 6

For each of the classes listed in Drugs at a Glance, know representative drugs, and explain the mechanism of drug action, primary actions, and important adverse effects.

Concepts for Lecture

1. **Agents for HIV-AIDS—Nucleoside and Nucleotide Reverse Transcriptase Inhibitors.** Prototype drug: zidovudine (Retrovir, AZT). Mechanism of action: As the reverse transcriptase enzyme begins to synthesize viral DNA, it mistakenly uses zidovudine as one of the nucleosides, thus creating a defective DNA strand. Primary use: in combination with other antiretrovirals for both symptomatic and asymptomatic HIV-infected patients, as well as for postexposure prophylaxis in HIV-exposed health care workers. An important indication is to reduce the transmission rate of HIV from an HIV-positive mother to her fetus. Adverse effects: severe toxicity to blood cells at high doses; anemia and neutropenia are common and may limit therapy. Many patients experience anorexia, nausea, and diarrhea. Patients may report fatigue and generalized weakness.

2. **Agents for HIV-AIDS—Nonnucleoside Reverse Transcriptase Inhibitors.** Prototype drug: nevirapine (Viramune). Mechanism of action: to bind directly to reverse transcriptase, disrupting the enzyme's active site. Primary use: always used in combination with other antivirals in treatment using HAART. Adverse effects: GI-related effects such as nausea, diarrhea, and abdominal pain are experienced by some patients, and skin rashes, fever, and fatigue are frequent side effects.

3. **Agents for HIV-AIDS—Protease Inhibitors.** Prototype drug: saquinavir mesylate (Fortovase, Invirase). Mechanism of action: to inhibit HIV protease. Primary use: in combination with other antiretrovirals for HIV-infected patients. Adverse effects: nausea, vomiting, dyspepsia, and diarrhea. General fatigue and headache are possible. (See Table 36.1.)

4. **Agents for Herpesviruses.** Prototype drug: acyclovir (Zovirax). Mechanism of action: to prevent viral DNA synthesis. Primary use: limited to the herpesviruses, for which it is a drug of choice. Adverse effects: nephrotoxicity when the medication is given IV. (See Table 36.2.)

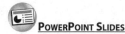

PowerPoint Slides

Table 36.1 Antiretroviral Drugs for HIV-AIDS
Table 36.2 Drugs for Herpesviruses

Prototype Drug
- zidovudine (Retrovir, AZT)
- nevirapine (Viramune)
- saquinavir mesylate (Fortovase, Invirase)
- acyclovir (Zovirax)

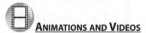

Animations and Videos

- Mechanism in Action: Zidovudine (Retrovir, AZT)
- Mechanism in Action: Acyclovir (Zovirax)
- Mechanism in Action: Saquinavir Mesylate (Fortovase, Invirase)

Suggestions for Classroom Activities

- Have each student make drug cards for each classification of drug used to treat viral infections. Use two different drugs for each classification. The card should include actions, uses, routes of administration, dosages, and adverse effects.
- Divide students into small groups, and have each group develop a teaching plan for a patient receiving medications for viral infections.

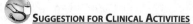

Suggestion for Clinical Activities

- Direct students to bring their drug cards to clinical, and assign the students to administer antiviral medications.

© 2011 Pearson Education, Inc.

LEARNING OUTCOME 7

Use the nursing process to care for patients receiving drug therapy for viral infections.

Concepts for Lecture

1. **Patients receiving pharmacotherapy for HIV-AIDS—Assessment:** Obtain a complete health history including neurologic, cardiovascular, respiratory, hepatic or renal disease, and the possibility of pregnancy. Obtain a drug history including allergies and possible drug interactions. Assess signs and symptoms of current infection noting onset, duration, characteristics, presence or absence of fever or pain. Evaluate: CBC, CD-4 count, HIV RNA assay, culture and sensitivity for any concurrent infections, hepatic and renal function studies, lipid levels, serum amylase, and glucose. Assess patient's ability to receive and understand instruction. Assess for adverse effects.

2. **Patients receiving pharmacotherapy for HIV-AIDS—Nursing diagnoses:** *Infection; Activity Intolerance; Fatigue; Anxiety; Imbalanced Nutrition, Less than Body Requirements; Deficient Fluid Volume; Diarrhea; Impaired Oral Mucus Membranes; Impaired Skin Integrity; Insomnia; Social Isolation; Confusion* (acute or chronic); *Ineffective Therapeutic Regimen Management*, related to complex medication regimen and disease treatment; *Deficient Knowledge*, related to disease process, transmission, and drug therapy; *Hopelessness; Spiritual Distress; Risk for Injury, Risk for Falls*, related to adverse drug effects or disease; *Risk for Caregiver Role Strain.*

3. **Patients receiving pharmacotherapy for HIV-AIDS—Planning:** The patient will experience CD-4 counts and HIV RNA assays within acceptable limits, absence of signs and symptoms of concurrent infection, ability to maintain ADLs; be free from or experience minimal adverse effects. Verbalize an understanding of the drug's use, adverse effects and required precautions. Demonstrate proper self-administration of the medication (e.g., dose, timing, when to notify provider).

4. **Patients receiving pharmacotherapy for HIV-AIDS—Implementation:** Monitor vital signs, especially temperature if fever is present. Monitor for symptoms of hypersensitivity and allergic reactions. Continue to monitor periodic lab work: hepatic and renal function tests, CBC, CD-4 counts, HIV RNA assays, lipid levels, serum amylase, culture and sensitivity if concurrent infections are present, glucose. Monitor patient for signs of stomatitis. Continue to monitor for hepatic and renal, toxicities (e.g., jaundice, RUQ pain, darkened urine, diminished urine output). Monitor for dermatologic effects including red or purplish skin rash, blisters, or peeling skin, including oral mucus membranes. Monitor for signs and symptoms of neurotoxicity (e.g., drowsiness, dizziness, mental changes, insomnia, delusions, paresthesias, headache, changes in level of consciousness, seizures). Monitor for signs and symptoms of blood dyscrasias (e.g., low-grade fevers, bleeding, bruising, significant fatigue). Monitor for significant GI effects, including nausea, vomiting, abdominal pain or cramping, and diarrhea. Administer drugs as per guidelines. Ensure adequate nutrition and caloric intake. Monitor for symptoms of pancreatitis, including severe abdominal pain, nausea, vomiting, and abdominal distension. Monitor blood glucose in patients taking antiretrovirals Encourage infection control and good hygiene measures. Provide resources for medical and emotional support. Instruct the patient and/or family in proper self-administration techniques followed by return demonstration.

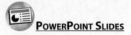

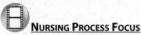

NURSING PROCESS FOCUS

- Care for Patients Receiving Drug Therapy for Viral Infections

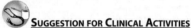

SUGGESTION FOR CLASSROOM ACTIVITIES

- Divide students into small groups, and have each group develop a teaching plan for a patient receiving drug therapy for viral infections.

SUGGESTION FOR CLINICAL ACTIVITIES

- Direct students to analyze the care plans for their patients with viral infections. Ask them to make contributions to the current care plans.

5. **Patients receiving pharmacotherapy for HIV-AIDS—Evaluation:** The patient will experience CD-4 counts and HIV-RNA assays within acceptable limits, absence of signs and symptoms of concurrent infection, ability to maintain ADLs; be free from or experience minimal adverse effects. Verbalize an understanding of the drug's use, adverse effects, and required precautions. Demonstrate proper self-administration of the medication (e.g., dose, timing, when to notify provider).

6. **Patients receiving anti-viral pharmacotherapy for infections other than HIV-AIDS—Assessment:** Obtain a complete health history including neurologic, cardiovascular, respiratory, hepatic or renal disease, and the possibility of pregnancy. Obtain a drug history including allergies and possible drug interactions. Assess signs and symptoms of current infection noting onset, duration, characteristics, presence or absence of fever or pain. Evaluate appropriate laboratory findings (e.g., CBC, hepatic and renal function studies, viral cultures). Assess patient's ability to receive and understand instruction. Assess for adverse effects.

7. **Patients receiving anti-viral pharmacotherapy for infections other than HIV-AIDS—Nursing diagnoses:** *Impaired Oral Mucus Membranes; Impaired Skin Integrity; Fatigue; Activity Intolerance; Social Isolation; Deficient Knowledge,* related to disease process, transmission, and drug therapy; *Risk for Deficient Fluid Volume,* related to disease process or adverse drug reactions; *Risk for Imbalanced Nutrition, Less than Body Requirements,* related to disease process or adverse drug reactions.

8. **Patients receiving anti-viral pharmacotherapy for infections other than HIV-AIDS—Planning:** The patient will experience therapeutic effects (e.g., diminished or absence of signs and symptoms of infection, able to maintain nutrition and hydration, activity level increased); be free from or experience minimal adverse effects. Verbalize an understanding of the drug's use, adverse effects and required precautions. Demonstrate proper self-administration of the medication (e.g., dose, timing, when to notify provider).

9. **Patients receiving anti-viral pharmacotherapy for infections other than HIV-AIDS—Implementation:** Monitor vital signs, especially temperature if fever is present. Monitor for symptoms of hypersensitivity and allergic reactions. Continue to monitor periodic lab work: CBC, hepatic and renal function tests, viral cultures. Continue to monitor for hepatic and renal, toxicities (e.g., jaundice, RUQ pain, darkened urine, diminished urine output). Monitor for signs and symptoms of neurotoxicity, particularly in patients on IV acyclovir (e.g., drowsiness, dizziness, tremors, headache, confusion, changes in level of consciousness, seizures). Ensure patient safety and have patient rise slowly from lying or sitting to standing. Monitor for signs and symptoms of blood dyscrasias (e.g., bleeding, bruising, significant fatigue, increasing signs of infection). Monitor for significant GI effects, including nausea, vomiting, and diarrhea. Ensure adequate nutrition and caloric intake. Encourage infection control and good hygiene measures based on disease condition. Maintain hydration during acyclovir therapy, providing pre-administration hydration if the drug is given IV. Monitor intake and output in the hospitalized patient. Instruct patient and/or family in proper self-administration techniques followed by return demonstration.

10. **Patients receiving anti-viral pharmacotherapy for infections other than HIV-AIDS—Evaluation:** The patient will experience therapeutic effects (e.g., diminished or absence of signs and symptoms of infection, able to maintain nutrition and hydration, activity level increased); be free from or experience minimal adverse effects. Verbalize an understanding of the drug's use, adverse effects and required precautions. Demonstrate proper self-administration of the medication (e.g., dose, timing, when to notify provider).

GENERAL CHAPTER CONSIDERATIONS

1. Have students study and learn key terms listed at the beginning of the chapter.
2. Have students complete end-of-chapter exercises either in their book or on the MyNursingKit website.
3. Use the Classroom Response Questions provided in PowerPoint to assess students prior to lecture.

MyNursingKit
(www.mynursingkit.com)

- Websites
- NCLEX® questions
- Critical Thinking Questions
- Case Studies
- Animations and Videos
- Drug Prototype Questions

MyNursingLab
(www.mynursinglab.com)

- Knowledge Quick Check
- Pre/Posttests
- Customized study plans
- *Separate purchase*

STUDENT WORKBOOK AND RESOURCE GUIDE

- Chapter 36 activities
- *Separate purchase*

PEARSON NURSE'S DRUG GUIDE

- *Separate purchase*

PEARSON eTEXT

- Students can search, highlight, take notes, and more all in electronic format.
- *Separate purchase*

CLASSROOM RESPONSE QUESTION POWERPOINTS

TESTBANK

© 2011 Pearson Education, Inc.

CHAPTER 37
DRUGS FOR NEOPLASIA

LEARNING OUTCOME 1

Explain differences between normal cells and cancer cells.

Concepts for Lecture

Cancer (carcinoma) is characterized by rapid, uncontrolled cell division. Cells lose normal functions and invade normal surrounding tissues. Metastasize means to travel to another location. A tumor (neoplasm) is named according to tissue of origin. (See Table 37.1 for classification and naming of tumors.) (Figure 37.1 illustrates invasion and metastasis by cancer cells.)

 POWERPOINT SLIDES

Table 37.1 Classification and Naming of Tumors
Figure 37.1 Invasion and Metastasis by Cancer Cells

 SUGGESTION FOR CLASSROOM ACTIVITIES

• Direct students to make a table comparing normal cells and cancer cells.

 SUGGESTION FOR CLINICAL ACTIVITIES

• Assign students to the pathology lab to observe types of cancer tissue.

LEARNING OUTCOME 2

Identify factors associated with an increased risk of cancer.

Concepts for Lecture

Causes of cancer can be chemical, physical, and biological. Chemical causes include tobacco (responsible for one-third of all cancers), asbestos (lung cancer), and benzene (leukemia). Physical causes can be x-rays (leukemia) or ultraviolet (UV) light from the sun (skin cancer). Biological causes can be viruses (associated with 15% of all cancers). Examples of viruses are herpes simplex viruses, Epstein-Barr, papillomavirus, and cytomegalovirus. Other biological factors that contribute to the formation of cancer are those that suppress the immune system, such as HIV and immunosuppressant medications given after transplants. Oncogenes (genetic predisposition) and damage to tumor suppressor genes are also biological factors that contribute to cancer formation. (Table 37.2 shows agents associated with an increased risk of cancer.)

 POWERPOINT SLIDES

Table 37.1 Classification and Naming of Tumors

 SUGGESTION FOR CLASSROOM ACTIVITIES

• Direct students to develop concept maps explaining how chemical, physical, or biological factors can cause cancer.

 SUGGESTION FOR CLINICAL ACTIVITIES

• Direct students to research their oncology patients' charts for possible chemical, physical, or biological causes for cancer.

LEARNING OUTCOME 3

Describe lifestyle factors associated with a reduced risk of acquiring cancer.

Concepts for Lecture

Many environmental and lifestyle factors are associated with a higher risk of cancer. Nurses encourage people to adopt healthy lifestyle habits. Some of those habits are to eliminate use and exposure to tobacco, limit alcohol use, reduce animal fats in the diet, increase plant fiber in the diet, choose most foods from plant sources, exercise regularly, keep weight

 POWERPOINT SLIDES

Table 37.2 Agents Associated with an Increased Risk of Cancer

 SUGGESTION FOR CLASSROOM ACTIVITIES

• Have students identify their own lifestyle habits, and discuss which of these habits may be predisposing them to develop cancer.

within normal guidelines, use protection from the sun, self-examine body for abnormal lumps and skin lesions, and have periodic screenings (mammogram, prostate exam, fecal occult blood test, colonoscopy, Pap test, and pelvic exam). (Table 37.2 illustrates agents associated with increased risk of cancer.)

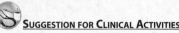

SUGGESTION FOR CLINICAL ACTIVITIES

• Direct students to educate their patients about healthy lifestyle habits.

LEARNING OUTCOME 4

Identify the three primary therapies for cancer.

Concepts for Lecture

1. Cancer may be treated using surgery, radiation therapy, and drugs. Chemotherapy may be used for cure, palliation, or prophylaxis.
2. Surgery is performed to remove a tumor when it is localized or pressing on nerves, airways, or other vital tissues. Surgery is not an option when tumors affect blood cells or when it would not extend lifespan or improve quality of life. Radiation and drug therapy is generally more successful.
3. Radiation can destroy tumor cells. Ionizing radiation is aimed directly at a tumor and may follow surgery. It is used as palliation for inoperable cancers to shrink the size of a tumor and to relieve pain or difficulty breathing or swallowing.
4. Chemotherapy is transported through the blood and has the potential to reach each cancer cell. Some drugs can cross the blood–brain barrier. Some drugs are distilled directly into body cavities (for example, the bladder). Chemotherapy is often combined with or done after surgery and radiation to increase the chance of a cure; this is called adjuvant therapy.

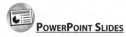

POWERPOINT SLIDES

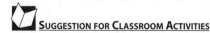

SUGGESTION FOR CLASSROOM ACTIVITIES

• Direct students to make a table showing the types of cancer therapies and the rationale for each.

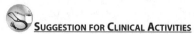

SUGGESTION FOR CLINICAL ACTIVITIES

• Direct students to research chemotherapy protocols and policies in the clinical area.

LEARNING OUTCOME 5

Explain the significance of growth fraction and the cell cycle to the success of chemotherapy.

Concepts for Lecture

1. The **growth fraction,** the percentage of cancer cells undergoing mitosis at any given time, is the ratio of replicating cells to resting cells. It is a major factor determining success of chemotherapy. Antineoplastics are more effective against cells that are rapidly dividing. A high growth fraction means there are many replicating cells. Solid tumors have a low growth fraction; thus, they are less sensitive to chemotherapy. Leukemias and lymphomas have a high growth fraction; thus, chemotherapy is more effective. Hair follicles, bone marrow, and gastrointestinal tissue have a high growth factor; this explains many adverse effects.
2. The cell cycle proceeds as follows: G0 Phase is the resting stage, G1 Phase is when the cell synthesizes material needed to duplicate DNA, S Phase is when the cell duplicates DNA, G2 Phase is the premitotic phase, M Phase is when mitosis occurs, and then the cell returns to the G0 phase. (See Figure 37.2.)
3. To achieve a total cure, every malignant cell must be removed or killed through surgery, radiation, or drugs or by the patient's immune system. Even one cell could reproduce and continue the cancer. The immune system eliminates a very small number of cancer cells, so it is important

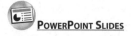

POWERPOINT SLIDES

Figure 37.2 Antineoplastic Agents and the Cell Cycle Cell
Figure 37.3 Cell Kill and Chemotherapy

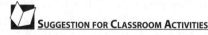

SUGGESTION FOR CLASSROOM ACTIVITIES

• Direct students to do concept mapping of the cell cycle and chemotherapy.

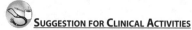

SUGGESTION FOR CLINICAL ACTIVITIES

• Assign students to take care of patients undergoing chemotherapy.

© 2011 Pearson Education, Inc.

to diagnose cancer early and treat with surgery, radiation, and/or drugs (chemotherapy). (See Figure 37.3 for an illustration of cell kill and chemotherapy.)

LEARNING OUTCOME 6

Describe the nurse's role in the pharmacologic management of cancer.

Concepts for Lecture

1. The role of the nurse in the pharmacologic management of cancer involves careful monitoring of a patient's condition and providing education as it relates to the prescribed drug treatment. Obtain baseline medical, surgical, and drug history; lifestyle and dietary habits, including use of herbal or alternative therapies; and a detailed description of symptomology and current therapies.

2. **Alkylating agents:** These drugs may be withheld if RBC, WBC, and platelet counts fall below a predetermined limit during therapy. Administer with caution to patients with hepatic or renal impairment, recent steroid therapy, leukopenia, or thrombocytopenia. Hydrate patients with IV or oral fluids before starting chemotherapy. Advise patients to avoid crowds and those who have respiratory infections. Remain alert to the possible development of blood dyscrasias. Monitor nutritional intake. Assess for nausea and vomiting. Be prepared to administer antiemetic drugs. Offer ice chips or ice pops to relieve mouth pain. Assess skin integrity. Monitor for signs of hearing loss. Patients of childbearing age should be informed of the potential adverse impact on fertility. Alkylating agents range from pregnancy category C (streptozocin, cyclophosphamide) to category X (estramustine). Maintain strict medical asepsis.

3. **Antimetabolites:** Many antimetabolites are contraindicated in pregnancy; for example, methotrexate (Mexate) is a category X drug, and pregnancy should be avoided for at least 6 months following termination of therapy. Further contraindications include hepatic, cardiac, and renal insufficiency; myelosuppression; and blood dyscrasias. Antimetabolites cause many of the adverse effects common to other antineoplastics, including alopecia, fatigue, nausea, vomiting, diarrhea, bone-marrow depression, and blood dyscrasias. These drugs may also cause photosensitivity and idiosyncratic pneumonitis. Teach patients to use good oral hygiene, and encourage mouth rinses every 2 hours with normal saline. Patients should brush teeth with soft toothbrush. Monitor IV site frequently for extravasation. Patients should apply ice pack and notify health care provider if this occurs.

4. **Antitumor antibiotics:** Assess cardiac status—and obtain a baseline ECG to rule out signs of cardiac abnormality or heart failure. Assess for pregnancy and lactation because antitumor antibiotics range from pregnancy category C to category D. These drugs produce the same general cytotoxic effects as other antineoplastics, including alopecia, fatigue, nausea, vomiting, diarrhea, bone-marrow suppression, and blood dyscrasias. The risk of hypersensitivity reactions such as life-threatening angioedema exists, as with other antibiotics. Changes in the rectal mucosa contraindicate suppositories or rectal temperatures. Protect yourself and use extreme caution when administering antitumor antibiotics. Doxorubicin is easily absorbed through the skin and by inhalation and may cause fetal death or birth defects as well as liver disease. Wear protective clothing (gloves, mask, and apron) when preparing the drug. Monitor IV site because doxorubicin is a severe vesicant. Give drug through a large-bore, quickly running IV. Monitor for extravasation.

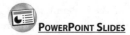
POWERPOINT SLIDES

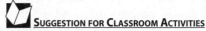
SUGGESTION FOR CLASSROOM ACTIVITIES

- Discuss the role of the nurse in monitoring patients who are taking chemotherapy.

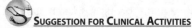
SUGGESTION FOR CLINICAL ACTIVITIES

- Direct students to create a teaching plan for the patient taking chemotherapy.

5. **Hormones and hormone antagonists:** Because hormone antagonists are given to block the growth of hormone-dependent tumors, assess for pregnancy and breast-feeding because both are contraindicated with the antitumor hormones and hormone antagonists. Therapy using hormones other than tamoxifen (Nolvadex) may be palliative rather than curative; it is important that both patient and family understand this limitation before beginning chemotherapy. One of the most common, yet distressing, side effects of sex-hormone therapy is the development of cross-gender secondary sexual characteristics. Fertility is sometimes affected. Discuss these effects frankly with the patient and offer support and simple interventions to increase self-esteem.

6. **Natural products:** Interview the patient regarding any allergy to plants or flowers, including herbs or foods, which may provide clues to possible hypersensitivity to these drugs. Vincristine (Oncovin) may produce acute bronchospasm and skin rashes. Inquire if female patients are pregnant or breast-feeding because many of these agents are contraindicated in pregnancy and lactation. These drugs produce many of the same cytotoxic effects as other antineoplastics, including alopecia, fatigue, nausea, vomiting, diarrhea, bone-marrow suppression, and blood dyscrasias. Emphasize the need to establish a nutritional plan to combat constipation, including high fluid and fiber intake. Natural-product antineoplastics can affect blood pressure, causing either hypotension or hypertension. Observe patients for symptoms such as headache, dizziness, or syncope. These drugs may produce severe mental depression; thus, remain alert to the possibility of suicidal ideation.

LEARNING OUTCOME 7

Explain how combination therapy and special dosing protocols increase the effectiveness of chemotherapy.

Concepts for Lecture

Multiple drugs from different classes affect different stages in the cell cycle. The different mechanisms of action increase the cell kill. These combinations allow for lower doses, which reduce toxicity and slow the development of resistance. Specific dosing protocols depend on type of tumor, stage of disease, and overall condition of patient. The drugs can be given as a single dose or several doses and may be given within several days or after several weeks have passed. This gives normal cells a chance to recover. Sometimes, the optimum dose must be delayed to let the patient recover from drug toxicities; for example, in the case of bone-marrow depression.

LEARNING OUTCOME 8

Describe the general adverse effects of chemotherapeutic agents.

Concepts for Lecture

It is difficult to kill cancer cells without killing normal cells. Serious toxicity limits therapy. Some of the adverse effects are alopecia and mucositis (severe nausea, vomiting, and diarrhea). Those drugs with high emetic potential are pretreated with antiemetics (Compazine, Reglan, Ativan). Another adverse effect is bone-marrow depression (anemia, leukopenia, and thrombocytopenia); it is treated with bone-marrow transplantation, platelet infusions, or growth factors. Infection risk grows if the absolute neutrophil count (ANC) falls below 500 mm³. Drugs that

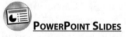

POWERPOINT SLIDES

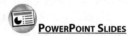

SUGGESTION FOR CLASSROOM ACTIVITIES
- Discuss multiple dosing and dosing schedules.

SUGGESTION FOR CLINICAL ACTIVITIES
- Direct students to observe the medication-administration records of patients taking chemotherapy. What type of dosing schedules do you see?

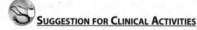

POWERPOINT SLIDES

Table 37.3 List of Adverse Effects

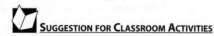

SUGGESTION FOR CLASSROOM ACTIVITIES
- Show students pictures of patients who have extravasation after a vesicant medication infiltrated. Discuss how extravasation may be prevented.

© 2011 Pearson Education, Inc.

are vesicants can cause tissue injury (extravasation). Know the emergency treatment before giving vesicants intravenously. Long-term consequences for some of the drugs are possible infertility and increased risk for secondary tumors. (See Table 37.3 for a list of adverse effects of cancer drugs.)

LEARNING OUTCOME 9

For each of the drug classes listed in Drugs at a Glance, know representative drugs, and explain their mechanism of drug action, primary actions, and important adverse effects.

Concepts for Lecture

1. **Alkylating Agents.** Prototype drug: cyclophosphamide (Cytoxan). Mechanism of action: attaches to DNA and disrupts replication, particularly in rapidly dividing cells. Primary use: alone or in combination with other drugs, against a wide variety of cancers, including Hodgkin's disease, lymphoma, multiple myeloma, breast cancer, and ovarian cancer. Adverse effects: rapid and powerful immunosuppressant effects. Leukocyte counts often serve as a guide to dosage adjustments during therapy. Thrombocytopenia is common, though less severe than with many other alkylating agents. Nausea, vomiting, anorexia, and diarrhea are frequently experienced. Cyclophosphamide causes alopecia, although this effect is usually reversible. Several metabolites of cyclophosphamide may cause hemorrhagic cystitis. (See Figure 37.4 for the mechanism of action of the alkylating agents.)

2. **Antimetabolites.** Prototype drug: methotrexate (Folex, Mexate, others). Mechanism of action: by blocking the synthesis of folic acid (vitamin B_9), methotrexate inhibits replication, particularly in rapidly dividing cells. Primary use: to treat choriocarcinoma, osteogenic sarcoma, leukemias, head and neck cancers, breast carcinoma, and lung carcinoma. Adverse effects: fatal bone-marrow toxicity at high doses. Hemorrhage and bruising are often observed, due to low platelet counts. Nausea, vomiting, and anorexia are common, and GI ulceration may result in serious intestinal bleeding. (See Figure 37.5 for the structural similarities between antimetabolites and their natural counterparts.)

3. **Antitumor Antibiotics.** Prototype drug: doxorubicin (Adriamycin). Mechanism of action: attaches to DNA, distorting its double helical structure and preventing normal DNA and RNA synthesis. It is used in solid tumors of the lung, breast, ovary, and bladder, and for various leukemias and lymphomas. Adverse effects: cardiotoxicity. Acute effects include dysrhythmias; delayed effects may include irreversible heart failure. Like many of the anticancer drugs, doxorubicin may profoundly lower blood-cell counts. Acute nausea and vomiting are common.

4. **Natural Products.** Prototype drug: vincristine (Oncovin). Mechanism of action: This is a cell-cycle-specific (M-phase) agent that kills cancer cells by preventing their ability to complete mitosis. Primary use: in treatment of Hodgkin's and non-Hodgkin's lymphomas, leukemias, Kaposi's sarcoma, Wilms' tumor, bladder carcinoma, and breast carcinoma. Adverse effects: nervous-system toxicity. Children are particularly susceptible. Symptoms include numbness and tingling in the limbs, muscular weakness, loss of neural reflexes, and pain. Paralytic ileus may occur in young children. Severe constipation is common. Reversible alopecia occurs in most patients.

- Direct students to use the clinical resources to find the antidotes and procedures a nurse would use in the case of extravasation with a vesicant medication.

POWERPOINT SLIDES

Figure 37.4 Mechanism of Action of the Alkylating Agents
Figure 37.5 Structural Similarities Between Antimetabolites and Their Natural Counterparts

Prototype Drug
- cyclophosphamide (Cytoxan)
- methotrexate (Folex, Mexate, others)
- doxorubicin (Adriamycin)
- vincristine (Oncovin)
- tamoxifen (Nolvadex)

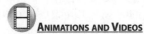

ANIMATIONS AND VIDEOS

- Mechanism in Action: Methotrexate (Folex, Mexate, others)
- Mechanism in Action: Cyclophosphamide (Cytoxar, Neosar)

SUGGESTIONS FOR CLASSROOM ACTIVITIES

- Have each student make drug cards for each classification of drug used to treat neoplasia. Use two different drugs for each classification. The card should include actions, uses, routes of administration, dosages, and adverse effects.
- Divide students into small groups, and have each group develop a teaching plan for a patient receiving medications for neoplasia.

SUGGESTION FOR CLINICAL ACTIVITIES

- Instruct students to bring drug cards to the clinical site, and have students use them to explain chemotherapy drugs to the clinical instructor before administering them.

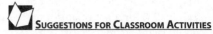

5. **Hormones/Hormone Antagonists.** Prototype drug: tamoxifen (Nolvadex). Mechanism of action: blocks estrogen receptors on breast cancer cells. It is used in patients with breast cancer and also given to high-risk patients to prevent the disease. Adverse effects: Other than nausea and vomiting, tamoxifen produces little serious toxicity. Of concern, however, is the association of tamoxifen therapy with an increased risk of endometrial cancer and thromboembolic disease. Hot flashes, fluid retention, and vaginal discharges are relatively common.

LEARNING OUTCOME 10

Categorize anticancer drugs based on their classification and mechanism of action.

Concepts for Lecture

1. **Alkylating agents** have a broad spectrum of activity and act by changing the structure of DNA in cancer cells. Their use is limited because they can cause significant bone-marrow suppression. (See Table 37.4 for a list of alkylating agents.)
2. **Antimetabolites** act by disrupting critical pathways in cancer cells, such as folate metabolism or DNA synthesis. The three types of antimetabolites are purine analogs, pyrimidine analogs, and folate inhibitors. (See Table 37.5 for a list of antimetabolites.)
3. Due to their cytotoxicity, a few antibiotics are used to treat cancer by inhibiting cell growth. They have a narrow spectrum of clinical activity, and their actions are similar to alkylating agents. Cardiotoxicity is a major limiting factor that may occur within minutes or years later. (See Table 37.6 for a list of anti-tumor antibiotics.)
4. Some plant extracts have been isolated that are structurally different but have the common ability to kill cancer cells by preventing cell division. These are called **mitotic inhibitors** and include the vinca alkaloids, taxanes, topoisomerase inhibitors, and camptothecins. (See Table 37.7 for a list of natural products.)
5. Some **hormones** and **hormone antagonists** are antineoplastic agents that are effective against reproductive-related tumors such as breast, prostate, or uterine. They are less cytotoxic than other antineoplastics. (See Table 37.8 for a list of hormones.)
6. **Biologic response modifiers** and some additional antineoplastic drugs have been found to be effective against tumors by stimulating or assisting the patient's immune system. They are less toxic than other classes of antineoplastics and include interferons, interleukins, and monoclonal antibodies. They are given concurrently with other neoplastics to limit immunosuppressive effects. (See Table 37.9 for a list of biologic response modifiers.)
7. **Miscellaneous antineoplastics** include the following: Asparaginase deprives cancer cells of an essential amino acid. Mitotane (Lysodren) is similar to the insecticide DDT. Two new antineoplastics, Imatinib (Gleevec) and sorafenib, inhibit the enzyme tyrosine kinase in tumor cells. (See Table 37.9 for a list of the miscellaneous antineoplastics.)

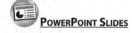

POWERPOINT SLIDES

Table 37.4 Alkylating Agents
Table 37.5 Antimetabolites
Table 37.6 Antitumor Antibiotics
Table 37.7 Natural Products with Antineoplastic Activity
Table 37.8 Hormone and Hormone Antagonists Used for Neoplasia
Table 37.9 Selected Biologic Response Modifiers and Miscellaneous Antineoplastics

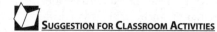

SUGGESTION FOR CLASSROOM ACTIVITIES

- Divide the students into small groups, and have them prepare questions and answers for different categories of drugs used to treat neoplasia. Include questions on each drug's classification and mechanisms of action.

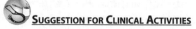

SUGGESTION FOR CLINICAL ACTIVITIES

- Assign students to care for patients receiving pharmacotherapy for neoplasia.

© 2011 Pearson Education, Inc.

LEARNING OUTCOME 11

Use the nursing process to care for patients who are receiving antineoplastic medications as part of their treatment of cancer.

Concepts for Lecture

1. **Patients receiving antineoplastic therapy—Assessment:** Obtain a complete health history including neurologic, cardiovascular, respiratory, hepatic or renal disease, and the possibility of pregnancy. Assess for signs and symptoms of current infections, for history of herpes zoster or chickenpox and immunization history, especially recent vaccinations with live vaccines, particularly varicella. Evaluate appropriate laboratory findings (e.g., CBC, platelet count, urinalysis, hepatic and renal function studies, uric acid, electrolytes, glucose). Obtain baseline weight and vital signs. Assess level of fatigue and presence of pain. Assess deep tendon reflexes—DTRs. Assess findings from other diagnostic tests specific to planned type of antineoplastic therapy regimen (e.g., audiology or cardiac testing, ECG, EMG). Assess patient's ability to receive and understand instruction. Obtain a drug history to determine possible drug interactions and allergies. Assess for adverse effects: nausea, vomiting, dysrhythmias, diminished or absent deep tendon reflexes, hypotension, hyperglycemia, bruising, bleeding, fever, severe diarrhea, decreased urine output or hematuria.

2. **Patients receiving antineoplastic therapy—Nursing diagnoses:** *Infection; Activity Intolerance; Fatigue; Anxiety; Imbalanced Nutrition, Less than Body Requirements; Deficient Fluid Volume; Diarrhea; Impaired Oral Mucus Membranes; Impaired Oral Mucus Membranes; Impaired Skin Integrity; Pain* (acute or chronic); *Social Isolation; Ineffective Therapeutic Regimen Management,* related to complex medication regimen and disease treatment; *Deficient Knowledge,* related to disease process and drug therapy; *Hopelessness; Spiritual Distress; Risk for Decreased Cardiac Output,* related to adverse drug effects; *Risk for Injury; Risk for Falls,* related to adverse drug effects or disease; *Risk for Caregiver Role Strain.*

3. **Patients receiving antineoplastic therapy—Planning:** The patient will experience therapeutic effects (e.g., reduction in tumor mass or decreased progression of abnormal cell growth, absence of signs and symptoms of concurrent infection, able to maintain ADLs); be free from or experience minimal adverse effects. Verbalize an understanding of the drug's use, adverse effects, and required precautions. Demonstrate proper self-administration of the medication (e.g., dose, timing, when to notify provider).

4. **Patients receiving antineoplastic therapy—Implementation:** Monitor CBC and temperature. Collect stool samples for guaiac testing of occult blood. Monitor vital signs, cardiorespiratory status, including dyspnea, pitting edema, heart and chest sounds, and ECG, especially for T-wave flattening, ST depression, or voltage reduction. Monitor renal status, urine, intake and output, and daily weight. Monitor GI status and nutrition, and administer antiemetics 30–45 minutes prior to antineoplastic administration or at the first sign of nausea. Monitor for constipation. Monitor neurological/sensory status. Monitor genitourinary status. Monitor for hypersensitivity or other adverse reactions. Monitor hair and skin status. Monitor for conjunctivitis. Monitor liver-function tests. Administer with caution to patients with diabetes mellitus. Provide for adequate pain medication and rest. Provide emotional support for patient.

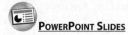
POWERPOINT SLIDES

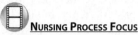
NURSING PROCESS FOCUS

• Care for patients who are receiving antineoplastic medications as part of their treatment of cancer.

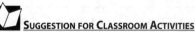
SUGGESTION FOR CLASSROOM ACTIVITIES

• Divide students into small groups, and have each group develop a teaching plan for a patient receiving antineoplastic medications as part of the treatment of cancer.

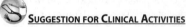
SUGGESTION FOR CLINICAL ACTIVITIES

• Invite an oncology nurse to speak to the class about patients who are receiving antineoplastic medications as part of their treatment of cancer.

5. **Patients receving antineoplastic therapy—Evaluation:** The patient will experience therapeutic effects (e.g., reduction in tumor mass or decreased progression of abnormal cell growth, absence of signs and symptoms of concurrent infection, able to maintain ADLs); will free from or experience minimal adverse effects. Verbalize an understanding of the drug's use, adverse effects and required precautions. Demonstrate proper self-administration of the medication (e.g., dose, timing, when to notify provider).

GENERAL CHAPTER CONSIDERATIONS

1. Have students study and learn key terms listed at the beginning of the chapter.
2. Have students complete end-of-chapter exercises either in their book or on the MyNursingKit website.
3. Use the Classroom Response Questions provided in PowerPoint to assess students prior to lecture.

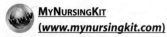

MYNURSINGKIT (*www.mynursingkit.com*)

- Websites
- NCLEX® questions
- Critical Thinking Questions
- Case Studies
- Animations and Videos
- Drug Prototype Questions

MYNURSINGLAB (*www.mynursinglab.com*)

- Knowledge Quick Check
- Pre/Posttests
- Customized study plans
- *Separate purchase*

STUDENT WORKBOOK AND RESOURCE GUIDE

- Chapter 37 activities
- *Separate purchase*

PEARSON NURSE'S DRUG GUIDE

- *Separate purchase*

PEARSON eTEXT

- Students can search, highlight, take notes, and more all in electronic format.
- *Separate purchase*

CLASSROOM RESPONSE QUESTION POWERPOINTS

TESTBANK

© 2011 Pearson Education, Inc.

CHAPTER 38
DRUGS FOR ALLERGIC RHINITIS AND THE COMMON COLD

LEARNING OUTCOME 1

Identify major functions of the upper respiratory tract.

Concepts for Lecture

The upper respiratory tract warms, humidifies, and cleans incoming air. The upper respiratory tract traps particulate matter and many pathogens, preventing them from being carried to bronchioles and alveoli. The nasal mucosa is richly supplied with vascular tissue and is controlled by the autonomic nervous system. This first line of immunological defense incorporates ciliated epithelium, nasal mucus, and the mast cells that line the nasal mucosa to protect the body. The respiratory tract provides the body with the oxygen critical for all cells to carry on normal activities. The respiratory system also provides a means by which the body can rid itself of excess acids and bases.

LEARNING OUTCOME 2

Describe common causes and symptoms of allergic rhinitis.

Concepts for Lecture

Allergic rhinitis or hay fever is inflammation of the nasal mucosa resulting from exposure to allergens. Allergic rhinitis is characterized by sneezing, watery eyes, and nasal congestion. It is caused by exposure to an antigen (allergen), which causes histamine release. The most common allegens include: pollens from weeds, grasses, and trees; mold spores; dust mites; certain foods; and animal dander. Chemical fumes, tobacco smoke, or air pollutants such as ozone are nonallergenic factors that may worsen symptoms. Pharmacotherapy is targeted at *preventing* the disorder or *relieving* its symptoms. (Figure 38.2 illustrates the mechanism of allergic rhinitis.)

LEARNING OUTCOME 3

Differentiate between H_1 and H_2 histamine receptors.

Concepts for Lecture

Histamine is a chemical mediator of the inflammatory response. H_1 histamine receptors are found in the smooth muscle of the vascular system and bronchial tree and are responsible for many of the symptoms of allergic rhinitis. The other major histamine receptor, H_2, is found in the gastric mucosa and is responsible for peptic ulcers.

POWERPOINT SLIDES

Figure 38-1 The Respiratory System

SUGGESTION FOR CLASSROOM ACTIVITIES

- Direct students to diagram the upper respiratory tract.

SUGGESTION FOR CLINICAL ACTIVITIES

- Direct students to do a complete respiratory assessment on their patient this week in clinical.

POWERPOINT SLIDES

Figure 38.2 Mechanism of Allergic Rhinitis

SUGGESTION FOR CLASSROOM ACTIVITIES

- Discuss the causes of allergic rhinitis and how these sources may be identified in a patient with symptoms of allergic rhinitis.

SUGGESTION FOR CLINICAL ACTIVITIES

- Assign students to a clinic setting and have them care for patients with allergic rhinitis.

POWERPOINT SLIDES

SUGGESTION FOR CLASSROOM ACTIVITIES

- Discuss the difference in H_1 and H_2 receptors.

SUGGESTION FOR CLINICAL ACTIVITIES

- Assign students to administer antihistamines during clinical. Direct them to report indications and reactions of patients to the drugs.

LEARNING OUTCOME 4

Compare and contrast the oral and intranasal decongestants.

Concepts for Lecture

1. Intranasal glucocorticoids have become drugs of choice in treating allergic rhinitis due to their high efficacy and wide margin of safety. For maximum effectiveness, they must be administered 2 to 3 weeks prior to allergen exposure. Intranasal glucocorticoids decrease the secretion of inflammatory mediators, reduce tissue edema, and cause mild vasoconstriction. Alternative therapy is with mast cell stabilizers such as intranasal cromolyn (Nasalcrom). (See Table 38.3.)
2. The most commonly used decongestants are oral and intranasal sympathomimetics, which alleviate the nasal congestion associated with allergic rhinitis and the common cold. (See Table 38.4.)
3. Intranasal drugs are more efficacious but should only be used for 3 to 5 days due to rebound congestion. Intranasal preparations are available over the counter in sprays and drops. They affect a local action within minutes and have few systemic effects.
4. Oral preparation decongestants have more systemic effects, response time is slower, and they are less effective at relieving severe congestion. These drugs are often combined with antihistamine preparations.

LEARNING OUTCOME 5

Discuss the pharmacotherapy of cough.

Concepts for Lecture

1. Cough is a natural reflex mechanism that serves to forcibly remove excess secretions and foreign material from the respiratory system. Common colds and allergies create cough. Antitussives are effective at relieving cough due to the common cold. Opioids are used for severe cough. Nonopioids such as dextromethorphan are used for mild or moderate cough. (See Table 38.5.)
2. Expectorants promote mucus secretion, making it thinner and easier to remove by coughing. Mucolytics directly break down mucous molecules.

LEARNING OUTCOME 6

Describe the role of expectorants and mucolytics in treating bronchial congestion.

Concepts for Lecture

1. **Expectorants** are drugs that reduce the thickness or viscosity of bronchial secretions. They increase mucus flow that can then be removed more easily by coughing. The most effective OTC expectorant is guaifenesin (Mucinex, Robitussin, others). Guaifenesin has fewer adverse effects and is a common ingredient in many OTC multisymptom cold and flu preparations. It is most effective in treating dry, nonproductive cough, but may also be of benefit for patients with productive cough.

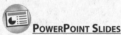
POWERPOINT SLIDES

Table 38.3 Intranasal Glucocorticoids
Table 38.4 Nasal Decongestants

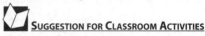
SUGGESTION FOR CLASSROOM ACTIVITIES

• Bring various inhalers to the classroom for the students to look at.

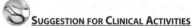
SUGGESTION FOR CLINICAL ACTIVITIES

• Assign the students to patients who are using inhalers.

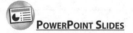
POWERPOINT SLIDES

Table 38.5 Selected Antitussives and Expectorants

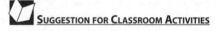
SUGGESTION FOR CLASSROOM ACTIVITIES

• Discuss over-the-counter availability and use of antitussives and expectorants.

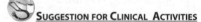
SUGGESTION FOR CLINICAL ACTIVITIES

• Assign students to care for patients who are exhibiting cough. Have them compare and contrast the treatments for cough related to underlying diagnosis and patient age.

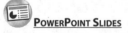
POWERPOINT SLIDES

Table 38.5 Selected Antitussives and Expectorants

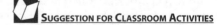
SUGGESTION FOR CLASSROOM ACTIVITIES

• Describe the role of expectorants and mucolytics in treating bronchial congestion.

© 2011 Pearson Education, Inc.

2. **Mucolytics** break down the chemical structure of mucus molecules. Mucolytics help loosen thick bronchial secretions. The mucus becomes thinner, and can be removed more easily by coughing. Acetylcysteine is delivered by the inhalation route and is used in patients who have cystic fibrosis, chronic bronchitis, or other diseases that produce large amounts of thick bronchial secretions. Mucomyst can trigger brochospasm and has an offensive odor resembling rotten eggs. A second mucolytic, dornase alfa (Pulmozyme), is approved for maintenance therapy in the management of thick bronchial secretions. Dornase alfa breaks down DNA molecules in the mucus, causing it to become less viscous. These agents are listed in Table 38.5.

Learning Outcome 7

For each of the classes listed in Drugs at a Glance, know representative drugs, and explain their mechanism of drug action, primary actions on the respiratory system, and important adverse effects.

Concepts for Lecture

1. **H₁ Receptor Antagonists (Antihistamines).** Prototype drug: diphenhydramine (Benadryl). Mechanism of action: as a histamine (H₁) receptor blocker (first generation). Primary use: to treat minor symptoms of allergy and the common cold, such as sneezing, runny nose, and tearing of the eyes. Adverse effects: drowsiness—occasionally, paradoxical CNS stimulation and excitability will be observed, rather than drowsiness. Anticholinergic effects such as dry mouth, tachycardia, and mild hypotension occur in some patients. Diphenhydramine may cause photosensitivity. (See Table 38.1.)

2. **H₁ Receptor Antagonists (Antihistamines).** Prototype drug: fexofenadine (Allegra). Mechanism of action: as a histamine (H₁) receptor blocker (second generation). Primary use: most effective when taken *before* symptoms develop. It reduces the severity of nasal congestion, sneezing, and tearing of the eyes. Adverse effects: drowsiness (less than first-generation H₁ blockers), headache, and upset stomach. (See Table 38.2.)

3. **Intranasal Glucocorticoids.** Prototype drug: fluticasone (Flonase). Mechanism of action: decreases local inflammation in the nasal passages, thus reducing nasal stuffiness. Primary use: to treat seasonal allergic rhinitis. Adverse effects: nasal irritation and epistaxis. (See Table 38.3.)

4. **Decongestants.** Prototype drug: oxymetazoline (Afrin). Mechanism of action: stimulates alpha-adrenergic receptors in the sympathetic nervous system. This causes arterioles in the nasal passages to constrict, thus drying the mucous membranes. Primary use: to treat nasal congestion. Adverse effects: rebound congestion, which is common when oxymetazoline is used for longer than 3 to 5 days. Minor stinging and dryness in the nasal mucosa may be experienced. (Table 38.4.)

5. **Antitussives.** Prototype drug: dextromethorphan (Delsym, Robitussin). Mechanism of action: acts in the medulla to inhibit cough reflex. Primary use: as a component in most OTC severe cold and flu preparations. Adverse effects: dizziness, drowsiness, and GI upset. (See Table 38.5.)

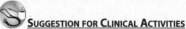

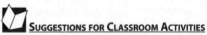 **Suggestion for Clinical Activities**

- Assign students to care for patients who are taking expectorants and mucolytics.

 PowerPoint Slides

Table 38.1 H₁ Receptor Antagonists
Table 38.2 Selected Antihistamine Combinations Available OTC for Allergic Rhinitis
Table 38.3 Intranasal Glucocorticoids
Table 38.4 Nasal Decongestants
Table 38.5 Selected Antitussives and Expectorants
Table 38.6 Selected Opioid Combination Drugs for Severe Cold Symptoms

Prototype Drug
- diphenhydramine (Benadryl)
- fexofenadine (Allegra)
- fluticasone (Flonase)
- oxymetazoline (Afrin)
- dextromethorphan (Benylin)

 Animations and Videos

- Mechanism in Action: Diphenhydramine (Benadryl, others)

Suggestions for Classroom Activities

- Have each student make drug cards for each classification of drug used to treat allergic rhinitis and the common cold. The card should include actions, uses, routes of administration, dosages, and adverse effects.
- Divide students into small groups, and have each group develop a teaching plan for a patient receiving medications for allergic rhinitis and the common cold.

 Suggestion for Clinical Activities

- Direct students to bring the medication cards they made for drugs used to treat allergic rhinitis and the common cold to clinical. Assign the students to administer medications discussed in this chapter; quiz them on the information contained on the medication cards.

LEARNING OUTCOME 8

Use the nursing process to care for patients who are receiving pharmacotherapy for allergic rhinitis and the common cold.

Concepts for Lecture

1. **Patients Receiving Antihistamine Therapy—Assessment:** Obtain a complete health history including previous history of symptoms and association to seasons, foods, or environmental exposures, existing cardiovascular, respiratory, hepatic, renal, or neurologic disease, glaucoma, prostatic hypertrophy or difficulty with urination, presence of fever or active infections, pregnancy or breast-feeding, alcohol use, or smoking. Obtain drug history noting type of adverse reaction or allergy, and possible drug interactions. Assess for any recent changes in diet, soaps including laundry detergent or softener, cosmetics, lotions, environment, or recent carpet-cleaning, particularly in infants and young children if allergy symptoms are of new onset. Obtain baseline ECG and vital signs, especially pulse rate and rhythm. Assess for adverse effects: dizziness, drowsiness, dry mouth, blurred vision, or headache. Evaluate appropriate laboratory findings (e.g., CBC, hepatic and renal labs). Assess respiratory status and breathing pattern. Assess neurologic status and level of consciousness. Report immediately any increasing fever, confusion, muscle weakness, tachycardia, palpitations, hypotension, syncope, dyspnea, pulmonary congestion, urinary retention, sudden severe eye pain or rainbow halos around lights.

2. **Patients Receiving Antihistamine Therapy—Nursing diagnoses:** *Ineffective Airway Clearance; Ineffective Breathing Pattern; Disturbed Sleep Pattern,* related to adverse drug effects; *Fatigue; Deficient Knowledge* (drug therapy); *Risk for Injury; Risk for Falls,* related to adverse drug effects.

3. **Patients Receiving Antihistamine Therapy—Planning:** The patient will experience therapeutic effects (e.g., decreased nasal congestion and drainage, decreased eye watering and itching); be free from or experience minimal adverse effects. Verbalize an understanding of the drug's use, adverse effects, and required precautions. Demonstrate proper self-administration of the medication (e.g., dose, timing, when to notify provider).

4. **Patients Receiving Antihistamine Therapy—Implementation:** Start therapy before beginning of allergy season and appearance of symptoms. Ensure patient safety, especially in the elderly. Monitor ambulation until effects of drug are known. Auscultate breath sounds before administering. Use with extreme caution in patients with asthma, COPD, and a history of cardiovascular disease. Keep resuscitative equipment accessible. Monitor vital signs especially pulse rate and rhythm (including ECG) for patients with existing cardiac disease before administering. Monitor for persistent dry cough, increasing cough severity, increasing congestion, or dyspnea. Monitor thyroid function. Use with caution in patients with a history of hyperthyroidism. Monitor for vision changes. Use with caution in patients with: narrow-angle glaucoma, history of kidney or urinary-tract disease, diabetes mellitus, history of seizure disorder; history of hyperthyroidism. Monitor neurologic status, especially LOC. Assess for urinary retention, especially in males over 40 or with a history of prostatic hypertrophy. Observe for signs of renal toxicity. Measure intake and output. Monitor periodic hepatic and renal function labs, especially in patients on long-term antihistamine use or those with previous history of hepatic or renal impairment. Monitor serum-glucose levels with increased frequency.

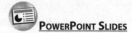

POWERPOINT SLIDES

NURSING PROCESS FOCUS

- Patients Receiving Antihistamine Therapy
- Patients Receiving Symptomatic Cold Relief: Antitussive, Nasal Decongestant, and Expectorant Therapy

SUGGESTION FOR CLASSROOM ACTIVITIES

- Divide students into small groups, and have each group develop a teaching plan for a patient receiving pharmacotherapy for allergic rhinitis and the common cold.

SUGGESTION FOR CLINICAL ACTIVITIES

- Assign students to care for patients receiving pharmacotherapy for allergic rhinitis or the common cold.

© 2011 Pearson Education, Inc.

Use with caution in patients with a history of GI disorders, especially peptic ulcers or liver disease. Monitor for GI side effects. Monitor for side effects, such as dry mouth; observe for signs of anticholinergic crisis. Instruct patient and/or family in proper self-administration of drug.

5. **Patients Receiving Antihistamine Therapy—Evaluation:** The patient will experience therapeutic effects (e.g., decreased nasal congestion and drainage, decreased eye watering and itching); be free from or experience minimal adverse effects. Verbalize an understanding of the drug's use, adverse effects, and required precautions. Demonstrate proper self-administration of the medication (e.g., dose, timing, when to notify provider).

6. **Patients Receiving Symptomatic Cold Relief: Antitussive, Nasal Decongestant, and Expectorant Therapy—Assessment:** Obtain a complete health history, including previous history and length of symptoms, existing cardiovascular, respiratory, hepatic, or renal disease, presence of fever, pregnancy or breast-feeding, alcohol use, or smoking; data on anaphylaxis, asthma, or and allergies, drug history, and possible drug interactions. Evaluate appropriate laboratory findings (e.g., CBC, hepatic and renal labs). Obtain vital signs, especially pulse rate and rhythm in patients with existing cardiac disease. Assess for adverse effects: dizziness, drowsiness, blurred vision, headache, epistaxis.

7. **Patients Receiving Symptomatic Cold Relief: Antitussive, Nasal Decongestant, and Expectorant Therapy—Nursing diagnoses:** *Ineffective Airway Clearance; Ineffective Breathing Pattern; Disturbed Sleep Pattern,* related to somnolence or agitation; *Deficient Knowledge* (drug therapy); *Risk for Injury,* related to adverse drug effects; *Risk for Injury,* related to adverse drug effects; *Risk for Falls,* related to adverse drug effects.

8. **Patients Receiving Symptomatic Cold Relief: Antitussive, Nasal Decongestant, and Expectorant Therapy—Planning:** The patient will experience therapeutic effects (e.g., decreased nasal congestion and drainage, increased ease in expectorating mucus, thinner secretions, breath sounds clear). Be free from, or experience minimal adverse effects. Verbalize an understanding of the drug's use, adverse effects and required precautions. Demonstrate proper self-administration of the medication (e.g., dose, timing, when to notify provider).

9. **Patients Receiving Symptomatic Cold Relief: Antitussive, Nasal Decongestant, and Expectorant Therapy—Implementation:** Monitor for persistent dry cough, increasing cough severity, increasing congestion, or dyspnea. Assess color and consistency of any expectorated sputum. Monitor for GI effects. Use decongestant nasal spray first followed in 5 to 10 minutes by the glucocorticoid. Instruct patient and/or family in proper self-administration of drug. Auscultate breath sounds before administering. Use with extreme caution in patients with: asthma, COPD, and a history of cardiovascular disease. Keep resuscitative equipment accessible. Monitor vital signs especially pulse rate and rhythm. Monitor for vision changes. Use with caution in patients with: narrow-angle glaucoma, history of kidney or urinary-tract disease, diabetes mellitus, history of seizure disorder, history of hyperthyroidism. Monitor neurologic status, especially LOC. Observe for signs of renal toxicity. Measure intake and output. Monitor serum glucose levels with increased frequency. Monitor for GI side effects. Use with caution in patients with a history of GI disorders, especially peptic ulcers or liver disease. Monitor for side effects, such as dry mouth; observe for signs of anticholinergic crisis. Report immediately any increasing fever, tachycardia, palpitations, syncope, dyspnea, pulmonary congestion, or confusion.

© 2011 Pearson Education, Inc.

10. **Patients Receiving Symptomatic Cold Relief: Antitussive, Nasal Decongestant, and Expectorant Therapy—Evaluation:** The patient will experience decreased nasal congestion and drainage, increased ease in expectorating mucus, thinner secretions, clear breath sounds; be free from or experience minimal adverse effects. Verbalize an understanding of the drug's use, adverse effects and required precautions. Demonstrate proper self-administration of the medication (e.g., dose, timing, when to notify provider).

GENERAL CHAPTER CONSIDERATIONS

1. Have students study and learn key terms listed at the beginning of the chapter.
2. Have students complete end-of-chapter exercises either in their book or on the MyNursingKit website.
3. Use the Classroom Response Questions provided in PowerPoint to assess students prior to lecture.

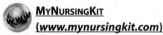

MYNURSINGKIT
(*www.mynursingkit.com*)

- Websites
- NCLEX® questions
- Critical Thinking Questions
- Case Studies
- Animations and Videos
- Drug Prototype Questions

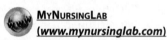

MYNURSINGLAB
(*www.mynursinglab.com*)

- Knowledge Quick Check
- Pre/Posttests
- Customized study plans
- *Separate purchase*

STUDENT WORKBOOK AND RESOURCE GUIDE

- Chapter 38 activities
- *Separate purchase*

PEARSON NURSE'S DRUG GUIDE

- *Separate purchase*

PEARSON eTEXT

- Students can search, highlight, take notes, and more all in electronic format.
- *Separate purchase*

CLASSROOM RESPONSE QUESTION POWERPOINTS

TESTBANK

© 2011 Pearson Education, Inc.

CHAPTER 39
DRUGS FOR ASTHMA AND OTHER PULMONARY DISORDERS

LEARNING OUTCOME 1

Identify anatomical structures associated with the lower respiratory tract and their functions.

Concepts for Lecture

The bronchial tree ends in dilated sacs called *alveoli*. An extremely thin membrane in the alveoli, allows gases to readily move between the internal environment of the blood and the inspired air. The membrane allows oxygen to enter the blood and carbon dioxide, and cellular waste products to move out of the blood to the air. Bronchioles are muscular, elastic structures whose diameter, or lumen, varies with the contraction or relaxation of smooth muscle. Dilation of bronchioles opens the lumen, allowing air to enter the lungs more freely, thus increasing the supply of oxygen to the body's tissues. Constriction of the bronchioles closes the lumen, resulting in less airflow. Respiration is the process of bringing O_2 into the body and moving carbon dioxide out of the body. The physiology of the respiratory system involves two main processes. Ventilation moves air into and out of the lungs, and perfusion—the flow of blood through the lungs—allows for gas exchange across capillaries. (Figure 39.1 illustrates the structure of the lower respiratory tract.)

 POWERPOINT SLIDES

Figure 39.1 The Lower Respiratory Tract

 SUGGESTION FOR CLASSROOM ACTIVITIES

- Direct students to draw a diagram of the respiratory system from nose to alveoli.

 SUGGESTION FOR CLINICAL ACTIVITIES

- Direct students to do a complete respiratory assessment on their patient during clinical.

LEARNING OUTCOME 2

Explain how the autonomic nervous system regulates airflow in the lower respiratory tract, and how this can be modified with drugs.

Concepts for Lecture

Bronchioles are lined with smooth muscle that controls the amount of air entering the lungs. Bronchodilation and bronchoconstriction are regulated by the two branches of the autonomic nervous system. The sympathetic branch activates beta$_2$-adrenergic receptors, which causes bronchiolar smooth muscle to relax, the airway diameter to increase, and bronchodilation to occur, allowing air to enter the lungs more freely, thus increasing the supply of oxygen to the body's tissues. The parasympathetic branch causes bronchiolar smooth muscle to contract, the airway diameter to narrow, and bronchoconstriction to occur, resulting in less airflow.

 POWERPOINT SLIDES

 SUGGESTION FOR CLASSROOM ACTIVITIES

- Discuss the autonomic nervous system, and compare actions of the sympathetic and parasympathetic branches.

 SUGGESTION FOR CLINICAL ACTIVITIES

- Assign students to the clinic setting. Have them research the types of drugs given in the event of a bronchospasm.

LEARNING OUTCOME 3

Compare the advantages and disadvantages of using the inhalation route of drug administration for pulmonary drugs.

Concepts for Lecture

1. Advantages of aerosol therapy are: Inhalation is a common route of administration for pulmonary drugs because it rapidly and efficiently

 POWERPOINT SLIDES

 SUGGESTION FOR CLASSROOM ACTIVITIES

- Do a case study on a patient who suffers a bronchospasm.

© 2011 Pearson Education, Inc.

delivers drugs directly to the sites of action. The lungs' rich blood supply allows for quick absorption and onset of action. Aerosol therapy is the suspension of droplets or particles in a gas; onset of action is almost immediate. Aerosol therapy causes immediate relief of bronchospasm, and thick mucus is loosened. Side effects are reduced, but systemic effects can still occur.

2. Disadvantages of aerosol therapy are difficulty in measuring the precise dose (usually, only 10% to 50% of the drug is placed), instruction may be complicated for some patients, and side effects occur if the patient swallows the drug or does not rinse the mouth after inhalation.

LEARNING OUTCOME 4

Describe the types of devices used to deliver aerosol therapies via the inhalation route.

Concepts for Lecture

Nebulizers, metered dose inhalers (MDIs), and **dry powdered inhalers (DPIs)** are devices used for aerosol therapies. A nebulizer vaporizes a liquid drug into a fine mist using a small machine and face mask. An MDI uses a propellant to deliver a measured dose of drug. The patient times inhalation to puffs of the drug. The DPI causes the patient to inhale a powdered drug; the device is activated by inhalation. (See Figure 39.2.)

LEARNING OUTCOME 5

Compare and contrast the pharmacotherapy of acute and chronic asthma.

Concepts for Lecture

1. **Asthma** is a chronic pulmonary disease. It has both inflammatory and bronchospasm components, and symptoms occur with exposure to triggers or upon exertion (exercise induced). (See Table 39.1 for common causes of asthma.) Characterized by acute bronchospasm, asthma can cause intense breathlessness, coughing, and gasping for air. Status asthmaticus is a prolonged asthma attack. Drugs are used to prevent asthmatic attacks and to terminate an attack in progress. (Figure 39.3 shows the changes in bronchioles during an asthma attack.) Because asthma has both a bronchoconstriction component and an inflammation component, pharmacotherapy of the disease focuses on one or both of these mechanisms. The goals of drug therapy are twofold: to *terminate* acute bronchospasms in progress and to *reduce the frequency* of asthma attacks. Different medications are needed to achieve each of these goals. The patient with asthma can present with acute or chronic symptoms.

2. **Beta-adrenergic agonists** are the most effective drugs for relieving acute bronchospasm. They work by activating beta$_2$-receptors in bronchial smooth muscle to cause bronchodilation. There are fewer cardiac side effects than with older nonselective beta-adrenergics and can range from ultrashort to long acting. **Inhalation therapy** produces rapid bronchodilation with little systemic toxicity. Oral therapy has a longer duration of action but has frequent side effects, and tolerance may develop.

SUGGESTION FOR CLINICAL ACTIVITIES

- Assign students to observe in a respiratory-care department.

POWERPOINT SLIDES

Figure 39.2 Devices Used to Deliver Respiratory Drugs

SUGGESTION FOR CLASSROOM ACTIVITIES

- Have devices for inhalation therapy available for students to look at in the classroom.

SUGGESTION FOR CLINICAL ACTIVITIES

- Assign students to administer inhalation therapy during clinical.

POWERPOINT SLIDES

Table 39.1 Common Triggers of Asthma
Table 39.2 Bronchodilators
Table 39.3 Anti-inflammatory Drugs for Asthma

SUGGESTION FOR CLASSROOM ACTIVITIES

- Discuss the pharmacotherapy of acute and chronic asthma.

SUGGESTION FOR CLINICAL ACTIVITIES

- Direct students to assess a patient's lungs while patient is having an asthma attack and then after the patient has had a medication to treat that problem. Report the results at postclinical.

© 2011 Pearson Education, Inc.

3. **Anticholinergics** block the parasympathetic nervous system with a bronchodilator effect. They are occasionally used as an alternative to the beta-agonists in asthma therapy. Anticholinergics are used in the inhaled form and are most effective when used in combination with a beta-agonist; for example, Combivent (ipratropium and albuterol).

4. **Methylxanthines** are bronchodilators related to caffeine. They were once the mainstay of chronic asthma pharmacotherapy; for example, theophylline. There is a narrow margin of safety, and they interact with numerous drugs. Side effects are common and include nausea, vomiting, and central nervous system (CNS) stimulation. They are administered by intravenous or oral routes. Methylxanthines are primarily for long-term prophylaxis of asthma that is unresponsive to beta-agonists or glucocorticoids.

5. **Glucocorticoids** are potent anti-inflammatory drugs. Inhaled, they are often drugs of choice for the long-term prophylaxis of asthma and must be taken daily. Systemic side effects are rarely observed. Oral drugs are used for the short-term therapy of severe, acute asthma. Systemic side effects occur with these, and therapy should be limited to under 10 days.

6. Leukotrienes are mediators of immune response. They are involved in allergic and asthmatic reactions. **Leukotriene modifiers** are primarily used for asthma prophylaxis and for reducing the inflammatory component of asthma. They are an oral medication used when persistent asthma is not controlled with other drugs.

7. **Mast-cell stabilizers** inhibit mast cells from releasing histamine and other chemical mediators. They are safe drugs for the prophylaxis of asthma but less effective than the inhaled glucocorticoids and ineffective at relieving acute bronchospasm.

LEARNING OUTCOME 6

Describe the nurse's role in the pharmacologic treatment of lower respiratory tract disorders.

Concepts for Lecture

1. The role of the nurse in the pharmacologic management of inflammatory disorders and fever involves careful monitoring of a patient's condition and providing education as it relates to the prescribed drug treatment. Obtain baseline medical, surgical, and drug history; lifestyle and dietary habits, including use of herbal or alternative therapies; and a detailed description of symptomology and current therapies.

2. **Beta-adrenergic agonist therapy for asthma:** Assess the patient's vital signs, especially respiratory and pulse rate, lung sounds, respiratory effort, skin color, and oxygen-saturation level prior to administration of beta-adrenergic agonists. These drugs should not be used if the patient has a history of dysrhythmia or MI. Use is limited in children younger than 6 years. Beta-adrenergic agonists are not recommended for use by women who are breast-feeding.

3. **Anticholinergic therapy for asthma:** Assess respiratory rate before and after the first dose of an MDI because the first dose may precipitate bronchospasm. Monitor vital signs, especially respiratory rate and pulse, respiratory effort, skin color, oxygen-saturation level, and lung sounds. Assess for history of narrow-angle glaucoma, benign prostatic hyperplasia, renal disorders, and urinary bladder neck obstruction. Anticholinergics should be used with caution in patients with a history of

POWERPOINT SLIDES

SUGGESTION FOR CLASSROOM ACTIVITIES

- Discuss the role of the nurse in the pharmacologic treatment of lower-respiratory-tract disorders.

SUGGESTION FOR CLINICAL ACTIVITIES

- Direct students to create a teaching plan for the patient using medications to treat lower-respiratory-tract conditions.

any of these disorders and in elderly patients. Ipratropium is not recommended in children younger than 12 years, and tiotropium is not recommended for use in patients younger than 18 years. Anticholinergics are not recommended for women who are breast-feeding.

4. **Methylxanthine therapy for asthma:** Assess the patient's vital signs, especially respiratory and pulse rate, cardiac rhythm, lung sounds, respiratory effort, skin color, and oxygen-saturation level prior to administration of methylxanthines. Assess for a history of coronary artery disease, angina pectoris, severe renal or liver disorders, peptic ulcer, benign prostatic hyperplasia, and diabetes mellitus. Methylxanthine use is contraindicated in patients with coronary artery disease or angina pectoris. Use is cautioned in elderly patients and children and not recommended in women who are breast-feeding.

5. **Glucocorticoid therapy for asthma:** Assess the patient for the presence and history of asthma, allergic rhinitis, hypertension, heart disease, blood clots, Cushing's syndrome, fungal infections, and diabetes mellitus. Monitor the patient's vital signs, especially respiratory and pulse rates, respiratory effort, lung sounds, skin color, oxygen-saturation level, and body weight. Assess for signs and symptoms of infection. Steroid inhalers should be used cautiously in patients with hypertension, GI disease, congestive heart failure, and thromboembolic disease. Use of glucocorticoids is not recommended for pregnant or breast-feeding women. Because the primary purpose of inhaled glucocorticoids is to *prevent* respiratory distress, advise the patient not to use this medication during an acute asthma attack. Additionally, alert the patient to watch for signs and symptoms of simple infections, to rinse the mouth after using steroid inhalers, and to closely monitor blood-glucose levels.

6. **Leukotriene therapy for asthma:** Monitor vital signs, especially respiratory and pulse rates, respiratory effort, lung sounds, skin color, and oxygen-saturation level. Monitor CBC and periodic liver-function tests. Closely monitor prothrombin time (PT) and international normalized ratio (INR) in patients concurrently taking warfarin (Coumadin). Closely monitor phenytoin level with concurrent phenytoin therapy; reduce theophylline dose and closely monitor levels (zileuton) if patient is using this therapy concurrently. Assess for signs and symptoms of infection, especially in patients older than 65 years. Because of their delayed onset, advise patients not to use leukotriene modifiers during an acute asthma attack.

LEARNING OUTCOME 7

For each of the classes listed in Drugs at a Glance, know representative drugs, and explain their mechanism of drug action, primary actions on the respiratory system, and important adverse effects.

Concepts for Lecture

1. **Bronchodilators—Beta-Adrenergic Agonists.** Prototype drug: salmeterol (Serevent). Mechanism of action: selectively binds to beta$_2$-adrenergic receptors in bronchial smooth muscle to cause bronchodilation. Primary use: When taken 30 to 60 minutes prior to physical activity, it can prevent exercise-induced bronchospasm. Its 12-hour duration of action is longer than many other bronchodilators, thus making it best suited for the management of chronic asthma. Because salmeterol takes 15 to 25 minutes to act, it is not indicated for the termination of acute bronchospasm. Adverse effects: Serious adverse effects from salmeterol are uncommon. Some patients

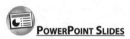

POWERPOINT SLIDES

Prototype Drug
- salmeterol (Serevent)
- ipratropium (Atrovent)
- beclomethasone (Beclovent, Beconase, Vancenase, Vanceril)
- zafirlukast (Accolate)

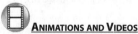

ANIMATIONS AND VIDEOS

- Mechanism in Action: Salmeterol (Serevent)
- Small-volume Nebulizer
- Metered Dose Inhaler (MDI)
- Dry Powder Inhaler (DPI)

© 2011 Pearson Education, Inc.

headaches, throat irritation nervousness, and restlessness. It also has the potential to cause tachycardia.

2. **Bronchodilators—Anticholinergic.** Prototype drug: ipratropium (Atrovent). Mechanism of action: causes bronchodilation by blocking cholinergic receptors in bronchial smooth muscle. Primary use: can relieve acute bronchospasm within minutes after administration, although peak effects may take 1 to 2 hours. Effects may continue for up to 6 hours. Ipratropium is less effective than the beta₂-agonists but is sometimes combined with beta-agonists or glucocorticoids for their additive effects. It is also prescribed for chronic bronchitis and for the symptomatic relief of nasal congestion. Adverse effects: Irritation of the upper respiratory tract may result in cough, drying of the nasal mucosa, or hoarseness. It produces a bitter taste, which may be relieved by rinsing the mouth after use.

3. **Anti-inflammatory Agents—Glucocorticoids.** Prototype drug: beclomethasone (Beclovent, Beconase, Vancenase, Vanceril). Mechanism of action: acts to reduce inflammation. Primary use: to decrease the frequency of asthma attacks. It is not a bronchodilator and should not be used to terminate asthma attacks in progress. It is available through aerosol inhalation (MDI) for asthma or as a nasal spray for allergic rhinitis. For asthma, two inhalations, two to three times per day, usually provide adequate prophylaxis. Adverse effects: oropharyngeal candidiasis.

4. **Leukotriene Modifiers.** Prototype drug: zafirlukast (Accolate). Mechanism of action: prevents airway edema and inflammation by blocking leukotriene receptors in the airways. Primary use: for the prophylaxis of persistent, chronic asthma. Adverse effects: Headache is the most common complaint; others are nausea and diarrhea.

LEARNING OUTCOME 8

Use the nursing process to care for patients who are receiving pharmacotherapy for lower respiratory tract disorders.

Concepts for Lecture

1. **Patients Receiving Bronchodilator Therapy—Assessment:** Obtain a complete health history including previous history of symptoms and association to seasons, foods, or environmental exposures, existing cardiovascular, respiratory, hepatic, renal, or neurologic disease, glaucoma, prostatic hypertrophy or difficulty with urination, presence of fever or active infections, pregnancy or breast-feeding, alcohol use, or smoking. If asthma symptoms are of new onset, assess for any recent changes in diet, soaps including laundry detergent or softener, cosmetics, lotions, environment, or recent carpet-cleaning, particularly in young children that may correlate with onset of symptoms. Assess pulmonary function with pulse oximeter, peak expiratory flow meter, and/or arterial blood gases to establish baseline levels. Assess for symptoms related to respiratory deficiency, such as dyspnea, orthopnea, cyanosis, nasal flaring, wheezing, and weakness. Obtain vital signs especially respiratory rate and depth. Auscultate bilateral breath sounds for air movement and adventitious sounds (rales, rhonchi, wheezes). Assess for adverse effects: dizziness, tachycardia, palpitations, blurred vision, or headache.

2. **Patients Receiving Bronchodilator Therapy—Nursing diagnoses:** *Impaired Gas Exchange; Ineffective Tissue Perfusion; Anxiety, Related to Difficulty in Breathing; Disturbed Sleep Pattern,* related to

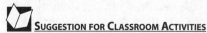
SUGGESTION FOR CLASSROOM ACTIVITIES

- Have each student make drug cards for each classification of drug used to treat lower-respiratory-tract disorders. Use two different drugs for each classification. The card should include actions, uses, routes of administration, dosages, and adverse effects. Divide students into small groups, and have each group develop a teaching plan for a patient receiving medications for lower-respiratory-tract disorders.

SUGGESTIONS FOR CLINICAL ACTIVITIES

- Have students administer medications for lower-respiratory-tract disorders.
- Quiz the students regarding the information on the medication cards.

POWERPOINT SLIDES

NURSING PROCESS FOCUS

- Care for patients who are receiving pharmacotherapy for lower-respiratory-tract disorders.

SUGGESTION FOR CLASSROOM ACTIVITIES

- Divide students into small groups, and have each group develop a teaching plan for a patient receiving pharmacotherapy for a lower-respiratory-tract disorder.

SUGGESTION FOR CLINICAL ACTIVITIES

- Assign students to care for patients receiving pharmacotherapy for a lower-respiratory-tract disorder.

adverse drug effects; *Activity Intolerance,* related to disease or ineffective drug therapy; *Deficient Knowledge,* related to drug therapy.

3. **Patients Receiving Bronchodilator Therapy—Planning:** The patient will experience therapeutic effects (e.g., increased ease of breathing, improvement in pulmonary function studies, able to experience normal sleep and eating periods, and to carry out ADLs to a level appropriate for condition); be free from or experience minimal adverse effects. Verbalize an understanding of the drug's use, adverse effects, and required precautions. Demonstrate proper self-administration of the medication (e.g., dose, timing, when to notify provider).

4. **Patients Receiving Bronchodilator Therapy—Implementation:** Monitor vital signs including pulse, blood pressure, respiratory rate and depth, and breath sounds. Monitor pulmonary function with pulse oximeter, peak expiratory flow meter, and/or arterial blood gases. Monitor the patient's ability to use the inhaler. Monitor eating and sleep patterns and ability to maintain functional ADLs. Provide for calorie-rich, nutrient-dense foods, frequent rest periods between eating or activity, and cool room for sleeping. Observe for side effects specific to the medication used. Start inhaler therapy at first sign of respiratory difficulty to abort the attack. Eliminate smoking, limit exposure to secondhand smoke, and limit caffeine intake, especially if taking methylxanthines. Maintain an environment free of respiratory contaminants, such as dust, dry air, and flowers. Maintain consistent dosing of long-acting bronchodilators. Utilize appropriate spacer between inhaler and mouth as appropriate and rinse mouth after using inhaler, especially after glucocorticoids. Instruct patient and/or family in proper self-administration of drug (e.g., take the drug at the first appearance of symptoms before symptoms are severe). Maintain a dietary intake that is adequate in essential nutrients and vitamins, and ensure adequate hydration (3–4 L/day). Provide emotional and psychosocial support during periods of shortness of breath. Monitor patient compliance with pharmacotherapy.

5. **Patients Receiving Bronchodilator Therapy—Evaluation:** The patient will experience increased ease of breathing, improvement in pulmonary function studies, reports normal sleep and eating periods, and ability to carry out ADLs to a level appropriate for condition; be free from or experience minimal adverse effects. Verbalize an understanding of the drug's use, adverse effects, and required precautions. Demonstrate proper self-administration of the medication (e.g., dose, timing, when to notify provider).

© 2011 Pearson Education, Inc.

GENERAL CHAPTER CONSIDERATIONS

1. Have students study and learn key terms listed at the beginning of the chapter.
2. Have students complete end-of-chapter exercises either in their book or on the MyNursingKit website.
3. Use the Classroom Response Questions provided in PowerPoint to assess students prior to lecture.

MyNursingKit
(www.mynursingkit.com)

- Websites
- NCLEX® questions
- Critical Thinking Questions
- Case Studies
- Animations and Videos
- Drug Prototype Questions

MyNursingLab
(www.mynursinglab.com)

- Knowledge Quick Check
- Pre/Posttests
- Customized study plans
- *Separate purchase*

STUDENT WORKBOOK AND RESOURCE GUIDE

- Chapter 39 activities
- *Separate purchase*

PEARSON NURSE'S DRUG GUIDE

- *Separate purchase*

PEARSON eTEXT

- Students can search, highlight, take notes, and more all in electronic format.
- *Separate purchase*

CLASSROOM RESPONSE QUESTION POWERPOINTS

TESTBANK

CHAPTER 40
DRUGS FOR PEPTIC ULCER DISEASE

LEARNING OUTCOME 1

Describe major anatomical structures of the upper gastrointestinal tract.

Concepts for Lecture

1. The digestive system consists of two basic anatomical divisions: the alimentary canal and the accessory organs. The accessory organs of the digestive system are the salivary glands, liver, gallbladder, and pancreas. (Figure 40.1 illustrates the digestive system.) The digestive system is responsible for breaking down food, absorbing nutrients, and eliminating wastes. A mucosa layer lines the alimentary canal and provides a surface area for breakdown and absorption of food. Peristalsis is the name for the rhythmic contractions of the smooth muscle in the gastrointestinal tract.

2. The stomach contains two muscular rings. First, the cardiac sphincter keeps food from moving back up the esophagus. The pyloric sphincter regulates the flow of food out of the stomach into the small intestine. The stomach's chief cells secrete enzymes, and its parietal cells secrete hydrochloric acid. Both of these accelerate the process of chemical digestion. A thick mucous layer and bicarbonate ion protect the stomach mucosa from the damaging effects of the acid. (Figure 40.2 illustrates the stomach's defenses.)

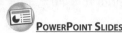

POWERPOINT SLIDES

Figure 40.1 The Digestive System
Figure 40.2 Natural Defenses Against Stomach Acid

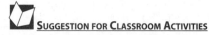

SUGGESTION FOR CLASSROOM ACTIVITIES

• Direct students to diagram the digestive system. Include the processes of food transportation, breakdown, absorption, and expulsion.

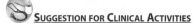

SUGGESTION FOR CLINICAL ACTIVITIES

• Direct students to perform a complete gastrointestinal assessment of their client.

LEARNING OUTCOME 2

Identify common causes, signs, and symptoms of peptic ulcer disease and gastroesophageal reflux disease.

Concepts for Lecture

1. The term *peptic ulcer* refers to a lesion located in either the stomach (gastric) or small intestine (duodenal). Peptic ulcer disease is associated with the following risk factors: close family history of PUD blood group; smoking tobacco; beverages and food containing caffeine; drugs, particularly glucocorticoids and nonsteroidal anti-inflammatory drugs (NSAIDs), including aspirin; excessive psychological stress; infection with *Helicobacter pylori*. The primary cause of PUD is infection by the gram-negative bacterium *Helicobacter pylori*. Secondary factors include secretion of excess gastric acid and hyposecretion of adequate mucous protection. The characteristic symptom of *duodenal* ulcer is a gnawing or burning, upper abdominal pain that occurs 1 to 3 hours after a meal. The pain is worse when the stomach is empty and often disappears on ingestion of food. Erosion into the mucosa may lead to bleeding that may be evident as either bright red blood in vomit or black, tarry stools. *Gastric* ulcers are less common than the duodenal type and have different symptoms. Loss of appetite, known as anorexia, as well as weight loss and vomiting are more common.

2. **Gastroesophageal reflux disease (GERD)** is a common condition in which the acidic contents of the stomach move upward into the

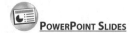

POWERPOINT SLIDES

Figure 40.3 Peptic Ulcer Formation

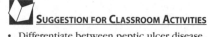

SUGGESTION FOR CLASSROOM ACTIVITIES

• Differentiate between peptic ulcer disease and gastroesophageal reflux disease.

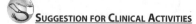

SUGGESTION FOR CLINICAL ACTIVITIES

• Assign students to care for clients who have either a peptic ulcer or gastroesophageal reflux disease. Ask the students to present the similarities and differences in postclinical.

© 2011 Pearson Education, Inc.

esophagus. GERD causes an intense burning (heartburn) sometimes accompanied by belching. In severe cases, untreated GERD can lead to complications such as esophagitis, or esophageal ulcers or strictures. The cause of GERD is usually a weakening of the lower esophageal sphincter. The sphincter may no longer close tightly, allowing the contents of the stomach to move upward when the stomach contracts. GERD is associated with obesity, and losing weight may eliminate the symptoms. Other lifestyle changes that can improve GERD symptoms include elevating the head of the bed, avoiding fatty or acidic foods, eating smaller meals at least 3 hours before sleep, and eliminating tobacco and alcohol use.

LEARNING OUTCOME 3

Compare and contrast duodenal ulcers and gastric ulcers.

Concepts for Lecture

1. Peptic ulcer disease (PUD) is caused by an erosion of the mucosal layer of the stomach or duodenum. A duodenal ulcer is more common than a gastric ulcer. It occurs most commonly in the 30 to 50 age group. The usual symptom is a gnawing or burning upper abdominal pain from 1 to 3 hours after a meal. The pain is worse when the stomach is empty. Clients also complain of nocturnal pain, nausea, and vomiting. Bleeding may occur and exhibit itself as bright red blood in the vomit or black, tarry stools.
2. Gastric ulcers are the less common type of ulcer. They are more common in the over 60 age group. Symptoms include pain that may be relieved after food or may continue after a meal, anorexia, weight loss, and vomiting. Remissions are infrequent or absent. Gastric ulcers are more commonly associated with cancer and require longer follow-up.

LEARNING OUTCOME 4

Describe treatment goals for the pharmacotherapy of gastroesophageal reflux disease.

Concepts for Lecture

The treatment of gastroesophageal reflux disease and peptic ulcer disease is similar. The primary goal is to reduce gastric-acid secretion. Classifications of drugs used to treat these problems include H_2-receptor blockers, antacids, and proton pump inhibitors. Surgery may be necessary in some cases.

LEARNING OUTCOME 5

Identify the classification of drugs used to treat peptic ulcer disease.

Concepts for Lecture

Peptic ulcer disease is best treated by a combination of lifestyle changes and pharmacotherapy. Treatment goals are to eliminate infection by

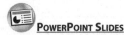**POWERPOINT SLIDES**

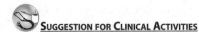**SUGGESTION FOR CLASSROOM ACTIVITIES**

- Differentiate between duodenal and gastric ulcers.

SUGGESTION FOR CLINICAL ACTIVITIES

- Assign students to observe an esophagastroduodenoscopy (EGD) procedure.

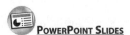**POWERPOINT SLIDES**

SUGGESTION FOR CLASSROOM ACTIVITIES

- Direct students to draw a concept map illustrating peptic ulcer disease and gastroesophageal reflux disease etiology, signs and symptoms, and treatment.

SUGGESTION FOR CLINICAL ACTIVITIES

- Direct students to access the care plans for clients with peptic ulcer disease or gastroesophageal reflux disease. Require each student to make a suggestion for one contribution to those care plans.

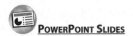**POWERPOINT SLIDES**

© 2011 Pearson Education, Inc.

H. pylori, promote ulcer healing, and prevent recurrence of symptoms. Drugs used in the treatment of peptic ulcer disease include H$_2$-receptor antagonists, proton pump inhibitors, antacids, antibiotics, and miscellaneous drugs.

SUGGESTION FOR CLASSROOM ACTIVITIES

- Have students search for a reputable Internet site that discusses the treatment guidelines for peptic ulcer disease. Have them submit a paper that summarizes the information they found.

SUGGESTION FOR CLINICAL ACTIVITIES

- Assign students to care for a client with peptic ulcer disease.

POWERPOINT SLIDES

LEARNING OUTCOME 6

Explain the pharmacologic strategies for eradicating *Helicobacter pylori*.

Concepts for Lecture

The primary goal of treatment for *H. pylori* is complete eradication of the bacteria. Other treatment goals include interventions that cause the ulcer to heal more rapidly and remain in remission longer. There is a very high reoccurrence of peptic ulcers when *H. pylori* is not completely eradicated. Infection can remain active for life if not treated.

SUGGESTION FOR CLASSROOM ACTIVITIES

- Direct students to research the history of how *H. pylori* was identified as a causative factor in ulcer formation. Discuss their research during the next class period.

SUGGESTION FOR CLINICAL ACTIVITIES

- Assign students to look at the medication administration records of clients who are newly diagnosed with *H. pylori*. What is the primary antibiotic used to eradicate *H. pylori* at your medical facility?

POWERPOINT SLIDES

LEARNING OUTCOME 7

Describe the nurse's role in the pharmacologic management of patients with peptic ulcer disease.

Concepts for Lecture

1. The role of the nurse in the pharmacologic management of peptic ulcer disease involves careful monitoring of a client's condition and providing education as it relates to the prescribed drug treatment. Obtain baseline medical, surgical, and drug history; lifestyle and dietary habits, including use of herbal or alternative therapies; and a detailed description of symptomology and current therapies.

2. **H$_2$-receptor antagonist therapy:** Assess the client's use of OTC formulations to avoid duplication of treatment. If using OTC formulations, clients should be advised to seek medical attention if symptoms persist or reoccur. Persistent epigastric pain or heartburn may be a symptom of more serious disease that requires different medical treatment. IV preparations of H$_2$-receptor antagonists are occasionally utilized. Because dysrhythmias and hypotension have occurred with IV cimetidine, ranitidine (Zantac) or famotidine (Pepcid) are administered if the IV route is necessary. Assess kidney and liver function. Evaluate the client's CBC for possible anemia during long-term use of these drugs.

3. **Proton pump inhibitor therapy for PUD:** Proton pump inhibitors are usually well tolerated for short-term use. With long-term use, liver function should be periodically monitored as well as serum gastrin,

SUGGESTION FOR CLASSROOM ACTIVITIES

- Direct students to concept map the role of the nurse in the pharmacologic treatment of clients with PUD.

SUGGESTION FOR CLINICAL ACTIVITIES

- Direct students to implement a teaching plan for clients with PUD.

© 2011 Pearson Education, Inc.

because oversecretion of gastrin occurs with constant acid suppression. Assess for drug–drug interactions. Proton pump inhibitors will affect the absorption of medications, vitamins, and minerals that need an acidic environment in the stomach. Obtain the client's history of smoking, because smoking increases stomach-acid production. These drugs should be taken 30 minutes prior to eating, usually before breakfast. These drugs may be administered at the same time as antacids. Proton pump inhibitors are often administered in combination with clarithromycin (Biaxin) for the treatment of *H. pylori*.

4. **Antacid therapy for PUD:** Obtain a medical history, including the use of OTC and prescription drugs. Assess the client for signs of renal insufficiency; magnesium-containing antacids should be used with caution in these clients. Hypermagnesemia may occur because the kidneys are unable to excrete excess magnesium. Magnesium- and aluminum-based products may cause diarrhea, and those with calcium may cause constipation.

LEARNING OUTCOME 8

For each of the classes listed in Drugs at a Glance, know representative drugs, and explain their mechanism of drug action, describe primary actions, and identify important adverse effects.

Concepts for Lecture

1. **H$_2$-Receptor Blockers:** Prototype drug: ranitidine (Zantac). Mechanism of action: acts by blocking H$_2$-receptors in the stomach to decrease acid production. Primary use: to treat peptic ulcer disease. Adverse effects: Although rare, severe reductions in the number of red and white blood cells and platelets are possible; thus, periodic blood counts may be performed. High doses may result in impotence or loss of libido in men. (See Table 40.2.)

2. **Proton Pump Inhibitors:** Prototype drug: omeprazole (Prilosec). Mechanism of action: reduces acid secretion in the stomach by binding irreversibly to the enzyme H^1, K^1-ATPase. Primary use: for the short-term, 4- to 8-week treatment of peptic ulcers and GERD. Adverse effects: generally minor and include headache, nausea, diarrhea, rash, and abdominal pain. The main concern with proton pump inhibitors is that long-term use has been associated with an increased risk of gastric cancer. (See Table 40.1.)

3. **Antacids:** Prototype drug: aluminum hydroxide (Amphojel). Mechanism of action: neutralizes stomach acid by raising the pH of the stomach contents. Primary use: most effectively used in combination with other anti-ulcer agents for the symptomatic relief of heartburn due to PUD or GERD. Adverse effects: minor; include constipation. (See Table 40.3.)

4. **Antibiotics:** These drugs are administered to treat *H. pylori* infections of the gastrointestinal tract. Two or more antibiotics are given concurrently to increase effectiveness and to lower the potential for resistance. The regimen often includes a proton pump inhibitor and/or bismuth compounds, which inhibit bacterial growth and prevent *H. pylori* from adhering to the gastric mucosa.

5. **Miscellaneous Drugs:** Several additional drugs are beneficial in treating peptic ulcer disease. Sucralfate coats the ulcer and protects it from further erosion. Misoprostol inhibits acid and stimulates production of mucus. Pirenzepine inhibits autonomic receptors responsible for gastric-acid secretion.

POWERPOINT SLIDES

Table 40.1 H$_2$-receptor Antagonists
Table 40.2 Proton Pump Inhibitors
Table 40.3 Antacids

Prototype Drug
- ranitidine (Zantac)
- omeprazole (Prilosec)
- aluminum hydroxide (Amphojel)

ANIMATIONS AND VIDEOS

- Mechanism in Action: Ranitidine (Zantac)
- Mechanism in Action: Omeprazole (Prilosec)

SUGGESTION FOR CLASSROOM ACTIVITIES

- Have each student make drug cards for each classification of drug used to treat PUD and GERD. Use two different drugs for each classification. The card should include actions, uses, routes of administration, dosages, and adverse effects.

SUGGESTION FOR CLINICAL ACTIVITIES

- Direct students to bring medication cards to clinical. Assign students to administer the medications discussed in this chapter. Quiz students on the information from the medication cards.

© 2011 Pearson Education, Inc.

LEARNING OUTCOME 9

Use the nursing process to care for patients who are receiving drug therapy for peptic ulcer disease.

Concepts for Lecture

1. **Patients Receiving Pharmacotherapy for PUD or GERD—Assessment:** Obtain a complete health history including gastrointestinal, hepatic, renal, respiratory, or cardiovascular disease, pregnancy or breast-feeding. Obtain drug history including allergies, and possible drug interactions. Obtain a history of past and current symptoms, noting any correlations between onset or presence of any pain related to meals, sleep, positioning or associated with other medications. Assess client for signs of GI bleeding. Note what measures have been successful to relieve the pain (e.g., eating). Obtain vital signs and weight. Evaluate appropriate laboratory findings (e.g., CBC, platelets, electrolytes, hepatic or renal function studies). Assess level of consciousness. Assess for adverse effects: nausea, vomiting, diarrhea, headache, drowsiness, dizziness. Severe abdominal pain, vomiting, coffee-ground or hematemesis, blood in stool or tarry stools should be reported immediately.

2. **Patients Receiving Pharmacotherapy for PUD or GERD—Nursing diagnoses:** *Acute Pain; Altered Nutrition, Less than Body Requirements; Deficient Knowledge* related to drug therapy; *Risk for Ineffective Health Maintenance* (individual or family; dietary and lifestyle changes).

3. **Patients Receiving Pharmacotherapy for PUD or GERD—Planning:** The client will experience therapeutic effects (e.g., diminished or absent gastric pain, absence of related symptoms such as bloating or belching); be free from or experience minimal adverse effects. Verbalize an understanding of the drug's use, adverse effects, and required precautions. Demonstrate proper self-administration of the medication (e.g., dose, timing, when to notify provider).

4. **Patients Receiving Pharmacotherapy for PUD or GERD—Implementation:** Monitor use of OTC drugs to avoid drug interactions, especially with cimetidine therapy. Monitor client use of alcohol. Discuss possible drug interactions. Institute effective safety measures regarding falls. Explain need for lifestyle changes. Observe client for signs of GI bleeding. Administer H_2-receptor blockers should be taken after meals; proton pump inhibitors before meals, antacids 2 hours before or after meals with a full glass of water. Monitor for any severe abdominal pain, vomiting, coffee-ground or hematemesis, blood in stool or tarry stools and report immediately. Monitor periodic hepatic and renal function tests and CBC, platelets, and electrolyte levels. Observe for dizziness and monitor ambulation until effects of drug are known. Instruct patient and/or family in proper self-administration of drug (e.g., during evening meal).

5. **Patients Receiving Pharmacotherapy for PUD or GERD—Evaluation:** The client will experiences diminished or absent gastric pain, absence of related symptoms such as bloating or belching; be free from or experience minimal adverse effects. Verbalize an understanding of the drug's use, adverse effects, and required precautions. Demonstrate proper self-administration of the medication (e.g., dose, timing, when to notify provider).

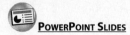
POWERPOINT SLIDES

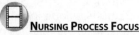
NURSING PROCESS FOCUS
- Patients Receiving Pharmacotherapy for PUD or GERD

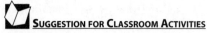
SUGGESTION FOR CLASSROOM ACTIVITIES
- Divide students into small groups, and have each group develop a teaching plan for a patient receiving medications for PUD.

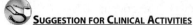
SUGGESTION FOR CLINICAL ACTIVITIES
- Invite an endoscopy nurse to postclinical to speak to the students after clinical. Meet in the endoscopy room for a tour.

© 2011 Pearson Education, Inc.

GENERAL CHAPTER CONSIDERATIONS

1. Have students study and learn key terms listed at the beginning of the chapter.
2. Have students complete end-of-chapter exercises either in their book or on the MyNursingKit website.
3. Use the Classroom Response Questions provided in PowerPoint to assess students prior to lecture.

MyNursingKit
(*www.mynursingkit.com*)

- Websites
- NCLEX® questions
- Critical Thinking Questions
- Case Studies
- Animations and Videos
- Drug Prototype Questions

MyNursingLab
(*www.mynursinglab.com*)

- Knowledge Quick Check
- Pre/Posttests
- Customized study plans
- *Separate purchase*

STUDENT WORKBOOK AND RESOURCE GUIDE

- Chapter 40 activities
- *Separate purchase*

PEARSON NURSE'S DRUG GUIDE

- *Separate purchase*

PEARSON eTEXT

- Students can search, highlight, take notes, and more all in electronic format.
- *Separate purchase*

CLASSROOM RESPONSE QUESTION POWERPOINTS

TESTBANK

CHAPTER 41
DRUGS FOR BOWEL DISORDERS AND OTHER GASTROINTESTINAL CONDITIONS

LEARNING OUTCOME 1

Identify the major anatomic structures of the lower gastrointestinal tract.

Concepts for Lecture

The small intestine is the location for most nutrient and drug absorption; peristalsis is controlled by the autonomic nervous system. Peptic ulcer is the most common disorder. The large intestine is responsible for the reabsorption of water and excretion of fecal matter.

LEARNING OUTCOME 2

Explain the pathogenesis of constipation and diarrhea.

Concepts for Lecture

1. Constipation is the infrequent passage of hard, small stools. It is a symptom of an underlying disorder and a common condition caused by lack of exercise; insufficient dietary fiber; diminished fluid intake; slow motility of waste material through the large intestine; and certain foods, medications, and diseases.
2. Diarrhea is the increase in the frequency and fluidity of bowel movements and occurs when the colon fails to reabsorb enough water. A type of body defense, diarrhea eliminates toxins and pathogens and certain medications and infections. Prolonged diarrhea can lead to fluid, electrolyte, and acid–base imbalance. Monitor diarrhea frequency and appearance, as it may be related to pseudomembranous colitis.

LEARNING OUTCOME 3

Discuss conditions in which the pharmacotherapy of bowel disorders is indicated.

Concepts for Lecture

1. Laxatives and cathartics are given to treat or prevent constipation and to prepare the bowel for surgery or diagnostic procedures. They promote emptying of the large intestine in several different ways. Stimulants and herbal agents stimulate peristalsis. Mineral oil lubricates the

POWERPOINT SLIDES

Figure 41.1 The Gastrointestinal Tract

SUGGESTION FOR CLASSROOM ACTIVITIES
- Direct students to diagram the lower GI tract and note the functions of each area.

SUGGESTION FOR CLINICAL ACTIVITIES
- Assign students to monitor all gastrointestinal output for a group of clients during their shift. This would include any bowel movements, colostomy drainage, nasogastric tube drainage, and vomitus. Direct them to document and report any abnormalities.

POWERPOINT SLIDES

SUGGESTION FOR CLASSROOM ACTIVITIES
- Direct students to research pseudomembranous colitis online and submit a paper summarizing what they have learned.

SUGGESTION FOR CLINICAL ACTIVITIES
- Assign students to observe gastrointestinal procedures and diagnostic studies in the radiology department.

POWERPOINT SLIDES

SUGGESTION FOR CLASSROOM ACTIVITIES
- Compare and contrast inflammatory bowel disease and irritable bowel syndrome.

© 2011 Pearson Education, Inc.

fecal mass. Bulk-forming agents, stool softeners or surfactants, saline or osmotic laxatives add more bulk or water to the colon contents.

2. Treatment for diarrhea depends on the severity and etiology. Opioids are administered for severe diarrhea; they are the most effective and work by slowing peristalsis. Over-the-counter medications are given for simple diarrhea; this group includes loperamide, bismuth compounds, psyllium preparations, and probiotic supplements.

3. Inflammatory bowel disease (IBD) includes both ulcerative colitis (erosions in the large intestine) and Crohn's disease (ulceration in the distal part of the small intestine). Symptoms of inflammatory bowel disease range from mild to acute abdominal cramping and diarrhea. There are periods of remissions and exacerbations.

4. Treatment of inflammatory bowel disease includes 5-aminosalicylic acid (5-ASA) agents such as sulfonamide sulfasalazine (Azulfidine), olsalazine (Dipentum), and mesalamine (Asacol). Glucocorticoids such as prednisone, methylprednisolone, and hydrocortisone are also used to treat this disease. The treatment may also include immunosuppressant drugs such as azathioprine (Imuran), methotrexate (MTX), and ifliximab (Remicade), a monoclonal antibody.

5. Irritable bowel syndrome (IBS) is also known as spastic colon or mucous colitis; it is a common disorder of the lower gastrointestinal tract. Symptoms include abdominal pain, cramping, bloating, gas, and constipation, alternating with diarrhea. It is a functional bowel disorder with no presence of detectable disease. Stress and dietary factors precipitate symptoms.

6. Treatment of irritable bowel syndrome is supportive and treats the symptoms. Medications used are bulk laxatives such as psyllium; anticholinergic medications to reduce bowel spasm, such as dicyclomine (Bentyl); Tegaserod, which is one of only a few drugs approved for irritable bowel syndrome with constipation; and serotonin agonists, which stimulate peristaltic reflex.

LEARNING OUTCOME 4

Explain conditions in which the pharmacotherapy of nausea and vomiting is indicated.

Concepts for Lecture

1. Vomiting is a defense mechanism used by the body to rid itself of toxic substances. It is controlled by the "vomiting center" located in the medulla of the brain. Vomiting is associated with many conditions, including infection, poisoning, psychological factors, pain, and changes in body position. Many drugs can cause nausea and vomiting as side effects, and this is a common reason to discontinue a drug. Emetogenic potential is the capacity of a drug to induce vomiting.

2. Nausea and vomiting are treated with antiemetics. Simple nausea is treated with over-the-counter drugs and herbal options. Serious nausea is treated with prescription drugs from many different classes, including phenothiazines, antihistamines, anticholinergics, cannabinoids, glucocorticoids, benzodiazepines, and serotonin receptor antagonists.

SUGGESTION FOR CLINICAL ACTIVITIES
• Assign students to tour the pharmacy, and have the pharmacy staff speak about medications used to treat gastrointestinal conditions.

POWERPOINT SLIDES

SUGGESTION FOR CLASSROOM ACTIVITIES
• Discuss prophylactic antiemetics and chemotherapy.

SUGGESTION FOR CLINICAL ACTIVITIES
• Assign students to care for clients experiencing nausea and vomiting. Direct the students to present the types of treatments used.

© 2011 Pearson Education, Inc.

LEARNING OUTCOME 5

Describe the types of drugs used in the short-term management of obesity.

Concepts for Lecture

Anorexiants are drugs that affect hunger and/or appetite and are used for the short-term management of obesity. These drugs produce only modest effects. In the 1970s amphetamine and dextroamphetamine were widely used; however, they are addictive and now are rarely prescribed. Fen-phen in the 1990s and ephedra products in 2004 were taken off the market after causing heart problems. There are two anorexiants used today: orlistat, which blocks lipid absorption in the gastrointestinal tract, and sibutramine, which is a selective serotonin reuptake inhibitor (SSRI).

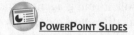
POWERPOINT SLIDES

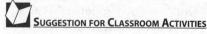
SUGGESTION FOR CLASSROOM ACTIVITIES

- Discuss the use of anorexiants in today's society.

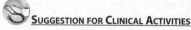
SUGGESTION FOR CLINICAL ACTIVITIES

- Assign students to create educational materials on lifestyle modifications that are necessary, in addition to use of anorexiants, for sustained weight loss.

LEARNING OUTCOME 6

Explain the use of pancreatic enzyme replacement in the pharmacotherapy of pancreatitis.

Concepts for Lecture

Pancreatitis results when pancreatic enzymes (amylase and lipase) are trapped in the pancreas and not released into the duodenum. It is associated with gallstones in women and alcoholism in men. Pharmacotherapy includes replacement enzymes and supportive drugs for reduction of pain and gastric-acid secretion.

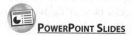
POWERPOINT SLIDES

SUGGESTION FOR CLASSROOM ACTIVITIES

- Direct students to concept map the etiology and treatment of pancreatitis.

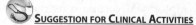
SUGGESTION FOR CLINICAL ACTIVITIES

- Assign students to care for a client with pancreatitis.

LEARNING OUTCOME 7

Describe the nurse's role in the pharmacologic management of bowel disorders, nausea and vomiting, and other GI conditions.

Concepts for Lecture

1. The role of the nurse in the pharmacologic management of bowel disorders, nausea and vomiting, and other GI conditions involves careful monitoring of a client's condition and providing education as it relates to the prescribed drug treatment. Obtain baseline medical, surgical, and drug history; lifestyle and dietary habits, including use of herbal or alternative therapies; and a detailed description of symptomology and current therapies.

2. Laxative therapy for bowel evacuation: Assess the abdomen for distension, bowel sounds, and bowel patterns. If there is absence of bowel sounds, peristalsis must be restored prior to laxative therapy. Assess for colon cancer, esophageal obstruction, intestinal obstruction, fecal impaction, and undiagnosed abdominal pain. If diarrhea occurs, discontinue laxative use. Use with caution during pregnancy and lactation. Take with one to two glasses of water. Assess the client's ability to swallow. Assess for the development of diarrhea and cramping. Assess for and educate clients about the proper use of laxatives and stool softeners.

3. Antidiarrheal therapy: Assess hydration status, serum potassium, magnesium, and bicarbonate. Also assess for blood in the stool. Antidiarrheals should not be used if constipation should be avoided, such as in pseudomembranous colitis or severe ulcerative colitis. Assess the

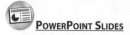
POWERPOINT SLIDES

SUGGESTION FOR CLASSROOM ACTIVITIES

- Discuss the role of the nurse in the pharmacologic treatment of clients with bowel disorders, nausea and vomiting, and other GI conditions.

SUGGESTION FOR CLINICAL ACTIVITIES

- Assign students to care for clients with a bowel disorder.

© 2011 Pearson Education, Inc.

client's ability to get out of bed safely. Antidiarrheals are contraindicated in clients with severe dehydration, electrolyte imbalance, liver and renal disorders, and glaucoma.

4. Tegaserod (Zelnorm) therapy for IBD: Prior to and during therapy, monitor liver and renal function. Monitor cardiovascular status, especially in clients with preexisting cardiovascular disease. Tegaserod is contraindicated in severe hepatic or renal impairment, bowel obstruction, gallbladder disease, and abdominal pain. Administer the drug just prior to a meal with a full glass of water. Tablets may be crushed. Do not give the drug to clients with frequent diarrhea because tegaserod accelerates gastric emptying.

5. **Antiemetic therapy:** Assess symptoms that precipitated the vomiting or that are occurring concurrently. If a client becomes sedated and continues to vomit, a nasogastric tube with suction may be indicated. Client safety is a concern because drowsiness is a frequent side effect. Clients may be at risk for falls because of medication side effects and the sensation of weakness from vomiting. Immediately report vomiting of blood, or if the vomiting is associated with severe abdominal pain. Do not use OTC antiemetics for prolonged periods; vomiting may be a symptom of a serious disorder that requires medical attention.

6. Drugs used to stimulate emesis should only be used in emergency situations under the direction of a health care provider. They are used only when the client is alert because of the risk of aspiration. When the client is comatose, a gastric lavage tube is placed and attached to suction to empty gastric contents. Before inducing vomiting with an OTC emetic, check with the health care provider; some poisons and caustic chemicals should not be vomited.

7. **Anorexiant therapy:** When administering anorexiants, focus on lifestyle changes that will have a greater effect on weight reduction in the long term. Drugs for weight loss have limited effectiveness and potentially serious side effects. Education of clients is essential; clients should not take OTC medications or herbal medications without notifying their health care provider. If taking orlistat, the client should also take a multivitamin each day but omit a dose if there is no fat present in the meal or if the meal is skipped. Client should know that excessive flatus and fecal leaking may occur when a high-fat meal is consumed.

8. **Pancreatic-enzyme replacement therapy:** Assess dietary habits for use of foods that stimulate gastric and pancreatic secretions. Assess for and monitor the presence, amount, and type of pain. Assess the symmetry of the chest wall and the movement of the chest and diaphragm. Monitor for other abnormal findings, such as elevated serum and urinary amylase and elevated serum bilirubin. Also monitor the client's nutritional and hydration status and for signs of infection. Check for pork allergy.

LEARNING OUTCOME 8

For each of the drug classes listed in Drugs at a Glance, know representative drugs, and explain the mechanism of drug action, describe primary actions, and identify important adverse effects.

Concepts for Lecture

1. **Laxatives:** Prototype drug: psyllium mucilloid (Metamucil). Mechanism of action: swells and increases the size of the fecal mass. Primary use: to promote the passage of stool. The larger the size of the fecal

 POWERPOINT SLIDES

Prototype Drug
- psyllium mucilloid (Metamucil)
- diphenoxylate with atropine (Lomotil)
- tegaserod (Zelnorm)
- prochloperazine (Compazine)
- sibutramine (Meridia)
- pancrelipase (Lipancreatin, Pamcrease, Zymase)

mass, the more the defecation reflex will be stimulated. Adverse effects: rarely produces side effects. It causes less cramping than stimulant-type laxatives and results in a more natural bowel movement. If taken with insufficient water, it may cause obstructions in the esophagus or intestine.

2. **Antidiarrheals, Opioids:** Prototype drug: diphenoxylate with atropine (Lomotil). Mechanism of action: slows peristalsis, allowing time for additional water reabsorption from the colon and more solid stools. Primary use: for moderate to severe diarrhea. Adverse effects: dizziness and drowsiness.

3. **Drugs for Inflammatory Bowel Disease and Irritable Bowel Syndrome:** Prototype drug: tegaserod (Zelnorm). Mechanism of action: as a serotonin receptor agonist that causes an increase in stool formation and the number of bowel movements. Primary use: for clients who have the constipation-dominant form of irritable bowel syndrome. Adverse effects: There are no serious adverse effects. The most common side effect is diarrhea, which usually occurs as a single episode and resolves as therapy progresses.

4. **Antiemetics, Phenothiazines, and Phenothiazide-like Drugs:** Prototype drug: prochloperazine (Compazine). Mechanism of action: blocks dopamine receptors in the brain, which inhibits signals to the vomiting center in the medulla. Primary use: for severe nausea and vomiting. Adverse effects: Dose-related anticholinergic side effects such as dry mouth, sedation, constipation, orthostatic hypotension, and tachycardia may occur. When used for prolonged periods at higher doses, extrapyramidal symptoms are a serious concern.

5. **Anorexiants:** Prototype drug: sibutramine (Meridia). Mechanism of action: as a selective serotonin reuptake inhibitor (SSRI). Primary use: most widely prescribed appetite suppressant for the short-term control of obesity. Adverse effects: Headache is the most common complaint reported during sibutramine therapy, although insomnia and dry mouth also occur. It should be used with great care in clients with cardiac disorders, as it may cause tachycardia and raise blood pressure.

6. **Pancreatic-Enzyme Replacement:** Prototype drug: pancrelipase (Lipancreatin, Pamcrease, Zymase). Mechanism of action: contains lipase, protease, and amylase of pork origin, which facilitates the breakdown and conversion of lipids into glycerol and fatty acids, starches into dextrin and sugars, and proteins into peptides. Primary use: as replacement therapy for clients with insufficient pancreatic exocrine secretions. Adverse effects: gastrointestinal symptoms of nausea, vomiting, and/or diarrhea; can cause metabolic symptom of hyperuricosuria.

LEARNING OUTCOME 9

Use the nursing process to care for patients who are receiving drug therapy for bowel disorders, nausea and vomiting, and other GI conditions.

Concepts for Lecture

1. Laxatives are drugs that promote bowel movements. Many are available over the counter for the self-treatment of simple constipation. (Doses of laxatives are identified in Table 41.1.) There are several types of laxative: Bulk-forming agents absorb water, thus adding size to the fecal mass. Stool softeners or surfactants cause more water and fat to be absorbed into the stools. Stimulants irritate the bowel to increase peristalsis. Saline or osmotic laxatives are not absorbed in the intestine; they pull water into the fecal mass to create a more watery stool.

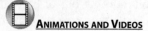

ANIMATIONS AND VIDEOS
- Mechanism of Action: Tegaserod (Zelnorm)

SUGGESTION FOR CLASSROOM ACTIVITIES
- Have each student make drug cards for each classification of drug used to treat bowel disorders, nausea, and vomiting. Use two different drugs for each classification. The card should include actions, uses, routes of administration, dosages, and adverse effects.

SUGGESTION FOR CLINICAL ACTIVITIES
- Divide students into small groups, and have each group develop a teaching plan for a patient receiving medications for bowel disorders, nausea, and vomiting.

POWERPOINT SLIDES

Table 41.1 Laxatives and Cathartics
Table 41.2 Antidiarrheals
Table 41.3 Selected Antiemetics

SUGGESTION FOR CLASSROOM ACTIVITIES
- Divide students into small groups, and have them prepare questions and answers for different categories of drugs used to treat bowel disorders, nausea and vomiting, and other GI conditions. Include questions on each drug's classification and mechanisms of action.

© 2011 Pearson Education, Inc.

Herbal agents are natural products available OTC that are widely used for self-treatment of constipation. The most commonly used herbal laxative is senna, a potent herb that irritates the bowel and increases peristalsis. Miscellaneous agents include mineral oil, which acts by lubricating the stool and the colon mucosa.

2. For mild diarrhea, OTC products are effective at returning elimination patterns to normal. For chronic or severe cases, the opioids are the most efficacious of the antidiarrheal agents. (The antidiarrheals are shown in Table 41.2.)

3. Drugs for inflammatory bowel disease and irritable bowel syndrome are from several classifications. Mild-to-moderate IBD is treated with 5-aminosalicylic acid (5-ASA) agents. Corticosteroids are used in more persistent cases. Particularly severe disease may require immunosuppressant drugs. Treatment of IBS is supportive, with drug therapy targeted at symptomatic treatment, depending on whether constipation or diarrhea is the predominant symptom. Medications include bulk laxatives, anticholinergic drugs, and serotonin agonists.

4. Antiemetic drugs from at least eight different classes are used to prevent nausea and vomiting. Many of these act by inhibiting dopamine or serotonin receptors in the brain. (The antiemetics are shown in Table 41.3.)

5. Anorexiants are drugs used to induce weight loss by suppressing appetite and hunger. Despite the public's desire for effective drugs to promote weight loss, however, there are few such drugs on the market. The approved agents produce only modest effects.

6. The pancreas secretes essential digestive enzymes. The enzymatic portion of pancreatic juice contains carboxypeptidase, chymotrypsin, and trypsin, which are converted to their active forms once they reach the small intestine. Three other pancreatic enzymes—lipase, amylase, and nuclease—are secreted in their active form but require the presence of bile for optimum activity. Because lack of secretion will result in malabsorption disorders, replacement therapy is sometimes warranted.

LEARNING OUTCOME 10

Use the nursing process to care for clients who are receiving drug therapy for bowel disorders, nausea and vomiting, and other GI conditions.

Concepts for Lecture

1. **Assessment:** Prior to administration, obtain a complete health history, including allergies, drug history, and possible drug interactions. Assess sodium, chloride, and potassium levels. Evaluate results of stool culture. Assess for presence of dehydration. Obtain vital signs and ECG.

2. **Nursing Diagnoses:** *Risk for Imbalanced Fluid Volume: Less Than Body Requirements* related to fluid loss secondary to diarrhea; *Risk for Injury (Falls)* related to drowsiness secondary to drug therapy.

3. **Planning:** The client will report relief of diarrhea; demonstrate an understanding of the drug's action by accurately describing drug side effects and precautions; immediately report effects such as persistent diarrhea, constipation, abdominal pain, blood in stool, confusion, dizziness, or fever.

4. **Implementation:** Monitor frequency, volume, and consistency of stools. Minimize the risk of dehydration and electrolyte imbalance. Prevent accidental overdosage. Monitor for dry mouth. Initiate safety measures to prevent falls. Monitor electrolyte levels.

SUGGESTION FOR CLINICAL ACTIVITIES

- Assign students to care for patients receiving pharmacotherapy for bowel disorders, nausea and vomiting, and other GI conditions.

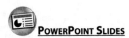

POWERPOINT SLIDES

NURSING PROCESS FOCUS

- Care for clients who are receiving drug therapy for bowel disorders, nausea and vomiting, and other GI conditions.

SUGGESTION FOR CLASSROOM ACTIVITIES

- Direct students to concept map the care of a client with a bowel disorder, nausea and vomiting, or any other gastrointestinal condition.

SUGGESTION FOR CLINICAL ACTIVITIES

- Direct the students to implement a teaching plan for clients with bowel disorders, nausea and vomiting, and other gastrointestinal conditions.

5. **Evaluation:** The client reports relief of diarrhea. The client accurately states the drug's action and side effects. The client accurately states signs and symptoms to be reported to the health care provider.

GENERAL CHAPTER CONSIDERATIONS

1. Have students study and learn key terms listed at the beginning of the chapter.
2. Have students complete end-of-chapter exercises either in their book or on the MyNursingKit website.
3. Use the Classroom Response Questions provided in PowerPoint to assess students prior to lecture.

MyNursingKit
(*www.mynursingkit.com*)

- Websites
- NCLEX® questions
- Critical Thinking Questions
- Case Studies
- Animations and Videos
- Drug Prototype Questions

MyNursingLab
(*www.mynursinglab.com*)

- Knowledge Quick Check
- Pre/Posttests
- Customized study plans
- *Separate purchase*

STUDENT WORKBOOK AND RESOURCE GUIDE

- Chapter 41 activities
- *Separate purchase*

PEARSON NURSE'S DRUG GUIDE

- *Separate purchase*

PEARSON eTEXT

- Students can search, highlight, take notes, and more all in electronic format.
- *Separate purchase*

CLASSROOM RESPONSE QUESTION POWERPOINTS

TESTBANK

CHAPTER 42
DRUGS FOR NUTRITIONAL DISORDERS

LEARNING OUTCOME 1

Identify characteristics that differentiate vitamins from other nutrients.

Concepts for Lecture

Vitamins are organic substances needed in small amounts to promote growth and maintain health. Human cells cannot produce vitamins except vitamin D. Vitamins or provitamins must be supplied in the diet. Deficiency of a vitamin will result in disease.

POWERPOINT SLIDES

SUGGESTION FOR CLASSROOM ACTIVITIES

- Give a prequiz to access student knowledge of vitamins and minerals.

SUGGESTION FOR CLINICAL ACTIVITIES

- Direct students to survey the medication-administration records of their clients for use of vitamins in that hospitalized population.

LEARNING OUTCOME 2

Describe the functions of vitamins and minerals.

Concepts for Lecture

Vitamins serve many important roles in the function of the body: The vitamin B complex includes coenzymes essential to metabolic processes, vitamin A is a precursor of retinol needed for normal vision, vitamin D regulates calcium metabolism, and vitamin K is needed to produce prothrombin. (See Table 42.1 for a list of vitamins.)

POWERPOINT SLIDES

Table 42.1 Vitamins

SUGGESTION FOR CLASSROOM ACTIVITIES

- Direct students to develop a matching game to correlate vitamins and minerals with their functions in the body.

SUGGESTION FOR CLINICAL ACTIVITIES

- Assign students to the newborn nursery, and supervise them as they give vitamin K injections.

LEARNING OUTCOME 3

Compare and contrast the properties of water-soluble and fat-soluble vitamins.

Concepts for Lecture

1. Vitamins are classified as lipid soluble (A, D, E, and K) or water soluble (C and B complex). Lipid-soluble vitamins must be ingested with lipids to be absorbed in the small intestine. Excess lipid-soluble vitamins are stored in the liver and adipose tissue so they can be removed from the storage areas and used as needed. Excessive intake of lipid-soluble vitamins can lead to dangerously high levels. (See Table 42.2 for a list of lipid-soluble vitamins.)

POWERPOINT SLIDES

Table 42.2 Lipid-soluble Vitamins for Treating Nutritional Disorders
Table 42.3 Water-soluble Vitamins for Treating Nutritional Disorders

SUGGESTION FOR CLASSROOM ACTIVITIES

- Discuss differences and similarities between water-soluble and fat-soluble vitamins.

2. Water-soluble vitamins are absorbed with water in the digestive tract; they are easily dissolved in blood and body fluids. Excess water-soluble vitamins cannot be stored; they are excreted in the urine and must be ingested daily. (See Table 42.3 for a list of water-soluble vitamins.)

LEARNING OUTCOME 4

Identify diseases and conditions that may benefit from vitamin or mineral pharmacotherapy.

Concepts for Lecture

1. Failure to meet the Recommended Dietary Allowances (RDAs) for vitamins may result in deficiency disorders. The RDA is the amount of a vitamin needed to prevent symptoms of deficiency, but the need for vitamins and minerals varies among individuals. Supplements should never substitute for a healthy diet. (See Table 42.4 for a list of Recommended Dietary Allowances.) Vitamin therapy is indicated for conditions such as poor nutritional intake, pregnancy, and chronic-disease states. Symptoms of deficiency are usually nonspecific and occur over a prolonged period. Clients often present with multiple deficiencies. In the United States these deficiencies many times are the result of poverty, fad diets, chronic alcohol or drug abuse, or prolonged parenteral feeding.
2. Deficiencies of vitamins A, D, E, or K are indications for pharmacotherapy with lipid-soluble vitamins. Vitamin A (retinol) is obtained from foods containing carotenes. Vitamin D is obtained from dairy products (D_2, ergocalciferol) and from ultraviolet light (D_3). For vitamin E tocopherols are found in plant-seed oils, whole-grain cereals, eggs, and certain organ meats; it is a primary antioxidant. Vitamin K is a mixture of several chemicals—K_1 is obtained from plant sources and K_2 from microbial flora in the colon. Vitamin K is needed for clotting.
3. Deficiencies of vitamin C can cause scurvy, thiamine (B_1) deficiencies can cause beriberi, niacin (B_3) deficiencies can cause pellagra, and cyanocobalamin (B_{12}) deficiencies can cause pernicious or megaloblastic anemia. Riboflavin, folic acid, or pyridoxine can also cause problems because of deficiencies that are indications for pharmacotherapy with water-soluble vitamins.
4. Minerals are inorganic substances needed in very small amounts to maintain normal body metabolism. They constitute 4% of body weight. Because they are needed in such small amounts, most minerals can be obtained from a normal diet. An excess of minerals can be toxic.

LEARNING OUTCOME 5

Describe the nurse's role in the pharmacologic management of nutritional disorders.

Concepts for Lecture

1. The role of the nurse in the pharmacologic management of nutritional disorders involves careful monitoring of a client's condition and providing education as it relates to the prescribed drug treatment. Obtain baseline medical, surgical, and drug history; lifestyle and dietary habits, including use of herbal or alternative therapies; and a detailed description of symptomology and current therapies.

SUGGESTION FOR CLINICAL ACTIVITIES
- Direct students to visit the food-services area of the medical facility to observe meal preparation and to identify foods with water-soluble vitamin and lipid-soluble vitamin content.

POWERPOINT SLIDES

Table 42.4 List of Recommended Dietary Allowances

SUGGESTIONS FOR CLASSROOM ACTIVITIES
- Direct students to develop a matching game correlating vitamins, sources of vitamins, and functions of vitamins.
- Direct students to the FDA website. Have them search for information on the approval process for vitamins and minerals.

SUGGESTION FOR CLINICAL ACTIVITIES
- Invite a dietician to postclinical to talk about the clinical aspects of vitamin deficiencies.

POWERPOINT SLIDES

SUGGESTION FOR CLASSROOM ACTIVITIES
- Discuss the role of the nurse in the pharmacologic treatment of clients with nutritional disorders.

© 2011 Pearson Education, Inc.

2. **Drug therapy with fat-soluble vitamins:** Teach clients that excessive vitamin intake can be harmful. Begin with assessment for deficiency. Assess clients for impaired liver function. Assess for chronic overdose of vitamins. When performing dietary counseling, consider the socioeconomic status and culture of the client. Recommend foods that both treat the deficiency and are affordable for and liked by the client.

3. **Water-soluble vitamin therapy:** Thiamine is often administered to hospitalized clients who have severe liver disease. Both niacin and pyridoxine may cause severe flushing. Inform the client that this is an expected reaction and will not cause permanent harm. Be sure to assess menstruating women for folic acid deficiency, especially prior to their attempting pregnancy and during pregnancy. Recommend that adequate levels be obtained from a multivitamin to avoid overdose. Caution clients with a history of kidney stones against using vitamin C unless directed by a health care provider. Advise clients taking vitamin C to increase fluid intake. Be aware that water-soluble vitamins are not stored in the body and must be replenished daily.

4. **Macromineral therapy for mineral deficiencies or eclampsia:** Although minerals cause no harm in small amounts, larger doses can cause life-threatening adverse effects. Encourage a well-balanced diet to eliminate or reduce the need for mineral supplements. If calcium is prescribed, inform the health care provider of any use of glucocorticoids, thiazide diuretics, and tetracyclines. If the client is taking calcium, avoid zinc-rich foods such as legumes, nuts, sprouts, and soy that impair calcium absorption. If phosphorus has been prescribed, inform the health care provider of a sodium- or potassium-restricted diet, immediately report seizure activity, and stop the drug; also avoid antacids. If the client is taking magnesium sulfate, immediately report changes in consciousness, deep tendon reflexes, thirst, or confusion, and stop the drug.

LEARNING OUTCOME 6

Compare and contrast the properties of macrominerals and trace minerals.

Concepts for Lecture

1. Pharmacotherapy with seven macrominerals includes agents containing calcium, chlorine, magnesium, phosphorous, potassium, sodium, and sulfur. They must be obtained daily from dietary sources in amounts of 100 mg or greater. (See Table 42.5 for more information on macrominerals.)

2. Pharmacotherapy with the nine microminerals includes agents containing iron, iodine, fluorine, and zinc. The required daily amount is 20 mg or less. (See Table 42.5 for more information on the microminerals.)

 SUGGESTION FOR CLINICAL ACTIVITIES

- Direct students to inspect the admissions forms at the clinical sites. Discuss whether the form has specific questions regarding self-administration of vitamins, minerals, or nutritional supplements in the home environment.

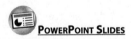 **POWERPOINT SLIDES**

Table 42.5 Macrominerals

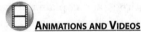 **ANIMATIONS AND VIDEOS**

- Lipid-soluble Vitamins for Treating Nutritional Disorders

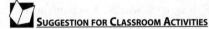 **SUGGESTION FOR CLASSROOM ACTIVITIES**

- Direct students to break into groups to compare and contrast the functions of minerals.

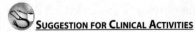 **SUGGESTION FOR CLINICAL ACTIVITIES**

- Direct students to differentiate between macrominerals and microminerals listed on the client's medication-administration record.

LEARNING OUTCOME 7

Identify differences among oligomeric, polymeric, modular, and specialized formulations for enteral nutrition.

Concepts for Lecture

1. Undernutrition may be caused by low dietary intake, malabsorption disorders, fad diets, or wasting disorders such as cancer or AIDS. Reasons for low dietary intake vary from poverty and depression to difficulty eating. Nutritional consultation is appropriate.
2. Enteral nutrition, provided orally or through a feeding tube, is a means of meeting a client's complete nutritional needs. Enteral products are classified as follows: oligomeric (Vivonex, T.E.N., Peptamen); polymeric, the most common type (Compeat, Sustacal, Ensure); modular, given to supplement a single nutrient (Casec, Polycose, Microlipid, MCT Oil); and specialized, given for special disease states (Amin-Aid, Hepatic-Aid II, Pulmocare).

LEARNING OUTCOME 8

Compare and contrast enteral and parenteral methods of providing nutrition.

Concepts for Lecture

Total parenteral nutrition (TPN), also known as hyperalimentation, is a means of supplying nutrition to clients via a peripheral vein (short term) or central vein (long term). It is administered through an infusion pump for precise monitoring.

LEARNING OUTCOME 9

For each of the drug classes listed in Drug at a Glance, know representative drugs, and explain the mechanism of drug action, describe primary actions, and identify important adverse effects.

Concepts for Lecture

1. **Vitamin Pharmacotherapy—Lipid-Soluble Vitamins:** Prototype drug: **vitamin A.** Mechanism of action: essential for general growth and development, particularly of the bones, teeth, and epithelial membranes. It is necessary for proper wound healing, is essential for the biosynthesis of steroids, and is one of the pigments required for night vision. Primary use: Vitamin A is indicated in deficiency states and during periods of increased need such as pregnancy, lactation, or undernutrition. Night blindness and slow wound healing can be effectively treated with as little as 30,000 units of vitamin A given daily over a week. It is also prescribed for GI disorders, when absorption in the small intestine is diminished or absent. Topical forms are available for acne, psoriasis, and other skin disorders. Doses of vitamin A are sometimes measured in retinoid equivalents (RE). In severe deficiency states, up to 500,000 units may be given per day for 3 days, gradually tapering off to 10,000 to 20,000 units/day.

 POWERPOINT SLIDES

 SUGGESTION FOR CLASSROOM ACTIVITIES

- Have examples of enteral feeding containers and feeding pumps available for students to look at.

 SUGGESTION FOR CLINICAL ACTIVITIES

- Assign students to a client having enteral feedings.

 POWERPOINT SLIDES

 SUGGESTION FOR CLASSROOM ACTIVITIES

- Discuss reasons why clients would have enteral instead of parenteral nutrition.

 SUGGESTION FOR CLINICAL ACTIVITIES

- Direct students to calculate how many calories and how much fluid the client had in enteral feedings on their shift.

 POWERPOINT SLIDES

 SUGGESTION FOR CLASSROOM ACTIVITIES

- Direct students to make a table of common vitamins and minerals.

SUGGESTION FOR CLINICAL ACTIVITIES

- Assign students to the clinic setting and have them prepare a teaching plan for a client taking vitamin or mineral replacement therapy.

© 2011 Pearson Education, Inc.

Adverse effects: Adverse effects are not observed with normal doses of vitamin A. Acute ingestion, however, produces serious CNS toxicity, including headache, irritability, drowsiness, delirium, and possible coma. Long-term ingestion of high amounts causes drying and scaling of the skin, alopecia, fatigue, anorexia, vomiting, and leukopenia.

2. **Vitamin Pharmacotherapy—Water-Soluble Vitamin:** Prototype drug: folic acid (Folacin). Mechanism of action: Folic acid is administered to reverse symptoms of deficiency, which most commonly occurs in patients with inadequate intake, such as with chronic alcohol abuse. Pregnancy markedly increases the need for dietary folic acid. Because this vitamin is destroyed at high temperatures, people who overcook their food may experience folate deficiency. Primary use: Folic acid is given during pregnancy to promote normal fetal growth. (Administration of 1 mg/day of oral folic acid often reverses the deficiency symptoms within 5 to 7 days. Because insufficient vitamin B_{12} creates a lack of activated folic acid, deficiency symptoms resemble those of vitamin B_{12} deficiency. The megaloblastic anemia observed in folate-deficient patients, however, does not include the severe nervous system symptoms seen in patients with B_{12} deficiency. Adverse effects during folic acid therapy are uncommon. Patients may feel flushed following IV injections. Allergic hypersensitivity to folic acid by the IV route is possible.

3. **Mineral Pharmacotherapy—Mineral Supplement:** Prototype drug: magnesium sulfate. Mechanism of action: It is essential for proper neuromuscular function. Magnesium also serves a metabolic role in activating certain enzymes in the breakdown of carbohydrates and proteins. Primary use: Severe hypomagnesemia can be rapidly reversed by the administration of IM or IV magnesium sulfate. Parenteral formulations include 4%, 8%, 12.5%, and 50% solutions. After administration, magnesium sulfate is distributed throughout the body, and therapeutic effects are observed within 30 to 60 minutes. Oral forms of magnesium sulfate are used as cathartics, when complete evacuation of the colon is desired. Magnesium sulfate is a CNS depressant and is sometimes given to prevent or terminate seizures associated with eclampsia as an anticonvulsant. Adverse effects: Early signs of magnesium overdose include flushing of the skin, sedation, confusion, intense thirst, and muscle weakness. Extreme levels cause neuromuscular blockade with resultant respiratory paralysis, heart block, and circulatory collapse. Because of these potentially fatal adverse effects, the use of magnesium sulfate is restricted to severe magnesium deficiency: Mild-to-moderate hypomagnesemia is treated with oral forms of magnesium such as magnesium gluconate or magnesium hydroxide.

LEARNING OUTCOME 10

Use the nursing process to care for patients who are receiving drug therapy for nutritional disorders.

Concepts for Lecture

1. **Patients Receiving Vitamin and Mineral Pharmacotherapy—Assessment:** Obtain a complete health history including cardiovascular, neurologic, endocrine, hepatic or renal disease. Obtain a drug history including allergies, current prescription and OTC drugs, and herbal preparations, alcohol use or smoking. Be alert to possible drug interactions. Obtain a history of any current symptoms that may indicate vitamin deficiencies or hypervitaminosis (e.g., dry itchy skin, alopecia, sore and reddened gums or tongue, tendency to bleed easily

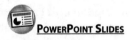

POWERPOINT SLIDES

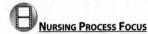

NURSING PROCESS FOCUS
- Patients Receiving Vitamin and Mineral Pharmacotherapy
- Clients Receiving Parenteral Nutrition

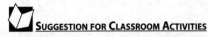

SUGGESTION FOR CLASSROOM ACTIVITIES
- Direct students to work in small groups to create teaching plans for patients receiving vitamin and mineral pharmacotherapy.

or excessive bruising, nausea or vomiting, excessive fatigue). Obtain a dietary history noting adequacy of essential vitamins, minerals, and nutrients obtained through food sources. Note sunscreen use and amount of sun exposure. Obtain baseline weight and vital signs. Evaluate appropriate laboratory findings (e.g., CBC, electrolytes, hepatic and renal function studies, ferritin and iron levels). Assess for and promptly report adverse effects: nausea, vomiting, excessive fatigue, tachycardia, palpitations, hypotension, constipation, drowsiness, dizziness, disorientation, hyperreflexia, electrolyte imbalances.

2. **Patients Receiving Vitamin and Mineral Pharmacotherapy— Nursing diagnoses:** *Imbalanced Nutrition: Less than Body Requirements; Impaired Health Maintenance* related to dietary habits, deficient knowledge; *Readiness for Enhanced Therapeutic Regimen Management; Deficient Knowledge* related to drug therapy; *Risk for Injury* related to adverse drug effects, hypervitaminosis.

3. **Patients Receiving Vitamin and Mineral Pharmacotherapy— Planning:** The client will experience therapeutic effects (e.g., maintenance of overall health, symptoms of previous deficiency are absent). Be free from, or experience minimal adverse effects. Verbalize an understanding of the drug's use, adverse effects, and required precautions. Demonstrate proper self-administration of the medication (e.g., dose, timing, when to notify provider).

4. **Patients Receiving Vitamin and Mineral Pharmacotherapy— Implementation:** Treat the cause: If a definitive cause of vitamin or mineral deficiency is identified, correct the deficiency using dietary sources of the nutrient where possible. Review dietary and supplement history to correct any existing possibility for hypervitaminosis and adverse drug effects. Continue to monitor periodic lab work as needed. Monitor the use of fat-soluble vitamins [A, D, E, and K] for possible toxic effects. Monitor liver function studies and for symptoms such as nausea, vomiting, headache, fatigue, dry and itchy skin, blurred vision, or palpitations. Encourage adequate intake of vitamin and folic-acid rich foods *prior* to conception. Instruct patient to keep pre-natal vitamins in a secure location if young children are in the household to prevent accidental poisoning. Ensure adequate hydration if large doses of water-soluble vitamins are taken. Instruct patient and/or family in proper self-administration of drug (e.g., taken with additional fluids).

5. **Patients Receiving Vitamin and Mineral Pharmacotherapy— Evaluation:** The client will experience maintenance of overall health, and symptoms of previous deficiency are absent; the client is free from or experiences minimal adverse effects. Verbalizes an understanding of the drug's use, adverse effects, and required precautions. Demonstrates proper self-administration of the medication (e.g., dose, timing, when to notify provider).

6. **Clients Receiving Parenteral Nutrition—Assessment:** Prior to administration, obtain a complete health history including cardiovascular, neurologic, endocrine, hepatic or renal disease, and a complete physical examination. Obtain a drug history including allergies, current prescription and OTC drugs, and herbal preparations, alcohol use or smoking. Be alert to possible drug interactions. Obtain baseline height, weight, and vital signs. Evaluate appropriate laboratory findings (e.g., CBC, electrolytes, glucose, BUN, hepatic and renal function studies, total protein, serum albumin, lipid profile, serum iron levels). Assess for and promptly report adverse effects: fever, nausea, vomiting, tachycardia, palpitations, hypotension, dyspnea, drowsiness, dizziness, disorientation, hypo or hyperglycemia, and electrolyte imbalances. Assess for the presence or history of nutritional deficits such as inadequate oral intake, GI disease, and increased metabolic need.

SUGGESTION FOR CLINICAL ACTIVITIES
- Assign students to care for clients receiving parenteral nutrition.

© 2011 Pearson Education, Inc.

7. **Clients Receiving Parenteral Nutrition—Nursing diagnoses:** *Risk for Infection; Imbalanced Nutrition: Less than Body Requirements; Risk for Imbalanced Fluid Volume; Deficient Knowledge,* related to drug therapy.

8. **Clients Receiving Parenteral Nutrition—Planning:** The client will experience therapeutic effects (e.g., maintenance or improvement of overall health and nutritional status); The client will be free from or experience minimal adverse effects. Verbalize an understanding of the drug's use, adverse effects, and required precautions. Demonstrate proper self-administration of the medication (e.g., dose, timing, when to notify provider).

9. **Clients Receiving Parenteral Nutrition—Implementation:** Monitor vital signs, observing for signs of infection such as elevated temperature. Assess patient's ability to take oral nutrition and encourage small oral feedings if allowed. Assess all access sites (e.g., gastric tube site, IV or port sites) frequently for redness, streaking, swelling, or drainage. Report any fever, chills, malaise, or changes in mental status immediately. Use strict aseptic technique with all IV tubing or bag changes, site dressing changes.

   Refrigerate TPN solution until 30 minutes before using. Monitor blood glucose levels. Observe for signs of hyperglycemia or hypoglycemia and obtain capillary glucose levels as ordered. Monitor for signs of fluid overload. Monitor renal status—intake and output ratio, daily weight, and laboratory studies such as serum creatinine and BUN should be monitored. Maintain accurate enteral feeding or TPN infusion rate with infusion pump; make rate changes gradually; and avoid abruptly discontinuing TPN feeding. Assess for appropriate enteral tube placement before administering any feeding. Instruct patient and/or family in proper self-administration of drug.

10. **Clients Receiving Parenteral Nutrition—Evaluation:** The client experiences maintenance or improvement of overall health and nutritional status; the client is free from, or experiences minimal adverse effects; verbalizes an understanding of the drug's use, adverse effects, and required precautions; demonstrates proper self-administration of the medication (e.g., dose, timing, when to notify provider).

GENERAL CHAPTER CONSIDERATIONS

1. Have students study and learn key terms listed at the beginning of the chapter.
2. Have students complete end-of-chapter exercises either in their book or on the MyNursingKit website.
3. Use the Classroom Response Questions provided in PowerPoint to assess students prior to lecture.

MYNURSINGKIT
(*www.mynursingkit.com*)

- Websites
- NCLEX® questions
- Critical Thinking Questions
- Case Studies
- Animations and Videos
- Drug Prototype Questions

MYNURSINGLAB
(*www.mynursinglab.com*)

- Knowledge Quick Check
- Pre/Posttests
- Customized study plans
- *Separate purchase*

STUDENT WORKBOOK AND RESOURCE GUIDE

- Chapter 42 activities
- *Separate purchase*

PEARSON NURSE'S DRUG GUIDE

- *Separate purchase*

PEARSON eTEXT

- Students can search, highlight, take notes, and more all in electronic format.
- *Separate purchase*

CLASSROOM RESPONSE QUESTION POWERPOINTS

TESTBANK

© 2011 Pearson Education, Inc.

CHAPTER 43
DRUGS FOR PITUITARY, THYROID, AND ADRENAL DISORDERS

LEARNING OUTCOME 1

Describe the general structure and functions of the endocrine system.

Concepts for Lecture

The endocrine system consists of glands that secrete hormones. The endocrine system is a major controller of homeostasis. It maintains homeostasis by using hormones transported through the blood as chemical messengers that are secreted in response to changes in the internal environment. The release of hormones is commonly controlled by negative feedback, and one hormone may control another. (See Figure 43.1.)

POWERPOINT SLIDES

Figure 43.1 The Endocrine System

SUGGESTION FOR CLASSROOM ACTIVITIES

- Direct students to concept map the endocrine system glands and functions.

SUGGESTION FOR CLINICAL ACTIVITIES

- Direct students to discuss all the different diagnoses of endocrine disorders that they observed in the group's clients.

LEARNING OUTCOME 2

Through the use of a specific example, explain the concept of negative feedback in the endocrine system.

Concepts for Lecture

In negative-feedback loops it is common for the last hormone in a pathway to provide feedback to turn off the secretion from the first hormone. For example, as serum calcium levels fall, PTH is released; PTH causes an increase in serum calcium, which provides feedback to the parathyroid glands to shut off PTH secretion. This characteristic feature of endocrine homeostasis is known as **negative feedback.** Negative feedback helps to prevent excessive secretion of hormones thereby limiting their physiologic responses.

POWERPOINT SLIDES

SUGGESTION FOR CLASSROOM ACTIVITIES

- Discuss several examples of negative-feedback loops in the endocrine system.

SUGGESTION FOR CLINICAL ACTIVITIES

- During postclinical, have students each give an example of a negative-feedback loop they have seen in a client.

LEARNING OUTCOME 3

Describe the clinical applications of the hypothalamic and pituitary hormones.

Concepts for Lecture

1. The hypothalamus and pituitary glands control many other glands. The hypothalamus secretes releasing hormones, which direct the anterior pituitary gland as to which hormones should be released. The posterior pituitary releases its hormones in response to nerve signals from the hypothalamus. (See Figure 43.2 for an illustration of the hypothalamus and pituitary.)

POWERPOINT SLIDES

Figure 43.2 Hormones Associated with the Hypothalamus and the Pituitary Gland

SUGGESTION FOR CLASSROOM ACTIVITIES

- Discuss how the hypothalamus and posterior pituitary control other glands.

2. Hormones are used as replacement therapy, as antineoplastics, and for their natural therapeutic effects, such as their exaggerated response or suppression of body defenses. Hormone blockers are used to inhibit actions of certain hormones. (See Table 43.1 for examples of hormone pharmacotherapy.)

LEARNING OUTCOME 4

Explain the pharmacotherapy of diabetes insipidus.

Concepts for Lecture

Antidiuretic hormone (ADH) conserves water in the body. A deficiency in ADH results in **diabetes insipidus (DI)**, a rare condition characterized by the production of large volumes of very dilute urine, usually accompanied by increased thirst. Two ADH preparations are available for the treatment of diabetes insipidus: vasopressin (Pitressin) and desmopressin (DDAVP, Stimate). Vasopressin is a synthetic hormone that has a structure identical with that of human ADH. It acts on the renal collecting tubules to increase their permeability to water, thus enhancing water reabsorption. Although it acts within minutes, vasopressin has a short half-life requiring it to be administered 3 to 4 times per day. Vasopressin tannate is formulated in peanut oil to increase its duration of action. Vasopressin is usually given IM or IV, although an intranasal form is available for mild diabetes insipidus. Desmopressin is the most common form of antidiuretic hormone in use. Details regarding this drug may be found in the Prototype Drug feature.

LEARNING OUTCOME 5

Identify the signs and symptoms of hypothyroidism and hyperthyroidism.

Concepts for Lecture

1. The thyroid gland secretes thyroxine (T_4) and triiodothyronine (T_3), which control the basal metabolic rate and affect every cell in the body. Parafollicular cells in the thyroid secrete calcitonin, which is responsible for calcium homeostasis. Follicular cells secrete T_4 and T_3, and iodine is essential for the synthesis of T_4 and T_3. A negative-feedback loop controls secretion, and low thyroxine levels signal the hypothalamus to release thyroid-releasing hormone (TRH), which signals the pituitary to release thyroid-stimulating hormone (TSH). (This negative feedback for the thyroid is illustrated in Figure 43.3.)
2. Early symptoms of hypothyroidism in adults, or **myxedema,** include general weakness, muscle cramps, and dry skin. More severe symptoms include slurred speech, bradycardia, weight gain, decreased sense of taste and smell, and intolerance to cold environments. Lab results generally reveal elevated TSH with diminished T_3 and T_4 levels. Symptoms of hyperthyroidism are increased body metabolism, tachycardia, weight loss, elevated body temperature, and anxiety.

SUGGESTION FOR CLINICAL ACTIVITIES

- Direct students to study the medication-administration records of drugs that are used in hormone pharmacotherapy.

POWERPOINT SLIDES

Table 43.2 Selected Hypothalamic and Pituitary Agents

SUGGESTION FOR CLASSROOM ACTIVITIES

- Discuss the use of growth hormone in children, both in those with growth hormone deficiency and those with normal levels of growth hormone.

SUGGESTION FOR CLINICAL ACTIVITIES

- Direct students to administer drugs used in the pharmacotherapy related to growth hormone or antidiuretic hormone.

POWERPOINT SLIDES

Figure 43.3 Feedback Mechanisms of the Thyroid Gland

SUGGESTION FOR CLASSROOM ACTIVITIES

- Direct students to concept map the negative-feedback mechanism for the thyroid hormone.

SUGGESTION FOR CLINICAL ACTIVITIES

- Direct students to assess clients with hypothyroidism and hyperthyroidism. Discuss the differences in the assessment results in postclinical.

© 2011 Pearson Education, Inc.

Learning Outcome 6

Explain the pharmacotherapy of thyroid disorders.

Concepts for Lecture

1. The most common cause of hypothyroidism (myxedema) is chronic autoimmune thyroiditis (Hashimoto's disease). Lab studies reveal an elevated thyroid-stimulating hormone (TSH) level and decreased T_3 and T_4 levels. Hypothyroidism may be treated by administering natural or synthetic thyroid hormones, especially levothyroxine (T_4). (See Table 43.3 for a list of medications.)
2. The most common cause of hyperthyroidism is Graves' disease. The goal of pharmacotherapy is to lower the activity of the thyroid. Hyperthyroidism is treated by administering agents such as the thioamides, such as propylthiouracil (PTU) and methimazole (Tapazole), which decrease the activity of the thyroid gland; or by using a radioactive iodide that kills overactive thyroid cells, such as sodium iodide-131, Lugol's solution.

Learning Outcome 7

Describe the signs and symptoms of Addison's disease and Cushing's syndrome.

Concepts for Lecture

1. The adrenal cortex secretes glucocorticoids, gonadocorticoids, and mineralocorticoids. The glucocorticoids mobilize the body for long-term stress and influence carbohydrate, lipid, and protein metabolism in most cells. Mineralocorticoids promote sodium reabsorption and potassium secretion. Gonadocorticoids include male sex hormones (androgens).
2. Addison's disease is primary adrenocortical insufficiency. It is rare and includes a deficiency of both glucocorticoids and mineralocorticoids. Symptoms include nausea, vomiting, lethargy, confusion, and coma. Low plasma cortisol, accompanied by high plasma ACTH levels, is diagnostic because this indicates the adrenal gland is not responding to ACTH stimulation.
3. Cushing's syndrome occurs when high levels of glucocorticoids are present in the body over a prolonged period. Signs and symptoms include adrenal atrophy, osteoporosis, hypertension, increased risk of infections, delayed wound healing, acne, peptic ulcers, general obesity, and a redistribution of fat around the face (moon face), shoulders, and neck (buffalo hump). Mood and personality changes may occur.

Learning Outcome 8

Explain the pharmacotherapy of adrenal gland disorders.

Concepts for Lecture

1. Control of glucocorticoid levels in the blood begins with corticotropin-releasing factor (CRF), secreted by the hypothalamus. CRF travels to the pituitary, where it causes the release of adrenocorticotropic hormone (ACTH). ACTH then travels through the blood and reaches the adrenal cortex, causing it to release glucocorticoids. When

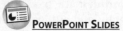

POWERPOINT SLIDES

Table 43.3 Thyroid and Antithyroid Drugs

SUGGESTION FOR CLASSROOM ACTIVITIES

- Discuss treatment for the thyroid from radiation damage after a nuclear bioterrorist act.

SUGGESTION FOR CLINICAL ACTIVITIES

- Direct students to administer medications used in the pharmacotherapy of thyroid disorders.

POWERPOINT SLIDES

SUGGESTION FOR CLASSROOM ACTIVITIES

- Discuss the functions of the three adrenal cortical hormones.

SUGGESTION FOR CLINICAL ACTIVITIES

- Direct students to assess clients who have been on long-term pharmacotherapy with glucocorticoids. Have them present results at postclinical.

POWERPOINT SLIDES

Figure 43.4 Feedback Control of the Adrenal Cortex
Table 43.4 Selected Glucocorticoids

ANIMATIONS AND VIDEOS

- Pharmacotherapy Illustrated 43.1

the level of cortisol in the blood rises, it provides negative feedback to the hypothalamus and pituitary to shut off further release of glucocorticoids. (This negative-feedback mechanism is shown in Figure 43.4.) Adrenocorticotropic hormone (ACTH) and related agents are rarely used as medications. They must be given parenterally and have many side effects. Their primary use is to diagnose adrenal disorders.

2. Adrenocortical insufficiency may be acute or chronic. Glucocorticoids are prescribed for primary (Addison's disease) and secondary adrenocortical insufficiency, allergies, neoplasms, and a wide variety of other conditions. (See Table 43.4 for a listing of medications.)

3. Antiadrenal drugs may be used to treat severe Cushing's syndrome, which occurs with prolonged glucocorticoid therapy by inhibiting corticosteroid synthesis. Antiadrenal drugs are not curative, and their use is usually limited to 3 months of therapy.

LEARNING OUTCOME 9

Describe the nurse's role in the pharmacologic management of pituitary, thyroid, and adrenal disorders.

Concepts for Lecture

1. The role of the nurse in the pharmacologic management of pituitary, thyroid, and adrenal disorders involves careful monitoring of a client's condition and providing education as it relates to the prescribed drug treatment. Obtain baseline medical, surgical, and drug history; lifestyle and dietary habits, including use of herbal or alternative therapies; and a detailed description of symptomology and current therapies.

2. **Antidiuretic hormone therapy for ADH deficiency:** Assess for electrolyte imbalances and changes in specific gravity and fluid intake. Monitor serum sodium and potassium levels. Monitor urinary specific gravity, routine urinalysis, body weight, and fluid intake and output. Assess vital signs, especially blood pressure and pulse. Assess neurological status for symptoms of headache and changes in mental status such as drowsiness and confusion. Advise clients to avoid alcohol.

3. **Thyroid hormone therapy:** Assess the client's weight and vital signs. Assess tachycardia, irregular heart rate, hypertension, nervousness, weight loss, diarrhea, and heat intolerance, which could indicate an overdose of thyroid hormone. Monitor clients with impaired renal function closely. Monitor for excess fatigue, slow speech, hoarseness or slow pulse, because these may indicate underdosage.

4. **Hypothyroidism therapy:** Assess for signs and symptoms of hypothyroidism, such as weight gain, hypotension, bradycardia, fatigue, depression, sensitivity to cold environments, hair loss, and dry skin. Assess for signs of jaundice, and monitor liver enzymes. Assess for bleeding and blood dyscrasias, such as agranulocytosis and jaundice. Clients should avoid children and pregnant women for one week after administration of radioactive iodine (I-131) and limit close physical contact with others for a few days.

5. **Glucocorticoid therapy for adrenocortical insufficiency:** Assess vital signs for temperature and blood-pressure elevations. Monitor potassium, T_3, T_4, and glucose levels. Monitor clients on long-term glucocorticoid therapy for osteoporosis and elevated serum cholesterol levels. Assess for signs and symptoms of Cushing's syndrome.

6. **Antiadrenal therapy for adrenocortical insufficiency:** Assess and monitor lab values, including platelet count, bilirubin, hepatic-function tests, and prothrombin. Assess for jaundice, bruising, and

SUGGESTION FOR CLASSROOM ACTIVITIES

• Compare and contrast etiology and treatment of Addison's disease and Cushing's syndrome.

SUGGESTION FOR CLINICAL ACTIVITIES

• Assign students to care for clients with Addison's disease or Cushing's syndrome.

POWERPOINT SLIDES

SUGGESTION FOR CLASSROOM ACTIVITIES

• Discuss the role of the nurse in the pharmacologic management of pituitary, thyroid, and adrenal disorders.

SUGGESTION FOR CLINICAL ACTIVITIES

• Direct students to observe carefully the implementations listed on the client's plan of care when caring for a client with endocrine disorders.

© 2011 Pearson Education, Inc.

bleeding. Monitor client's stress level, for orthostatic hypotension, and for dizziness and assist with ambulation. Caution client to change positions slowly.

LEARNING OUTCOME 10

For each of the classes listed in Drugs at a Glance, know representative drugs, and explain the mechanisms of drug action, primary actions, and important adverse effects.

Concepts for Lecture

1. **Anterior Pituitary Agents:** Prototype drug: vasopressin injection (Pitressin). Mechanism of action: to cause the renal collecting tubules to increase their permeability to water, thus enhancing water reabsorption. Primary use: for treatment of diabetes insipidus. Adverse effects: hypertension; it can precipitate angina episodes and myocardial infarction in clients with coronary artery disease. Excessive fluid retention can cause water intoxication.

2. **Thyroid Agents:** Prototype drug: levothyroxine (Synthroid). Mechanisms of action: same as those of thyroid hormone. Primary use: as the drug of choice for replacement therapy in clients with low thyroid function. Adverse effects: hyperthyroidism, palpitations, dysrhythmias, anxiety, insomnia, weight loss, and heat intolerance. Menstrual irregularities and osteoporosis can occur in women.

3. **Antithyroid Agents:** Prototype drug: propylthiouracil (PTU). Mechanism of action: to interfere with the synthesis of T_3 and T_4 in the thyroid gland. It also prevents the conversion of T_4 to T_3 in the target tissues. Primary use: for clients with hyperthyroidism. Adverse effects: symptoms of hypothyroidism. Rash and transient leucopenia are the most common side effects. A small percentage of clients experience agranulocytosis.

4. **Adrenal Drugs—Glucocorticoids:** Prototype drug: hydrocortisone (Aeroseb-HC, Alphaderm). Mechanism of action: acts as a synthetic corticosteroid. Primary use: as the drug of choice for treating adrenocortical insufficiency. Adverse effects: sodium and fluid retention; CNS effects, including insomnia, anxiety, headache, vertigo, confusion, and depression. Hypertension, tachycardia, peptic ulcer disease, and Cushing's syndrome can also occur with long-term therapy.

LEARNING OUTCOME 11

Use the nursing process to care for patients who are receiving drug therapy for pituitary, thyroid, and adrenal disorders.

Concepts for Lecture

1. **Clients receiving pharmacotherapy with hypothalamic and pituitary hormones—Assessment:** Obtain a complete health history and a complete physical examination. Obtain a drug history including allergies, current prescription and OTC drugs, herbal preparations, alcohol use or smoking. Be alert to possible drug interactions. Evaluate appropriate laboratory findings (e.g., urine and serum osmolality, urine specific gravity, serum protein, CBC, electrolytes, glucose, hepatic and renal function studies). Obtain baseline height, weight, and vital signs. Obtain ECG if needed on patients taking growth hormone antagonists. Assess for adverse effects: nausea, vomiting, diarrhea, headache.

 POWERPOINT SLIDES

Prototype Drug
- vasopressin injection (Pitressin)
- levothyroxine (Synthroid)
- propylthiouracil (PTU)
- hydrocortisone (Aeroseb-HC, Alphaderm)

 SUGGESTION FOR CLASSROOM ACTIVITIES

- Have each student make drug cards for each classification of drug used to treat pituitary, thyroid, and adrenal disorders. Use two different drugs for each classification. The card should include actions, uses, routes of administration, dosages, and adverse effects.

 SUGGESTION FOR CLINICAL ACTIVITIES

- Divide students into small groups, and have each group develop a teaching plan for a patient receiving medications for pituitary, thyroid, and adrenal disorders.

 POWERPOINT SLIDES

 NURSING PROCESS FOCUS

- Clients receiving pharmacotherapy with hypothalamic and pituitary hormones
- Clients receiving thyroid replacement and antithyroid drugs
- Clients receiving systemic glucocorticoid therapy

 SUGGESTION FOR CLASSROOM ACTIVITIES

- Develop concept maps based on the traditional nursing-care plans used for clients with drug therapy for pituitary, thyroid, and adrenal disorders.

2. **Clients receiving pharmacotherapy with hypothalamic and pituitary hormones—Nursing diagnoses:** *Deficient Fluid Volume; Diarrhea; Delayed Growth and Development; Situational Low Self-Esteem*, related to height, stature; *Impaired Urinary Elimination* (nocturnal enuresis); *Deficient Knowledge* (drug therapy).

3. **Clients receiving pharmacotherapy with hypothalamic and pituitary hormones—Planning:** The client will experience therapeutic effects (e.g., height increase measurable over time, diuresis slows with urine and serum osmolality within normal limits, return to normal bowel function, nocturnal enuresis has stopped); be free from or experience minimal adverse effects. Verbalize an understanding of the drug's use, adverse effects, and required precautions. Demonstrate proper self-administration of the medication (e.g., dose, timing, when to notify provider).

4. **Clients receiving pharmacotherapy with hypothalamic and pituitary hormones—Implementation:** Patients taking growth hormone: Monitor height and weight at each clinical visit. Report lack of growth to the health care provider. Patients taking growth hormone antagonists: Monitor levels of serum GH. Monitor bowel sounds and decreases in diarrhea. Patients taking antidiuretic hormones: For patients with diabetes insipidus, monitor urine output, urine and serum osmolality, and urine specific gravity for return to normal limits. Monitor for any complaints of muscle, joint or bone pain, particularly in the knee or hip, or any changes in gait. Monitor glucose levels, particularly in diabetic patients. Report consistent elevations to the health care provider. Monitor vital signs, especially pulse and blood pressure for patients with cardiac disease Monitor daily weight, output, lung sounds, and for peripheral edema. Monitor for signs of peripheral ischemia, or angina and report immediately. Monitor nutritional and fluid intake instruct patient or care giver in proper self-administration of drug (e.g., during evening meal).

5. **Clients receiving pharmacotherapy with hypothalamic and pituitary hormones—Evaluation:** The client will experience height increase measurable over time, diuresis slows with urine and serum osmolality within normal limits, return to normal bowel function, nocturnal enuresis has stopped; be free from or experience minimal adverse effects. Verbalize an understanding of the drug's use, adverse effects, and required precautions. Demonstrate proper self-administration of the medication (e.g., dose, timing, when to notify provider).

6. **Clients receiving thyroid replacement and antithyroid drugs—Assessment:** Obtain a complete health history including cardiovascular, gastrointestinal, hepatic, renal disease, pregnancy or breast-feeding. Obtain a drug history including allergies, current prescription and OTC drugs, herbal preparations, alcohol use or smoking. Be alert to possible drug interactions. Assess for the presence and history of symptoms of hypothyroidism. Evaluate appropriate laboratory findings (e.g., T_3, T_4, and TSH levels, CBC, platelets, electrolytes, glucose, and lipid levels). Obtain baseline height, weight, and vital signs. Obtain ECG as needed. Assess for adverse effects: Hypotension or hypertension, tachycardia, especially associated with angina should be reported immediately.

7. **Clients receiving thyroid replacement and antithyroid drugs—Nursing diagnoses:** *Activity Intolerance; Fatigue; Constipation; Deficient Knowledge* (drug therapy); *Risk for Infection* related to adverse drug effects.

8. **Clients receiving thyroid replacement and antithyroid drugs—Planning:** The client will experience therapeutic effects (e.g., decrease in symptoms, thyroid lab studies return to within normal limits); be free from or experience minimal adverse effects. Verbalize an understanding of the drug's use, adverse effects, and required precautions. Demonstrate

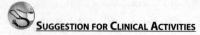

SUGGESTION FOR CLINICAL ACTIVITIES
- Assign students to care for patients receiving drug therapy for pituitary, thyroid, and adrenal disorders.

© 2011 Pearson Education, Inc.

proper self-administration of the medication (e.g., dose, timing, when to notify provider).

9. **Clients receiving thyroid replacement and antithyroid drugs—Implementation:** Monitor vital signs—appetite, weight, sensitivity to heat or cold, sleep patterns, and ADLs for return to normal limits. Monitor for decreasing symptoms related to hypothyroidism and to hyperthyroidism. Monitor T_3, T_4, and TSH levels. Avoid iodine-containing foods. Monitor for signs of infection: fever, rashes, sore throat, malaise, fatigue or weakness. Monitor CBC and platelet counts. Monitor blood-glucose levels, especially in individuals with diabetes mellitus. Ensure patient safety, especially in the elderly. Observe for dizziness and monitor ambulation until effects of drug are known. Ensure patient and care giver safety if radioactive iodine is used. Instruct the patient and/or family in proper self-administration of drug (e.g., take the drug in the morning at the same time each day).

10. **Clients receiving thyroid replacement and antithyroid drugs—Evaluation:** The client will experience a decrease in symptoms; thyroid lab studies return to within normal limits. The client will be free from or experience minimal adverse effects. Verbalize an understanding of the drug's use, adverse effects, and required precautions. Demonstrate proper self-administration of the medication (e.g., dose, timing, when to notify provider).

11. **Clients receiving systemic glucocorticoid therapy—Assessment:** Obtain a complete health history and a complete physical examination. Determine the reason the medication is being administered. Evaluate appropriate laboratory findings (e.g., CBC, platelets, electrolytes, glucose, lipid profile, hepatic or renal function studies). Obtain baseline vital signs and weight. Assess for and promptly report adverse effects.

12. **Clients receiving systemic glucocorticoid therapy—Nursing diagnoses:** *Deficient Knowledge* (drug therapy); *Risk for Fluid Volume Excess* related to fluid retention properties of glucocorticoids; *Risk for Injury* related to adverse drug effects; *Risk for Infections* related to adverse drug effects; *Risk for Impaired Skin Integrity* related to adverse drug effects.

13. **Clients receiving systemic glucocorticoid therapy—Planning:** The client will experience therapeutic effects (e.g., decreased signs and symptoms of inflammation or allergic response); be free from or experience minimal adverse effects. Verbalize an understanding of the drug's use, adverse effects and required precautions. Demonstrate proper self-administration of the medication (e.g., dose, timing, when to notify provider).

14. **Clients receiving systemic glucocorticoid therapy—Implementation:** Monitor vital signs, especially blood pressure and pulse. Report tachycardia or BP over 140/90. Monitor for abdominal pain, black or tarry stools, blood in the stool, hematemesis or coffee-ground emesis, dizziness, hypotension, especially if associated with tachycardia. Monitor for infection. Protect the client from potential infections. Monitor the client's compliance with drug regimen. Monitor for symptoms of Cushing's syndrome. Monitor blood-glucose levels. Monitor skin and mucous membranes for lacerations, abrasions, or break in integrity. Monitor GI status for peptic ulcer development. Monitor serum electrolytes. Monitor for osteoporosis (e.g., bone density testing) periodically in patients on long-term corticosteroids. Encourage adequate calcium intake, avoidance of carbonated sodas, and weight-bearing exercise. Monitor changes in musculoskeletal system. Monitor emotional stability. Weigh the patient daily and report weight gain or increasing peripheral edema. Measure intake and output in the hospitalized patient. Monitor vision periodically in patients on corticosteroids. Do not stop the drug abruptly. The drug must be

© 2011 Pearson Education, Inc.

tapered off if used longer than 1 or 2 weeks. Instruct the patient and/or family in proper self-administration of drug (e.g., with food or milk).

15. **Clients receiving systemic glucocorticoid therapy—Evaluation:** The client will experience decreased signs and symptoms of inflammation or allergic response; be free from or experience minimal adverse effects. Verbalize an understanding of the drug's use, adverse effects, and required precautions. Demonstrate proper self-administration of the medication (e.g., dose, timing, when to notify provider).

GENERAL CHAPTER CONSIDERATIONS

1. Have students study and learn key terms listed at the beginning of the chapter.
2. Have students complete end-of-chapter exercises either in their book or on the MyNursingKit website.
3. Use the Classroom Response Questions provided in PowerPoint to assess students prior to lecture.

 MYNURSINGKIT (*www.mynursingkit.com*)
- Websites
- NCLEX® questions
- Critical Thinking Questions
- Case Studies
- Animations and Videos
- Drug Prototype Questions

 MYNURSINGLAB (*www.mynursinglab.com*)
- Knowledge Quick Check
- Pre/Posttests
- Customized study plans
- *Separate purchase*

 STUDENT WORKBOOK AND RESOURCE GUIDE
- Chapter 43 activities
- *Separate purchase*

PEARSON NURSE'S DRUG GUIDE
- *Separate purchase*

 PEARSON ETEXT
- Students can search, highlight, take notes, and more all in electronic format.
- *Separate purchase*

 CLASSROOM RESPONSE QUESTION POWERPOINTS

 TESTBANK

© 2011 Pearson Education, Inc.

CHAPTER 44
DRUGS FOR DIABETES MELLITUS

LEARNING OUTCOME 1

Describe the endocrine and exocrine functions of the pancreas.

Concepts for Lecture

1. The pancreas is both an endocrine and an exocrine gland. It is responsible for the secretion of several enzymes into the duodenum that assist in the chemical digestion of nutrients. This is its exocrine function. The **islets of Langerhans** are responsible for its endocrine function: the secretion of glucagon and insulin.

2. Insulin is released when the blood-glucose level increases, and glucagon is released when the blood–glucose level decreases. Hormones and drugs can affect blood sugar (hyperglycemic or hypoglycemic effects). (See Figure 44.1 for an illustration of alpha and beta cells. See Figure 44.2 for an illustration of glucose, insulin, and glucagon action in the body.)

LEARNING OUTCOME 2

Compare and contrast type 1 and type 2 diabetes mellitus.

Concepts for Lecture

1. Type 1 DM is caused by an absolute lack of insulin secretion due to autoimmune destruction of pancreatic islet cells. If untreated, DM produces long-term damage to arteries, which leads to heart disease, stroke, kidney disease, and blindness.

2. Type 2 DM is **insulin resistance;** target cells become unresponsive to insulin due to a defect in insulin receptor function caused by a lack of sensitivity of insulin receptors at the target cells (insulin resistance) and a deficiency in insulin secretion. If untreated, the same chronic conditions result as in type 1 DM.

LEARNING OUTCOME 3

Compare and contrast types of insulin.

Concepts for Lecture

1. Type 1 DM is treated with dietary restrictions, exercise, and insulin therapy. The many types of insulin preparations vary as to their onset of action, time to peak effect, and duration. (See Table 44.1 for a list of types of insulin.)

2. Almost all insulin used today is human insulin made by recombinant DNA technology. It is more effective, causes fewer allergies, and creates less resistance. It is modified to be more rapid (Humalog) or have a prolonged action (Lantus). Insulin is administered by subcutaneous

 POWERPOINT SLIDES

Figure 44.1 Glucagon and Insulin-secreting Cells in the Islets of Langerhans
Figure 44.2 Insulin, Glucagon, and Blood Glucose

 SUGGESTION FOR CLASSROOM ACTIVITIES

- Direct students to diagram the endocrine and exocrine functions of the pancreas.

 SUGGESTION FOR CLINICAL ACTIVITIES

- Direct students to the pharmacy to view insulin and glucagon. Have the students research the routes and dosages of each.

 POWERPOINT SLIDES

 SUGGESTION FOR CLASSROOM ACTIVITIES

- Discuss the similarities and differences between type 1 and type 2 DM.

 SUGGESTION FOR CLINICAL ACTIVITIES

- Direct students to do a neurovascular assessment on a client with long-term diabetes and documented cardiovascular or nervous system damage.

 POWERPOINT SLIDES

Table 44.1 Insulin Preparations
Figure 44.3 An Illustration of an Insulin Pump

 SUGGESTION FOR CLASSROOM ACTIVITIES

- Discuss the route, onset, peak, and duration of the different types of insulin.

(SQ), inhaled (Exubera, approved in 2006), or intravenous routes. Only regular insulin can be given intravenously. (See Figure 44.3 for an illustration of an insulin pump.)

LEARNING OUTCOME 4

Describe the signs and symptoms of insulin overdose and underdose.

Concepts for Lecture

1. The most serious adverse effect from insulin therapy is hypoglycemia. Hypoglycemia can result from an overdose of insulin, improper timing of insulin dose, or skipping a meal. Signs and symptoms of hypoglycemia include tachycardia, confusion, sweating, drowsiness, convulsions, coma, and even death.
2. Hyperglycemia can result from an underdose of insulin or oral hypoglycemic. Signs and symptoms of hyperglycemia include fasting blood glucose greater than 126 mg/dL, polyuria, polydipsia, polyphagia, glucosuria, weight loss or gain, and fatigue.

LEARNING OUTCOME 5

Describe the nurse's role in the pharmacologic management of diabetes mellitus.

Concepts for Lecture

1. The role of the nurse in the pharmacologic management of diabetes mellitus involves careful monitoring of a client's condition and providing education as it relates to the prescribed drug treatment. Obtain baseline medical, surgical, and drug history; lifestyle and dietary habits, including use of herbal or alternative therapies; and a detailed description of symptomology and current therapies.
2. **Insulin therapy:** Be familiar with the onset, peak, and duration of action of the insulin(s) prescribed, as well as any other important aspects of the specific insulin, and convey this information to the client. It is important to understand that not all types of insulin are compatible and may not be mixed together in a single syringe. Clear insulin must be drawn into the syringe first to reduce the possible contamination of the clear insulin by the insulin containing a suspension. Know the signs and symptoms of hypoglycemia and hyperglycemia.
3. **Oral hypoglycemic therapy:** Assessment of the client with type 2 diabetes includes a physical examination, health history, psychosocial history, and lifestyle history. Provide clients with information about the importance of keeping blood-glucose levels within a normal range. Blood-glucose levels should be monitored daily; urinary ketones should be monitored if the blood-glucose level is over 300 mg/dL. Also monitor intake and output, and review lab studies for liver-function abnormalities. Monitor the client for signs and symptoms of illness or infection. Administer oral hypoglycemics as directed by the prescriber.

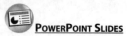 **SUGGESTION FOR CLINICAL ACTIVITIES**

- Assign students to care for clients who are receiving insulin therapy.

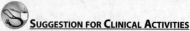 **POWERPOINT SLIDES**

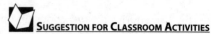 **SUGGESTION FOR CLASSROOM ACTIVITIES**

- Present case studies with clients suffering hypoglycemic or hyperglycemic episodes.

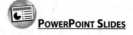 **SUGGESTION FOR CLINICAL ACTIVITIES**

- Direct students to research the clinical policies for treating hypoglycemia and hyperglycemia. Have them find the correct medications for each.

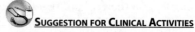 **POWERPOINT SLIDES**

SUGGESTION FOR CLASSROOM ACTIVITIES

- Discuss the role of the nurse in the pharmacologic treatment of clients with DM.

SUGGESTION FOR CLINICAL ACTIVITIES

- Direct students to assess the client who is taking insulin or oral hypoglycemic therapy for any contraindications to therapy.

© 2011 Pearson Education, Inc.

LEARNING OUTCOME 6

Identify drug classes used to treat type 2 diabetes mellitus.

Concepts for Lecture

1. Type 2 DM is controlled through lifestyle changes and oral hypoglycemic drugs. All oral hypoglycemics have the common action of lowering blood-glucose levels. Many have the potential to cause hypoglycemia. Oral hypoglycemics are not effective for type 1 DM. People with type 2 diabetes mellitus should have a preprandial blood sugar below 110 mg/dL. The six primary groups of oral antidiabetic drugs are classified by their chemical structures and their mechanisms of action. These include sulfonylureas, biguanides, meglitinides, thiazolidinediones (or glitazones), alpha-glucosidase inhibitors, and incretin therapies. (The oral hypoglycemics are shown in Table 44.2.)

2. **Sulfonylureas:** The first oral hypoglycemics available, sulfonylureas are divided into first- and second-generation categories. The sulfonylureas act by stimulating the release of insulin from pancreatic islet cells and by increasing the sensitivity of insulin receptors on target cells. The most common adverse effect of sulfonylureas is hypoglycemia, which is usually caused by taking too much medication or not eating enough food.

3. **Biguanides:** Metformin (Glucophage), the only drug in this class, acts by decreasing the hepatic production of glucose (gluconeogenesis) and reducing insulin resistance. It does not promote insulin release from the pancreas. Most side effects are minor and GI-related, such as anorexia, nausea, and diarrhea. A new extended-release formulations of metformin ((Fortamet, Glucophage XR, and Glumetza) approved in 2005, allow for once-daily dosing.

4. **Alpha-glucosidase inhibitors:** The alpha-glucosidase inhibitors such as acarbose (Precose) act by blocking enzymes in the small intestine that are responsible for breaking down complex carbohydrates into monosaccharides. Because carbohydrates must be in the monosaccharide form to be absorbed, digestion of glucose is delayed. These agents are usually well tolerated and have minimal side effects. The most common side effects are GI-related, such as abdominal cramping, diarrhea, and flatulence.

5. **Thiazolidinediones:** The thiazolidinediones, or glitazones, reduce blood glucose by decreasing insulin resistance and inhibiting hepatic gluconeogenesis. Optimal lowering of blood glucose may take 3 to 4 months of therapy. The most common adverse effects are fluid retention, headache, and weight gain. Hypoglycemia does not occur with drugs in this class.

6. **Meglitinides:** The meglitinides are a newer class of oral hypoglycemics that act by stimulating the release of insulin from pancreatic islet cells in a manner similar to that of the sulfonylureas. Both agents in this class have short durations of action of 2 to 4 hours. Their efficacy is equal to that of the sulfonylureas, and they are well tolerated. Hypoglycemia is the most common adverse effect.

7. **Newer agents:** These agents act by affecting the incretin–glucose control mechanism. Incretins are hormones secreted by the intestine following a meal when the blood-glucose level is elevated. Two new drugs with unique mechanisms entered the market in 2005. Exenatide (Byetta) is an injectable drug that belongs to a class of drugs called incretin mimetics. These drugs mimic the effects of incretins, which are hormones produced and released into the blood by the intestine in response to food. Sitaglipton inhibits DPP-4, thereby reducing the destruction of incretins. Levels of incretin hormones increase, thus

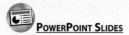
Table 44.2 Oral Hypoglycemics

SUGGESTION FOR CLASSROOM ACTIVITIES

- Divide students into small groups, and have them prepare questions and answers for different categories of drugs used to treat DM. Include questions on each drug's classification and mechanisms of action.

SUGGESTION FOR CLINICAL ACTIVITIES

- Assign students to care for patients receiving pharmacotherapy for DM.

decreasing blood-glucose levels in patients with type 2 diabetes. The drug is given once daily by the oral route. Pramlintide (Symlin) is a new injectable drug for type 1 and type 2 DM that resembles human amylin, a hormone produced by the pancreas after meals that helps the body to regulate blood glucose. In 2009, an old drug with a new use was approved to treat type 2 diabetes—bromocriptine (Parlodel) marketed as Cycloset, whose exact mechanism of action is still unclear.

LEARNING OUTCOME 7

For each of the drug classes listed in Drugs at a Glance, know representative drug examples, and explain the mechanisms of drug action, primary actions, and important adverse effects.

Concepts for Lecture

1. **Insulins:** Prototype drug: regular insulin. Mechanism of action: to promote the entry of glucose into cells. Primary use: This is a short-acting insulin, with an onset of 30 to 60 minutes, a peak effect at 2 to 3 hours, and a duration of 5 to 7 hours. It is used to quickly decrease blood glucose; also used in the emergency management of ketoacidosis. Adverse effects: hypoglycemia.

2. **Oral hypoglycemics:** Prototype drug: glipizide (Glucotrol, Glucotrol XL). Mechanism of action: to stimulate the pancreas to secrete more insulin. It also increases the sensitivity of insulin receptors at target tissues. Primary use: for treatment of type 2 diabetes. Adverse effects: hypoglycemia, rashes, and photosensitivity. Some clients experience mild, GI-related effects such as nausea, vomiting, or loss of appetite.

LEARNING OUTCOME 8

Use the nursing process to care for patients receiving drug therapy for diabetes mellitus.

Concepts for Lecture

1. **Clients receiving insulin therapy—Assessment:** Obtain a complete health history, including allergies, drug history, and possible drug interactions. Obtain a history of current symptoms, duration and severity, and other related signs or symptoms (e.g., paresthesias of hands or feet). Assess feet and lower extremities for possible ulcerations. Obtain a dietary history including caloric intake if on an ADA diet, number of meals and snacks per day. Assess fluid intake and type of fluids consumed. Obtain baseline vital signs, height, and weight. Evaluate appropriate laboratory findings (e.g., CBC, electrolytes, glucose, A1C level, lipid profile, osmolality, hepatic and renal function studies). Assess subcutaneous areas for potential insulin injection sites. Assess client's knowledge of insulin and ability to self-administer insulin.

2. **Clients receiving insulin therapy—Nursing diagnoses:** *Imbalanced Nutrition, Less than Body Requirements* (Type I diabetes, related to lack of insulin availability for normal metabolism); *Imbalanced Nutrition, More Than Body Requirements* (Type II diabetes, related to insulin resistance and intake more than body needs); *Deficient Knowledge*

POWERPOINT SLIDES

Prototype Drug
- regular insulin
- glipizide (Glucotrol, Glucotrol XL)

SUGGESTION FOR CLASSROOM ACTIVITIES

- Have each student make drug cards for each classification of drug used to treat DM. Use two different drugs for each classification. The card should include actions, uses, routes of administration, dosages, and adverse effects.

SUGGESTION FOR CLINICAL ACTIVITIES

- Divide students into small groups, and have each group develop a teaching plan for a patient receiving medications for DM.

ANIMATIONS AND VIDEOS

- Mechanism in Action: glipizide (Glucotrol)

POWERPOINT SLIDES

NURSING PROCESS FOCUS

- Clients receiving insulin therapy
- Clients receiving oral hypoglycemic therapy

SUGGESTION FOR CLASSROOM ACTIVITIES

- Invite a diabetes-educator nurse to the class to discuss pharmacotherapy for diabetes mellitus.

SUGGESTION FOR CLINICAL ACTIVITIES

- Assign students to care for clients taking insulin and oral hypoglycemic therapy.

© 2011 Pearson Education, Inc.

(drug therapy); *Ineffective Therapeutic Regimen Management* related to deficient knowledge or altered compliance with prescribed treatment *Altered Compliance, Noncompliance* related to complexity of treatment plan, deficient knowledge; *Risk for Deficient Fluid Volume* related to polyuria from hyperglycemia; *Risk for Injury* related to adverse drug effects, lack of sensation in extremities from neuropathies; *Risk for Infection* related to hyperglycemia, impaired circulation to extremities, neuropathies.

3. **Clients receiving insulin therapy—Planning:** The client will experience therapeutic effects (e.g., blood sugar within normal limits). The client will be free from or experience minimal adverse effects. Verbalize an understanding of the drug's use, adverse effects and required precautions. Demonstrate proper self-administration of the medication (e.g., dose, timing, when to notify provider).

4. **Clients receiving insulin therapy—Implementation:** Administer insulin correctly and per schedule ordered (e.g., routine dosing with or without sliding-scale coverage), planning insulin administration and peak times around meal times. Ensure dietary needs are met based on need to lose, gain, or maintain current weight and glucose levels. Hold insulin dose if blood sugar is less than 70 mg/dL and report to the health care provider. Continue to monitor periodic lab work: CBC, electrolytes, glucose, A1C level, lipid profile, osmolality, hepatic and renal function studies. Assess for symptoms of hypoglycemia, especially around time of insulin peak activity. Monitor blood-glucose levels more frequently during periods of illness or stress. Encourage increased physical activity but monitor blood–glucose levels before and after exercise and begin any new or increased exercise routine gradually. Rotate insulin administration sites weekly. Change insulin pump subcutaneous catheters every 2 to 3 days to prevent infections at the site of insertion. Ensure proper storage of insulin to maintain maximum potency. Instruct patient and/or family in proper self-administration of drug. Check urine for ketones if blood glucose is over 300 mg/dL.

5. **Clients receiving insulin therapy—Evaluation:** The client will experience blood sugar within normal limits) and be free from or experience minimal adverse effects. Verbalizes an understanding of the drug's use, adverse effects, and required precautions. Demonstrates proper self-administration of the medication (e.g., dose, timing, when to notify provider).

6. **Clients receiving oral hypoglycemic therapy—Assessment:** Obtain a complete health history including allergies, drug history, and possible drug interactions. Obtain a history of current symptoms, duration and severity, and other related signs or symptoms (e.g., paresthesias of hands or feet). Assess feet and lower extremities for possible ulcerations. Obtain a dietary history including caloric intake, number of meals and snacks per day. Assess fluid intake and type of fluids consumed. Obtain baseline vital signs, height, and weight. Evaluate appropriate laboratory findings (e.g., CBC, electrolytes, glucose, A1C level, lipid profile, hepatic and renal function studies). Assess for pain location and level. Assess client's knowledge of drug. Assess client's ability to conduct blood-glucose testing. Assess for and report promptly any adverse effects appropriate to type of oral agent signs of hypoglycemia and hyperglycemia.

7. **Clients receiving oral hypoglycemic therapy—Nursing diagnoses:** *Imbalanced Nutrition, More than Body Requirements* (Type II diabetes, related to insulin resistance and intake more than body needs); *Deficient Knowledge* (drug therapy); *Ineffective Therapeutic Regimen Management* related to deficient knowledge or altered compliance with prescribed treatment; *Altered Compliance, Noncompliance* related to complexity of treatment plan, deficient knowledge; *Risk for Injury* related to adverse drug effects, lack of sensation in

extremities from neuropathies; *Risk for Infection* related to hyper-glycemia, impaired circulation to extremities, neuropathies.

8. **Clients receiving oral hypoglycemic therapy—Planning:** The client will experience therapeutic effects (e.g., blood sugar within normal limits) and will be free from or experience minimal adverse effects. Verbalize an understanding of the drug's use, adverse effects, and required precautions. Demonstrate proper self-administration of the medication (e.g., dose, timing, when to notify provider).

9. **Clients receiving oral hypoglycemic therapy—Implementation:** Ensure dietary needs are met based on need to lose, gain, or maintain current weight and glucose levels. Consult with dietician as needed. Limit or eliminate alcohol use. Check with health care provider before giving oral hypoglycemic if blood sugar is less than 70 mg/dL and monitor periodic lab work: CBC, electrolytes, glucose, A1C level, lipid profile, hepatic and renal function studies. Assess for symptoms of hypoglycemia. If symptoms of hypoglycemia are noted, provide a quick-acting carbohydrate source (e.g., juice or other simple sugar), and then check capillary glucose level. Monitor blood-glucose levels more frequently during periods of illness or stress. Encourage increased activity but monitor blood-glucose levels before and after exercise and begin any new or increased exercise routine gradually. Monitor for signs of lactic acidosis if the client is receiving biguanide. Monitor for hypoglycemia up to 48 hours after exercise. Monitor for hypersensitivity and allergic reactions. Assess for pregnancy. Monitor for edema, BP, and lung sounds in patients taking thiazolidiones. Monitor for hypoglycemia more frequently in patients on concurrent beta-blocker therapy. Instruct patient and/or family in proper self-administration of drug.

10. **Clients receiving oral hypoglycemic therapy—Evaluation:** The client will experience therapeutic effects (e.g., blood sugar within normal limits) and will be free from or experience minimal adverse effects. Verbalize an understanding of the drug's use, adverse effects, and required precautions. Demonstrates proper self-administration of the medication (e.g., dose, timing, when to notify provider).

© 2011 Pearson Education, Inc.

GENERAL CHAPTER CONSIDERATIONS

1. Have students study and learn key terms listed at the beginning of the chapter.
2. Have students complete end-of-chapter exercises either in their book or on the MyNursingKit website.
3. Use the Classroom Response Questions provided in PowerPoint to assess students prior to lecture.

 MYNURSINGKIT
(www.mynursingkit.com)
- Websites
- NCLEX® questions
- Critical Thinking Questions
- Case Studies
- Animations and Videos
- Drug Prototype Questions

 MYNURSINGLAB
(www.mynursinglab.com)
- Knowledge Quick Check
- Pre/Posttests
- Customized study plans
- *Separate purchase*

 STUDENT WORKBOOK AND RESOURCE GUIDE
- Chapter 44 activities
- *Separate purchase*

PEARSON NURSE'S DRUG GUIDE
- *Separate purchase*

 PEARSON ETEXT
- Students can search, highlight, take notes, and more all in electronic format.
- *Separate purchase*

 CLASSROOM RESPONSE QUESTION POWERPOINTS

TESTBANK

CHAPTER 45
DRUGS FOR DISORDERS AND CONDITIONS OF THE FEMALE REPRODUCTIVE SYSTEM

LEARNING OUTCOME 1

Describe the roles of the hypothalamus, pituitary, and ovaries in maintaining female reproductive function.

Concepts for Lecture

1. Regulation of the female reproductive system is achieved by hormones from the hypothalamus, pituitary gland, and ovary. The hypothalamus secretes gonadotropin-releasing hormone (GnRH), which stimulates the pituitary to secrete follicle-stimulating hormone (FSH) and luteinizing hormone (LH). Both of these pituitary hormones act on the ovary and cause immature ovarian follicles to begin developing. The rising and falling levels of pituitary hormones create two interrelated cycles that occur on a periodic, monthly basis, the ovarian and uterine cycles. (The hormonal changes that occur during the ovarian and uterine cycles are illustrated in Figure 45.1.)
2. Estrogens are secreted by ovarian follicles and are responsible for maturation of the sex organs and the secondary sex characteristics of the female. Progestins are secreted by the corpus luteum and prepare the endometrium for implantation. High progesterone and estrogen levels in the final third of the uterine cycle provide negative feedback to shut off GnRH, FSH, and LH secretion.

LEARNING OUTCOME 2

Explain the mechanisms by which estrogens and progestins prevent conception.

Concepts for Lecture

1. Low doses of estrogens and progestins prevent conception by blocking ovulation. Oral contraceptives are drugs used to prevent pregnancy, which is the most common use for female sex hormones. Commonly referred to as "the pill," most oral contraceptives are a combination of estrogens and progestins. See Figure 45.3 for an illustration of the oral contraceptive packet. In small doses, they prevent fertilization by inhibiting ovulation. (Selected oral contraceptives are shown in Table 45.1.)
2. Estrogen-progestin oral contraceptives act by providing negative feedback to the pituitary to shut down the secretion of LH and FSH. The three types of estrogen-progestin formulations are monophasic, biphasic, and triphasic. The progestin-only oral contraceptives, sometimes called minipills, prevent pregnancy primarily by producing thick, viscous mucus at the entrance to the uterus that discourages penetration by sperm.

POWERPOINT SLIDES

Figure 45.1 Hormonal Changes During the Ovarian and Uterine Cycles
Figure 45.2 Negative Feedback Control of the Female Reproductive Hormones

SUGGESTION FOR CLASSROOM ACTIVITIES

- Direct students to draw a concept map of the functions of estrogen and progestin.

SUGGESTION FOR CLINICAL ACTIVITIES

- Assign students to observe in a fertility clinic. Direct them to correlate the ovarian and uterine cycles to the treatments they see.

POWERPOINT SLIDES

Table 45.1 Selected Oral Contraceptives
Figure 45.3 Illustration of Oral Contraception Packet

SUGGESTION FOR CLASSROOM ACTIVITIES

- Have available different types of contraceptives for the student to examine.

SUGGESTION FOR CLINICAL ACTIVITIES

- Invite a nurse from the women's health clinic to speak to the students about contraception during postclinical.

© 2011 Pearson Education, Inc.

LEARNING OUTCOME 3

Explain how drugs may be used to provide emergency contraception and to terminate early pregnancy.

Concepts for Lecture

Drugs for emergency contraception may be administered within 72 hours after unprotected sex to prevent implantation of the fertilized egg. Following are the two regimens approved by the FDA. First, Plan B: This regimen involves taking 0.75 mg of levonorgestrel in two doses, 12 hours apart. The alternative is Preven: A combination of ethinyl estradiol and levonorgestrel, Preven is effective, although nausea and vomiting are common. Once the ovum has been fertilized, several pharmacological choices are available to terminate the pregnancy. These agents are given to stimulate uterine contractions to expel the implanted embryo. A single dose of mifepristone (Mifeprex, RU486), followed 36 to 48 hours later by a single dose of misoprostol (Cytotec), is a frequently used regimen. (See Table 45.3.)

LEARNING OUTCOME 4

Describe the role of drug therapy in the treatment of menopausal and postmenopausal symptoms.

Concepts for Lecture

Estrogen-progestin combinations are used for hormone replacement therapy during and after menopause; however, their long-term use may have serious adverse effects. Over the past 20 years, health care providers have commonly prescribed hormone replacement therapy (HRT) to treat unpleasant symptoms of menopause and to prevent the long-term consequences of estrogen loss listed in Table 45.4. All this changed, however, in 2002 when the results of a large clinical study, the Women's Health Initiative (WHI), suggested increased risks of cardiac problems, stroke, and cancer. However, HRT appears to prevent osteoporotic bone fractures. Women are now encouraged to discuss alternatives with their health care provider.

LEARNING OUTCOME 5

Identify the role of the female sex hormones in the treatment of cancer.

Concepts for Lecture

When used alone, estrogen increases the risk of uterine cancer. Estrogen without progestin is only considered appropriate for clients who have had a hysterectomy. High doses of estrogen are sometimes used to treat prostate and breast cancer. Prostate cancer is usually dependent on androgens for growth; administration of estrogens will suppress androgen secretion. As an antineoplastic hormone, estrogen is rarely used alone. It is one of many agents used in combination for the chemotherapy of cancer.

 POWERPOINT SLIDES

Table 45.3 Drugs for Emergency Contraception and Pharmacological Abortion

 SUGGESTION FOR CLASSROOM ACTIVITIES

- Direct students to research emergency contraception and submit a paper summarizing that research.

 SUGGESTION FOR CLINICAL ACTIVITIES

- Assign students to observe in a women's health clinic. Direct them to submit a summary of the client care they see, especially in the area of emergency contraception.

 POWERPOINT SLIDES

Figure 45.4 Oxytocin and Breast-feeding
Table 45.4 Potential Consequences of Estrogen Loss Related to Menopause

 SUGGESTION FOR CLASSROOM ACTIVITIES

- Discuss how a woman can make an informed decision regarding HRT.

 SUGGESTION FOR CLINICAL ACTIVITIES

- Assign students to observe in a clinic that deals with women's menopausal problems.

 POWERPOINT SLIDES

 SUGGESTION FOR CLASSROOM ACTIVITIES

- Direct students to develop a poster that details the treatment of cancer with female hormones.

SUGGESTION FOR CLINICAL ACTIVITIES

- Assign students to care for a client undergoing the use of hormones as cancer therapy.

LEARNING OUTCOME 6

Discuss the uses of progestins in the therapy of dysfunctional uterine bleeding.

Concepts for Lecture

Dysfunctional uterine bleeding is a condition in which hemorrhage occurs on a noncyclic basis or in abnormal amounts. It is the health problem most frequently reported by women and a common reason for hysterectomy. The cause is often an imbalance between estrogen and progesterone. Whereas the function of estrogen is to cause proliferation of the endometrium, progesterone limits and stabilizes endometrial growth. Progestins are the drugs of choice for treating uterine abnormalities. (See Table 45.5.)

LEARNING OUTCOME 7

Compare and contrast the use of uterine stimulants and relaxants in the treatment of antepartum and postpartum patients.

Concepts for Lecture

Oxytocics are natural hormones secreted by the posterior pituitary; they stimulate uterine contractions to induce labor. Suckling stimulates release of oxytocin, which causes more milk ejection. (See oxytocin and breast-feeding illustrated in Figure 45.4.) Tocolytics slow uterine contractions to delay labor. They are used in clients with premature labor.

LEARNING OUTCOME 8

Explain how drug therapy may be used to treat female infertility.

Concepts for Lecture

Causes of female infertility are varied and include lack of ovulation, pelvic infection, and physical obstruction of the uterine tubes. For women whose infertility has been determined to have an endocrine etiology, pharmacotherapy may be of value. Endocrine disruption of reproductive function can occur at the level of the hypothalamus, the pituitary, or the ovary, and pharmacotherapy is targeted to the specific cause of the dysfunction. Lack of regular ovulation is a cause of infertility that can be successfully treated with drug therapy. Clomiphene (Clomid, Serophene) is a drug of choice for female infertility that acts as an antiestrogen. Clomiphene stimulates the release of LH, resulting in the maturation of more ovarian follicles than would normally occur. The rise in LH level is sufficient to induce ovulation in about 90% of treated women. (See Table 45.7.)

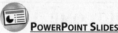

POWERPOINT SLIDES

Table 45.5 Selected Estrogens and Progestins

SUGGESTION FOR CLASSROOM ACTIVITIES

• Discuss pharmacotherapy choices and surgical alternatives for dysfunctional uterine bleeding.

SUGGESTION FOR CLINICAL ACTIVITIES

• Assign the students to a clinic that deals in women's health issues to care for women who are experiencing dysfunctional uterine bleeding.

POWERPOINT SLIDES

Figure 45.4. Oxytocin and Breast-feeding
Table 45.6 Uterine Stimulants and Relaxants

SUGGESTION FOR CLASSROOM ACTIVITIES

• Discuss case studies with students to illustrate situations in which either an oxytocic drug or a tocolytic drug would be most appropriate.

SUGGESTION FOR CLINICAL ACTIVITIES

• Assign students to an obstetrics department to observe women in labor and the oxytocic and tocolytic drugs used in these situations.

POWERPOINT SLIDES

Table 45.7 Agents for Female Infertility

SUGGESTION FOR CLASSROOM ACTIVITIES

• Discuss side effects of the fertility drugs.

SUGGESTION FOR CLINICAL ACTIVITIES

• Assign students to attend a conference dealing with female infertility.

© 2011 Pearson Education, Inc.

LEARNING OUTCOME 9

Describe the nurse's role in the pharmacologic management of disorders and conditions of the female reproductive system.

Concepts for Lecture

1. The role of the nurse in the pharmacologic management of disorders and conditions of the female reproductive system involves careful monitoring of a client's condition and providing education as it relates to the prescribed drug treatment. Obtain baseline medical, surgical, and drug history; lifestyle and dietary habits, including use of herbal or alternative therapies; and a detailed description of symptomology and current therapies.

2. **Oral contraceptive therapy:** Blood pressure should be monitored because these medications can cause mild to moderate hypertension. Assess vital signs frequently, and monitor for symptoms of thrombophlebitis, such as pain, redness, and tenderness of the calves. Oral contraceptives can mimic certain symptoms of pregnancy, including breast tenderness, nausea, bloating, and chloasma. Reassure the client that these side effects do not indicate pregnancy. Oral contraceptives may increase the risk of certain types of breast cancer; therefore, teach clients how to perform breast self-exams and provide information on routine scheduling of mammograms appropriate for their age bracket.

3. **Hormone replacement therapy:** Because of the risk of thromboembolism, monitor the client closely for signs and symptoms of thrombus or embolus, such as pain in calves, limited movement in legs, dyspnea, sudden severe chest pain, or anxiety. Encourage the client to report signs of depression, decreased libido, headache, fatigue, and weight gain. Because current controversy surrounds the long-term use of these drugs as hormone replacement therapy, it is imperative for women to be aware of current research and to discuss treatment alternatives with their health care provider before beginning pharmacotherapy. When using HRT to treat male clients, inform them that secondary female characteristics, such as a higher voice, sparse body hair, and increased breast size, may develop. Inform the client that impotence may also occur.

4. **Progestin therapy:** Assess for severe, colicky abdominal pain, vomiting, abdominal distension, diarrhea, and constipation. Common side effects of progesterone include breakthrough bleeding, nausea, abdominal cramps, dizziness, edema, and weight gain. Monitor for amenorrhea; sudden, severe headache; and signs of pulmonary embolism, such as sudden, severe chest pain and dyspnea; and report such symptoms to the health care provider immediately. Progesterone can cause photosensitivity and phototoxicity and monitor for pruritus, sensitivity to light, acne, rash, and alopecia. Phototoxic reactions cause serious sunburn within 5 to 18 hours after sun exposure.

5. **Uterine stimulant therapy:** Frequently assess the client in labor because oxytocin increases the frequency and force of uterine contractions. Discontinue the infusion if fetal distress is detected to prevent fetal anoxia. Hypertensive crisis may occur if local or regional anesthesia is used in combination with oxytocin. Monitor fluid balance, because prolonged IV infusion of oxytocin may cause water intoxication. Assess for symptoms of water intoxication, and report immediately. Symptoms include drowsiness, listlessness, headache, confusion, anuria, and weight gain. Side effects of oxytocin include anxiety, maternal dyspnea, hypotension or hypertension, nausea, vomiting, neonatal jaundice, and maternal or fetal dysrhythmias.

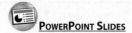
POWERPOINT SLIDES

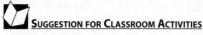
SUGGESTION FOR CLASSROOM ACTIVITIES

- Discuss the role of the nurse in the pharmacologic management of disorders and conditions of the female reproductive system.

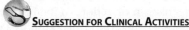
SUGGESTION FOR CLINICAL ACTIVITIES

- Direct students to create teaching plans for clients with disorders and conditions of the female reproductive system.

LEARNING OUTCOME 10

For each of the classes shown in Drugs at a Glance, know representative drugs, and explain the mechanisms of drug action, primary actions, and important adverse effects.

Concepts for Lecture

1. **Oral contraceptives, estrogen-progestin combinations.** Prototype drug: ethinyl estradiol with norethindrone (Ortho-Novum 1/35). Mechanism of action: to inhibit the release of FSH and LH, thus preventing ovulation. Primary use: as a contraceptive, for improvement in menstrual cycle regularity, and to decrease incidence of dysmenorrhea. Adverse effects: edema, nausea, abdominal cramps, dysmenorrhea, breast tenderness, fatigue, skin rash, acne, headache, weight gain, midcycle breakthrough bleeding, vaginal candidiasis, photosensitivity, and changes in urinary patterns. Serious cardiovascular side effects are more common in smokers and include hypertension and thromboembolic disorders.

2. **Hormone replacement therapy.** Prototype drug: conjugated estrogens (Premarin) and conjugated estrogens with medroxyprogesterone (Prempro). Mechanism of action: a replacement for female sex hormones used to exert several positive metabolic effects, including an increase in bone density and a reduction in LDL cholesterol. Primary use: for postmenopausal replacement therapy and to treat abnormal uterine bleeding due to hormonal imbalance. Adverse effects: nausea, fluid retention, edema, breast tenderness, abdominal cramps and bloating, acute pancreatitis, appetite changes, acne, mental depression, decreased libido, headache, fatigue, nervousness, and weight gain.

3. **Drugs for dysfunctional uterine bleeding—Progestins.** Prototype drug: medroxyprogesterone (Provera). Mechanism of action: to inhibit the effect of estrogen on the uterus, thus restoring normal hormonal balance. Primary use: for treatment of dysfunctional uterine bleeding, secondary amenorrhea, and contraception. Medroxyprogesterone may also be given IM for the palliation of metastatic uterine or renal carcinoma. Adverse effects: breakthrough bleeding and breast tenderness. Weight gain, depression, hypertension, nausea, vomiting, and dysmenorrhea and vaginal candidiasis may also occur. The most serious side effect is an increased risk for thromboembolic disease.

4. **Uterine stimulant—Oxytocics.** Prototype drug: oxytocin (Pitocin, Syntocinon). Mechanism of action: to induce labor by increasing the frequency and force of uterine contractions. Primary use: as the drug of choice for inducing labor. Adverse effects: complications in the fetus, such as dysrhythmias or intracranial hemorrhage. Serious complications in the mother may include uterine rupture, seizures, or coma.

LEARNING OUTCOME 11

Use the nursing process to care for patients who are receiving drug therapy for disorders and conditions of the female reproductive system.

Concepts for Lecture

1. **Patients Receiving Estrogen and Progestin Therapy (Oral Contraceptives, HRT, and Treatment of Dysfunctional Uterine Bleeding)—Assessment:** Obtain a complete health history including

POWERPOINT SLIDES

Prototype Drug
- ethinyl estradiol with norethindrone (Ortho-Novum 1/35)
- conjugated estrogens (Premarin)
- conjugated estrogens with medroxyprogesterone (Prempro)
- medroxyprogesterone (Provera)
- oxytocin (Pitocin, Syntocinon)

ANIMATIONS AND VIDEOS
- Mechanism in Action: Ethinyl estradiol with norethindrone (Ortho-Novum)

SUGGESTION FOR CLASSROOM ACTIVITIES
- During postclinical conference, divide students into small groups, and have each group discuss the client education they did or observed for women with reproductive disorders.

SUGGESTION FOR CLINICAL ACTIVITIES
- During postclinical conference, divide students into small groups, and have each group discuss the client education they did or observed for women with reproductive disorders.

POWERPOINT SLIDES

NURSING PROCESS FOCUS
- Care for clients who are receiving drug therapy for disorders and conditions of the female reproductive system.

© 2011 Pearson Education, Inc.

smoking, cardiovascular, peripheral vascular, migraine headaches, thyroid, hepatic or renal disease, diabetes, pregnancy or breast-feeding. Note personal or family history of thromboembolic disorders (e.g., MI, CVA, PVD) and of reproductive cancers (e.g., breast, uterine, or ovarian cancer). Evaluate appropriate laboratory findings (e.g., CBC, platelets, electrolytes, glucose, lipid, and thyroid function levels) and Pap test. Obtain baseline height, weight, and vital signs.

2. **Patients Receiving Estrogen and Progestin Therapy (Oral Contraceptives, HRT, and Treatment of Dysfunctional Uterine Bleeding)—Nursing diagnoses:** *Decisional Conflict* related to concerns about benefits and risks of drug therapy; *Disturbed Body Image* related to aging process, adverse effects of drug therapy; *Deficient Knowledge* (drug therapy); *Risk of Injury* related to adverse drug effects.

3. **Patients Receiving Estrogen and Progestin Therapy (Oral Contraceptives, HRT, and Treatment of Dysfunctional Uterine Bleeding)—Planning:** The client will experience therapeutic effects (e.g., effective birth control, decrease in symptoms of menopause, dysfunctional uterine bleeding and diminished). The client will be free from or experience minimal adverse effects. Verbalize an understanding of the drug's use, adverse effects and required precautions. Demonstrate proper self-administration of the medication (e.g., dose, timing, when to notify provider).

4. **Patients Receiving Estrogen and Progestin Therapy (Oral Contraceptives, HRT, and Treatment of Dysfunctional Uterine Bleeding)—Implementation:** Monitor appropriate medication administration for optimum results. Monitor for symptoms of thromboembolism. Monitor blood pressure at each clinical visit. Encourage smoking cessation and provide information about smoking cessation programs. Monitor blood-glucose levels in diabetic patients more frequently. Monitor hepatic function tests and symptoms of liver dysfunction, lipid profile studies, and thyroid levels periodically. Monitor concurrent drug therapy. Monitor yearly Pap tests and breast exams. Monitor the occurrence of any breakthrough bleeding. Report any continuous, unusual, or heavy bleeding. Instruct patient or caregiver in proper self-administration of drug (e.g., consistently at same time each day to help remember dose).

5. **Patients Receiving Estrogen and Progestin Therapy (Oral Contraceptives, HRT, and Treatment of Dysfunctional Uterine Bleeding)—Evaluation:** The client will experience therapeutic effects (e.g., effective birth control, decrease in symptoms of menopause, dysfunctional uterine bleeding and diminished). The client will be free from or experience minimal adverse effects. Verbalize an understanding of the drug's use, adverse effects, and required precautions. Demonstrate proper self-administration of the medication (e.g., dose, timing, when to notify provider).

6. **Patients Receiving Oxytocin—Assessment:** Obtain a complete health history, including past and present gynecologic and obstetric history, cardiovascular, neurologic, hepatic or renal disease, diabetes, or breast-feeding, Obtain drug history to determine possible drug interactions and allergies. Evaluate appropriate laboratory findings (e.g., CBC, platelets, coagulation studies, electrolytes, glucose, magnesium level, hepatic and renal function studies). Obtain baseline height, weight, and vital signs. Obtain fetal heart rate, intrauterine positioning. Check for postpartum bleeding and note number of pads saturated. Assess for and report adverse effects: nausea, vomiting, severe headache, tachycardia, hypertension, changes in LOC, and seizures.

7. **Patients Receiving Oxytocin—Nursing diagnoses:** *Pain* Acute, related to strong uterine contractions; *Ineffective Breast-feeding,*

SUGGESTION FOR CLASSROOM ACTIVITIES

- Invite a nurse from an OB/GYN clinical to discuss disorders and conditions of the female reproductive system.

SUGGESTION FOR CLINICAL ACTIVITIES

- Invite a nurse from an OB/GYN clinical to discuss disorders and conditions of the female reproductive system.

Potential for Effective Breast-feeding; Deficient Knowledge (drug therapy); *Risk of Injury Patient or Fetus* related to adverse drug effects, strong uterine contractions; *Risk for Imbalanced Fluid Volume, Excess* related to water intoxication from drug's antidiuretic hormone effects.

8. **Patients Receiving Oxytocin—Planning:** The client will experience therapeutic effects (e.g., strong labor contractions supportive of labor, adequate milk letdown supportive of breast-feeding, postpartum bleeding is diminished). The client will be free from or experience minimal adverse effects. Verbalize an understanding of the drug's use, adverse effects, and required precautions. Demonstrate proper self-administration of the medication (e.g., dose, timing, when to notify provider).

9. **Patients Receiving Oxytocin—Implementation:** Monitor fetal heart rate. Monitor maternal status, including blood pressure, pulse, and frequency, duration, and intensity of contractions. Monitor fluid balance. Monitor for postpartum/postabortion hemorrhage. Monitor lactation status. Periodically monitor of CBC, platelets, electrolytes, glucose, and magnesium level. Monitor postpartum bleeding and pad count. Monitor appropriate medication administration for optimum results. Monitor timing, quality, and duration of contractions continuously. Report any sustained uterine contractions immediately and stop the infusion, run normal saline, and place patient on her side. Continuously monitor fetal heart rate and response to contractions and report signs of fetal distress. Monitor vital signs and urine output frequently and report any BP above 140/90 or less than 90/60. Monitor fundal firmness and location, postpartum bleeding, and pad count. Monitor progress of labor—cervical dilation and effacement, quality and duration of any existing contractions, fetal response to contractions, noting any sign of fetal distress. Notify health care provider if more than 2 full-size pads are saturated in 2 hours time. Report sustained uterine contractions immediately to the health care provider.

10. **Patients Receiving Oxytocin—Evaluation:** The client will experience strong labor contractions supportive of labor, adequate milk letdown supportive of breast-feeding, postpartum bleeding is diminished. The client will be free from or experience minimal adverse effects. Verbalize an understanding of the drug's use, adverse effects, and required precautions. Demonstrate proper self-administration of the medication (e.g., dose, timing, when to notify provider).

© 2011 Pearson Education, Inc.

GENERAL CHAPTER CONSIDERATIONS

1. Have students study and learn key terms listed at the beginning of the chapter.
2. Have students complete end-of-chapter exercises either in their book or on the MyNursingKit website.
3. Use the Classroom Response Questions provided in PowerPoint to assess students prior to lecture.

 MyNursingKit
(www.mynursingkit.com)

- Websites
- NCLEX® questions
- Critical Thinking Questions
- Case Studies
- Animations and Videos
- Drug Prototype Questions

 MyNursingLab
(www.mynursinglab.com)

- Knowledge Quick Check
- Pre/Posttests
- Customized study plans
- *Separate purchase*

 Student Workbook and Resource Guide

- Chapter 45 activities
- *Separate purchase*

Pearson Nurse's Drug Guide

- *Separate purchase*

 Pearson eText

- Students can search, highlight, take notes, and more all in electronic format.
- *Separate purchase*

 Classroom Response Question PowerPoints

 Testbank

CHAPTER 46
DRUGS FOR DISORDERS AND CONDITIONS OF THE MALE REPRODUCTIVE SYSTEM

LEARNING OUTCOME 1

Describe the roles of the hypothalamus, pituitary, and testes in regulating male reproductive functions.

Concepts for Lecture

Gonadatropin-releasing hormone (GRH) is released from the hypothalamus and stimulates the release of hormones from the pituitary. Follicle-stimulating hormone (FSH) regulates sperm production in men. Luteinizing hormone (LH) regulates the production of testosterone, an androgen secreted by the testes and the primary hormone contributing to the growth, health, and maintenance of the male reproductive system; testosterone is also responsible for maturation of the male sex organs and the secondary sex characteristics of men. Hormonal control of the male reproductive hormones is illustrated in Figure 46.1.

LEARNING OUTCOME 2

Identify indications for pharmacotherapy with androgens.

Concepts for Lecture

Androgens include testosterone and related hormones that control many aspects of male reproductive function. Therapeutically, they are used to treat hypogonadism and certain cancers. Primary hypogonadism is due to testicular failure, and secondary hypogonadism is due to lack of follicle-stimulating hormone (FSH) or luteinizing hormone (LH). Pharmacotherapy with androgens increases libido and corrects erectile dysfunction. (These agents are shown in Table 46.1.)

LEARNING OUTCOME 3

Describe the misuse and dangers associated with the use of anabolic steroids to enhance athletic performance.

Concepts for Lecture

Anabolic steroids are testosterone-like compounds. Androgens are classified as Schedule III drugs. They are frequently abused by athletes even though they are illegal. Anabolic steroids can result in serious adverse effects with long-term use. Adverse effects include increased

POWERPOINT SLIDES

Figure 46.1 Hormonal Control of the Male Reproductive Hormones

SUGGESTION FOR CLINICAL ACTIVITIES
- Invite a nurse from a clinic specializing in men's health to speak at postclinical.

SUGGESTION FOR CLASSROOM ACTIVITIES
- Direct students to draw a concept map of the male reproductive system and include hormonal control with the functions of the male hormones.

POWERPOINT SLIDES

Table 46.1 Selected Androgens
Table 46.2 Androgen Formulations

SUGGESTION FOR CLASSROOM ACTIVITIES
- Discuss how successful pharmacotherapy of hypogonadism can help a person's psychosocial sense of self.

SUGGESTION FOR CLINICAL ACTIVITIES
- Direct students to tour the pharmacy to observe the drugs used for disorders and conditions of the male reproductive system.

POWERPOINT SLIDES

SUGGESTION FOR CLASSROOM ACTIVITIES
- Discuss the use of steroids by athletes.

SUGGESTION FOR CLINICAL ACTIVITIES
- Invite a sports trainer to talk to the students at postclinical about use of anabolic steroids.

© 2011 Pearson Education, Inc.

cholesterol levels, low sperm count, impotence, menstrual irregularities and the appearance of male characteristics in women, aggression, and psychological dependence.

LEARNING OUTCOME 4

Explain the role of medications in the treatment of male infertility.

Concepts for Lecture

It is estimated that 30% to 40% of infertility among couples is caused by difficulties with the male's reproductive system. Drug therapy for male infertility is not as successful as fertility pharmacotherapy in women, because only about 5% of infertile males have an endocrine etiology for their disorder. Because of the expense of pharmacotherapy and the large number of injections needed, other means of conception may be explored, such as in vitro fertilization or intrauterine insemination. Medications used in the treatment of male infertility include human chorionic gonadotropin (HCG), which increases testosterone and sperm production; menotropin (Pergonal), which is a mixture of follicle-stimulating hormone (FSH) and luteinizing hormone (LH); testolactone, for those exhibiting hypogonadism; and antiestrogens (tamoxifen, clomiphene) to block the negative feedback of estrogen.

LEARNING OUTCOME 5

Describe the etiology, pathogenesis, and pharmacotherapy of erectile dysfunction.

Concepts for Lecture

Erectile dysfunction is a common disorder associated with vascular diseases; with medications, including thiazide diuretics, beta blockers, selective serotonin reuptake inhibitors (SSRIs), and antidepressants; and with psychogenic causes, such as depression, fatigue, guilt, and fear of failure. Pharmacotherapy for erectile dysfunction includes the use of phosphodiesterase-5 inhibitors. Sildenafil (Viagra) does not cause an erection; it enhances it. Vardenafil (Levitra) has a faster onset and slightly longer duration than Viagra. Tadalafil (Cialis) acts within 30 minutes and lasts from 24 to 36 hours. (See Table 46.2 for a list of medications used for erectile dysfunction.)

LEARNING OUTCOME 6

Describe the pathogenesis and pharmacotherapy of benign prostatic hyperplasia.

Concepts for Lecture

1. Benign prostatic hyperplasia (BPH) is enlargement of the prostate. It is the most common benign neoplasm in men. The pathogenesis of BPH involves two components: static and dynamic. It obstructs the urethra and decreases flow. BPH is not a precursor to cancer. Symptoms include increased urinary frequency, urgency, leakage, nocturia, decreased force, and incomplete emptying of the bladder. Aggravating

POWERPOINT SLIDES

SUGGESTION FOR CLASSROOM ACTIVITIES

- Direct students to create several multiple-choice exam questions from the material discussed regarding medications for male infertility.

SUGGESTION FOR CLINICAL ACTIVITIES

- Assign students to a clinical in a clinic that works with men on fertility issues.

POWERPOINT SLIDES

Table 46.3 Drugs for Erectile Dysfunction

SUGGESTION FOR CLASSROOM ACTIVITIES

- Discuss advertising by pharmaceutical companies regarding the drugs for erectile dysfunction.
- Discuss client compliance with medications that may cause erectile dysfunction.

SUGGESTION FOR CLINICAL ACTIVITIES

- Create and implement a teaching plan for clients taking medications for erectile dysfunction.

POWERPOINT SLIDES

Figure 46.2 Benign Prostatic Hyperplasia: (a) Normal Prostate with Penis; (b) Benign Prostatic Hyperplasia
Table 46.4 Drugs for Benign Prostatic Hyperplasia

factors include alpha-adrenergic agonists; anticholinergics; testosterone; and caffeine, alcohol, and fluids at bedtime. (See an illustration of benign prostatic hyperplasia in Figure 46.2.)

2. Pharmacotherapy of static components of BPH relates to anatomical enlargement, and with dynamic components it relates to excessive numbers of alpha-adrenergic receptors compressing the urethra. Severe disease requires surgery. Drug options include alpha$_1$-adrenergic blockers, such as doxazosin (Cardura), terazosin (Hytrin), tamsulosin (Flomax), and 5-alpha-reductase inhibitors such as finasteride (Proscar). (See Table 46.4.)

LEARNING OUTCOME 7

Describe the nurse's role in the pharmacologic management of disorders and conditions of the male reproductive system.

Concepts for Lecture

1. The role of the nurse in the pharmacologic management of disorders and conditions of the male reproductive system involves careful monitoring of a client's condition and providing education as it relates to the prescribed drug treatment. Obtain baseline medical, surgical, and drug history; lifestyle and dietary habits, including use of herbal or alternative therapies; and a detailed description of symptomology and current therapies.

2. **Androgen therapy for hypogonadism:** Ask questions regarding the possibility of impaired sexual functioning and diminished libido. Conduct a physical assessment for evidence of decreased hormone production, such as decreased or absent body hair, small testes, or delayed signs of puberty. This assessment should also include the client's emotional status. Monitor lab results, especially liver enzymes, if the client has a history of anabolic steroid use. Also monitor serum cholesterol, especially in clients with a history of myocardial infarction or angina, as the drug can increase this lab value. Contraindications to androgen therapy include prostatic or male breast cancer, renal disease, cardiac and liver dysfunction, hypercalcemia, benign prostatic hyperplasia (BPH), and hypertension. Androgens must be used cautiously in prepubertal men, older adults, and in men with acute intermittent porphyria. Some adverse reactions found to occur in women as a result of androgen use include deepening of the voice, facial hair growth, enlarged clitoris, and irregular menses.

3. **Pharmacotherapy in erectile dysfunction therapy:** Obtain a complete physical examination including history of impaired sexual function, cardiovascular disease, and presence of emotional disturbances. Also obtain and monitor results of lab tests related to liver function. Laboratory tests may include testosterone, prolactin, and thyroxin levels. If hormones are the cause of the dysfunction, treatment will be aimed at correcting the abnormality. A nocturnal penile tumescence and rigidity (NPTR) test may be ordered. A blood-flow test is also used to determine if there is sufficient arterial and venous flow to the penis. Sildenafil, vardenafil, and tadalafil are contraindicated with the use of organic nitrates such as nitroglycerin and with alpha-adrenergic blockers.

4. **Drug therapy with antiprostatic agents for BPH:** Assess changes in urinary elimination, such as urine retention, nocturia, dribbling,

SUGGESTION FOR CLASSROOM ACTIVITIES

- Direct students to do an online search of guidelines of care for benign prostatic hyperplasia (BPH) and to bring that information to class for a discussion.

SUGGESTION FOR CLINICAL ACTIVITIES

- Assign students to care for an immediate postop transurethral resection of the prostate (TURP) client.

POWERPOINT SLIDES

SUGGESTION FOR CLASSROOM ACTIVITIES

- Discuss the role of the nurse in the pharmacologic management of disorders and conditions of the male reproductive system.

SUGGESTION FOR CLINICAL ACTIVITIES

- Direct students to find and analyze the nursing interventions noted on the care plans of clients taking medications for disorders and conditions of the male reproductive system.

© 2011 Pearson Education, Inc.

difficulty starting urinary stream, frequency, and urgency. The client may experience hypotension (first-dose phenomenon) with the initial doses, and orthostatic hypotension may persist throughout treatment. Alpha-blockers should be used cautiously in clients with asthma or heart failure because they cause bradycardia and bronchoconstriction. Monitor the emotional status of clients taking alpha blockers because depression is a common side effect. Inform the client that it may take 6 to 12 months of treatment before the maximum benefit from the drug is achieved. Monitor for side effects, including impotence, decreased volume of ejaculate, or decreased libido.

LEARNING OUTCOME 8

For each of the drug classes listed in Drugs at a Glance, know representative drugs, and explain the mechanism of drug action, primary actions, and important adverse effects.

Concepts for Lecture

1. **Androgens.** Prototype drug: testosterone base (Andro). Mechanism of action: stimulates RNA synthesis and protein metabolism. Primary use: for treatment of hypogonadism in males. Adverse effects: viralization; salt and water are often retained, causing edema, and a diuretic may be indicated. Liver damage is rare, although it is a potentially serious adverse effect with some of the orally administered androgens. Acne and skin irritation is common during therapy.

2. **Agents for erectile dysfunction—phosphodiesterase-5 inhibitor.** Prototype drug: sildenafil (Viagra). Mechanism of action: relaxes smooth muscle in the corpus cavernosum by blocking the enzyme phosphodiesterase-5, thus allowing increased blood flow into the penis. Primary use: to treat erectile dysfunction by causing a firmer and longer-lasting erection. Adverse effects: The most serious effect is hypotension. Common side effects include headache, dizziness, flushing, rash, nasal congestion, diarrhea, dyspepsia, UTI, chest pain, and indigestion. Other effects are blurred vision or changes in color perception and priapism.

3. **Agents for benign prostatic hyperplasia—5-alpha-reductase inhibitor.** Prototype drug: finasteride (Proscar). Mechanism of action: inhibits 5-alpha-reductase. Primary use: to promote shrinkage of enlarged prostate and to subsequently help to restore urinary function; it is also prescribed to promote hair regrowth in clients with male-pattern baldness. Adverse effects: various types of sexual dysfunction in up to 16% of clients, including impotence, diminished libido, and ejaculatory dysfunction.

LEARNING OUTCOME 9

Use the nursing process to care for patients who are receiving drug therapy for disorders and conditions of the male reproductive system.

Concepts for Lecture

1. **Patients receiving androgen therapy—Assessment:** Obtain a complete health history, including cardiovascular, peripheral vascular, thyroid, hepatic or renal disease, diabetes, prostatic hypertrophy, or prostatic or breast cancer. Obtain a drug history including allergies, possible drug interactions. Evaluate appropriate laboratory findings (e.g., CBC, electrolytes, glucose, lipid levels, PSA). Obtain baseline height, weight, and vital signs. Assess for adverse effects.

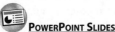
POWERPOINT SLIDES

Prototype Drug
- testosterone base (Andro)
- sildenafil (Viagra)
- finasteride (Proscar)

ANIMATIONS AND VIDEOS
- Mechanism in Action: Sildenafil (Viagra)

SUGGESTION FOR CLASSROOM ACTIVITIES
- Have each student make drug cards for each classification of drug used to treat disorders and conditions of the male reproductive system. Use two different drugs for each classification. The card should include actions, uses, routes of administration, dosages, and adverse effects.

SUGGESTION FOR CLINICAL ACTIVITIES
- Divide students into small groups, and have each group develop a teaching plan for a patient receiving medications for disorders and conditions of the male reproductive system.

POWERPOINT SLIDES

SUGGESTION FOR CLASSROOM ACTIVITIES
- Direct students to create a *Jeopardy*-like game using the classifications of drugs used to treat disorders and conditions of the male reproductive system.

2. **Patients receiving androgen therapy—Nursing diagnoses:** *Disturbed Body Image* related to related to drug effects, aging process; *Sexual Dysfunction* related to drug effects; *Fluid Volume Excess* related to adverse drug effects; *Deficient Knowledge* (drug therapy).

3. **Patients receiving androgen therapy—Planning:** The client will experience therapeutic effects (e.g., normal virility and development of secondary sex characteristics continues) and will be free from or experience minimal adverse effects. Verbalize an understanding of the drug's use, adverse effects, and required precautions. Demonstrate proper self-administration of the medication (e.g., dose, timing, when to notify provider).

4. **Patients receiving androgen therapy—Implementation:** Monitor appropriate medication administration for optimum results. Monitor blood pressure at each clinical visit. Check weight and for presence of edema. Monitor electrolytes, lipid levels, and hepatic function labs periodically. Monitor blood-glucose levels in diabetic patients more frequently. Monitor height and growth in children and adolescents. Monitor use in adolescent patients. Instruct patient or caregiver in proper self-administration of drug. Monitor serum cholesterol levels.

5. **Patients receiving androgen therapy—Evaluation:** The client will experience normal virility and development of secondary sex characteristics continues. is the client will be free from or experience minimal adverse effects. Verbalize an understanding of the drug's use, adverse effects, and required precautions. Demonstrate proper self-administration of the medication (e.g., dose, timing, when to notify provider).

6. **Patients receiving treatment for erectile dysfunction—Assessment:** Obtain a complete health history including cardiovascular, peripheral vascular, thyroid, hepatic or renal disease, diabetes, prostatic hypertrophy. Obtain a drug history including allergies, any antihypertensives, and any possible drug interactions. Evaluate appropriate laboratory findings (e.g., CBC, electrolytes, glucose, lipid levels, PSA). Obtain baseline vital signs, especially blood pressure. Assess for adverse effects.

7. **Patients receiving treatment for erectile dysfunction—Nursing diagnoses:** *Sexual Dysfunction; Disturbed Body Image; Deficient Knowledge* (drug therapy); *Risk for Injury* related to adverse drug effects.

8. **Patients Receiving Treatment for Erectile Dysfunction—Planning:** The client will experience therapeutic effects (e.g., ability to achieve and maintain an erection) and will be free from or experience minimal adverse effects. Verbalize an understanding of the drug's use, adverse effects and required precautions. Demonstrate proper self-administration of the medication (e.g., dose, timing, when to notify provider).

9. **Patients Receiving Treatment for Erectile Dysfunction—Implementation:** Monitor appropriate medication administration for optimum results. Monitor blood pressure at each clinical visit. Report any BP below 90/60. Assess for concurrent use of nitrates or antihypertensives and review any new prescription. Monitor for changes in vision, including blurred vision, changes in the ability to sense colors, especially blue or green, and for any sudden eye pain or lights or flashes in eyes. Monitor for the development of priapism and report occurrence. Monitor use in adolescent patients. Instruct patient or caregiver in proper self-administration of drug.

10. **Patients Receiving Treatment for Erectile Dysfunction—Evaluation:** The client will experience ability to achieve and maintain an erection. The client will be free from or experience minimal adverse effects. Verbalize an understanding of the drug's use, adverse effects,

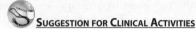

SUGGESTION FOR CLINICAL ACTIVITIES

- Direct students to implement a teaching plan for clients with a disorder or condition of the male reproductive system.

© 2011 Pearson Education, Inc.

and required precautions. Demonstrate proper self-administration of the medication (e.g., dose, timing, when to notify provider).

GENERAL CHAPTER CONSIDERATIONS

1. Have students study and learn key terms listed at the beginning of the chapter.
2. Have students complete end-of-chapter exercises either in their book or on the MyNursingKit website.
3. Use the Classroom Response Questions provided in PowerPoint to assess students prior to lecture.

MYNURSINGKIT
(www.mynursingkit.com)

- Websites
- NCLEX® questions
- Critical Thinking Questions
- Case Studies
- Animations and Videos
- Drug Prototype Questions

MYNURSINGLAB
(www.mynursinglab.com)

- Knowledge Quick Check
- Pre/Posttests
- Customized study plans
- *Separate purchase*

NURSING PROCESS FOCUS

- Clients receiving androgen therapy
- Clients receiving finasteride

PEARSON NURSE'S DRUG GUIDE

- *Separate purchase*

STUDENT WORKBOOK AND RESOURCE GUIDE

- Chapter 46 activities
- *Separate purchase*

PEARSON ETEXT

- Students can search, highlight, take notes, and more all in electronic format.
- *Separate purchase*

CLASSROOM RESPONSE QUESTION POWERPOINTS

TESTBANK

© 2011 Pearson Education, Inc.

CHAPTER 47
DRUGS FOR BONE AND JOINT DISORDERS

LEARNING OUTCOME 1

Describe the role of calcium in the body in maintaining homeostasis in the nervous, muscular, and cardiovascular systems.

Concepts for Lecture

Calcium is the primary mineral responsible for bone formation and for maintaining bone health throughout the lifespan. Adequate levels of calcium in the body are necessary to properly transmit nerve impulses, prevent muscle spasms, and provide stability and movement. This major mineral constitutes about 2% of our body weight and is also critical to proper functioning of the nervous, muscular, and cardiovascular systems. To maintain homeostasis, calcium balance in the body is regulated by parathyroid hormone (PTH), calcitonin, and vitamin D, as shown in Figure 47.1. Calcium ion influences the excitability of all neurons. When calcium concentrations are too high (hypercalcemia), sodium permeability decreases across cell membranes. This is a dangerous state, because nerve conduction depends on the proper influx of sodium into cells. When calcium levels in the bloodstream are too low (hypocalcemia), cell membranes become hyperexcitable. If this situation becomes severe, convulsions or muscle spasms may result. Calcium is also important for the normal functioning of other body processes such as blood coagulation and muscle contraction. It is, indeed, a critical mineral for life.

LEARNING OUTCOME 2

Identify the recommended dietary allowance and the normal serum levels of calcium.

Concepts for Lecture

Recommended dietary allowance (RDA) of calcium for adults is 800 to 1200 mg/day. Pregnant women, growing children, and menopausal women require increased amounts of calcium. Normal serum calcium range is 4.5 to 5.5 mEqL or 8.5 to 10.mg/dL. Serum calcium levels exceeding 5.5 mEq/L result in hypercalcemia. Hypocalcemia results from serum calcium levels below 4.5 mEq/L.

LEARNING OUTCOME 3

Explain the roles of parathyroid hormone, calcitonin, and vitamin D in maintaining calcium balance.

Concepts for Lecture

1. Adequate levels of calcium in the body are necessary to properly transmit nerve impulses, prevent muscle spasms, and provide stability and

PowerPoint Slides

Suggestion for Classroom Activities
- Discuss the role of calcium in maintaining homeostasis.

Suggestion for Clinical Activities
- Direct students to conduct an interview of a patient with a disorder related to calcium imbalance.

PowerPoint Slides

Suggestion for Classroom Activities
- Have students make a table of RDA and serum levels for other nutrients.

Suggestion for Clinical Activities
- Assign students to work with the dietician to learn about RDA requirements for patients with bone and joint disorders.

PowerPoint Slides

Figure 47.1 PTH and Calcitonin Action
Figure 47.2 Pathway for Vitamin D Activation and Action

© 2011 Pearson Education, Inc.

movement. Adequate levels of vitamin D, parathyroid hormone, and calcitonin are also necessary for these functions. Control of calcium by the endocrine system begins in the parathyroid, which secretes parathyroid hormone (PTH). PTH stimulates osteoclasts and accelerates bone resorption, which causes breakdown of the bone, and the calcium increases in the blood. The thyroid secretes calcitonin, which stimulates bone deposition and builds up the bone. This removes calcium from the blood. (Figure 47.1 shows PTH and Calcitonin Action.) Together PTH and calcitonin control calcium homeostasis; they influence three targets: bones, kidneys, and gastrointestinal tract. Calcium is also important for blood coagulation and myocardial activity. Vitamin D is necessary for effective absorption of calcium. It is synthesized from precursor molecules and introduced in two ways: Cholecalciferol in the skin is activated by sunlight (UV light), and cholecalciferol is also obtained in the gastrointestinal tract from dairy products and fortified foods. First, cholecalciferol is converted to an intermediate form, calcifediol. Then it is metabolized to calcitriol (the active form of vitamin D). (Figure 47.2 shows the pathway for Vitamin D.)

2. Hypercalcemia causes a decrease in sodium permeability across the cell membrane, which is dangerous for the nervous system. Hypocalcemia causes cell membranes to become excitable. It may produce convulsions or tetany.

LEARNING OUTCOME 4

Explain the pharmacotherapy of hypocalcemia, osteomalacia, osteoporosis, rickets, osteoarthritis, rheumatoid arthritis, and gout.

Concepts for Lecture

1. Hypocalcemia is not a disease but a sign of underlying pathology; therefore, diagnosis of the cause of hypocalcemia is essential. Many factors can cause hypocalcemia. Lack of sufficient dietary calcium and/or vitamin D is a common cause, and one that can be easily reversed by nutritional therapy. If hypocalcemia occurs with normal dietary intake, GI causes must be examined, such as excessive vomiting or malabsorption disorders. Chronic kidney disease may cause excessive loss of calcium in the urine. Another etiology for hypocalcemia is decreased secretion of PTH, as occurs when the thyroid and parathyroid glands are diseased or surgically removed. Drug therapy is occasionally a cause of hypocalcemia. Blood transfusions and certain anticonvulsants such as phenytoin can lower serum calcium levels. In addition, overtreatment with drugs used to *lower* serum calcium can result in "overshooting" normal levels. Some of these include furosemide (Lasix), phosphate therapy, or bisphosphonates (see Section 47.4). Of special concern is long-term therapy with corticosteroids, which is a very common cause of hypocalcemia and osteoporosis. To help prevent corticosteroid-induced osteoporosis, patients should receive daily supplements of calcium and vitamin D. Signs and symptoms of hypocalcemia are those of nerve and muscle excitability. Assessment may reveal muscle twitching, tremor, or abdominal cramping with hyperactive bowel sounds. Numbness and tingling of the extremities may occur, and convulsions are possible. Confusion and abnormal behavior may be observed.

2. **Pharmacotherapy of hypocalcemia:** Unless the hypocalcemia is life threatening, adjustments in diet should be attempted prior to initiating therapy with calcium supplements. Increasing the consumption of calcium-rich foods, especially dairy products, fortified orange juice, cereals, and green leafy vegetables is often sufficient to restore calcium

- Direct students to create concept maps showing the relationships between calcium, vitamin D, parathyroid hormone, and calcitonin.
- Discuss the role of the nurse in the pharmacologic management of disorders caused by calcium and vitamin D deficiencies.

SUGGESTIONS FOR CLINICAL ACTIVITIES

- Assign students to care for clients who are receiving calcium supplements.
- Direct students to study the liver-function tests and calcium, magnesium, and phosphate levels found in the lab area of the clients' charts.

POWERPOINT SLIDES

Figure 47.3 Calcium Metabolism in Osteoporosis
Figure 47.4 Client with Osteoarthritis
Figure 47.5 Client with Rheumatoid Arthritis
Table 47.1 Selected Calcium Salts and Vitamin D Therapy
Table 47.2 Selected Drugs for Osteoporosis and other Bone Disorders
Table 47.3 Selected Disease-modifying Antirheumatic Drugs (DMARDs)
Table 47.4 Drugs for Gout

SUGGESTIONS FOR CLASSROOM ACTIVITIES

- Direct students to develop a table showing pharmacotherapy for disorders related to bones and joints.
- Provide pictures or models of muscle, bone, and joint disorders for students to view.

SUGGESTION FOR CLINICAL ACTIVITIES

- Direct students to do an admission assessment on clients with bone or joint disorders.

balance. If a change in diet is not practical or has not proved adequate for reversing the hypocalcemia, effective and inexpensive calcium supplements are readily available over the counter (OTC) in a variety of formulations. Calcium supplements often contain vitamin D. Severe hypocalcemia requires the intravenous (IV) administration of calcium salts. (Table 47.1 lists calcium supplements.)

3. Osteoporosis is the most common metabolic bone disease; it is responsible for 1.5 million fractures per year. Osteoporosis is related to bone deterioration; bone resorption outpaces bone deposition. Etiology is related to lack of dietary calcium and vitamin D and disrupted bone homeostasis. (See Figure 47.3 for an illustration of Calcium Metabolism in Osteoporosis.) The most common risk factor for osteoporosis is the onset of menopause. Other risk factors include high alcohol or caffeine consumption, anorexia nervosa, tobacco use, physical inactivity, testosterone deficiency, and lack of vitamin D or calcium. Drugs that lower calcium in the blood include corticosteroids, anticonvulsants, and immunosuppressants.

4. Pharmacotherapy of osteoporosis includes calcium supplements and vitamin D, bisphosphonates, selective estrogen receptor modulators (SERMs), calcitonin, hormone replacement therapy (HRT), slow-release sodium fluoride, and parathyroid hormone (PTH) analog. Bisphosphonates are the most common treatment; they block bone resorption by inhibiting osteoclast activity. Adverse effects are usually gastrointestinal problems. However, they are recommended to be taken on an empty stomach as tolerated. Once-weekly dosing is effective because of their extended duration of action. Selective estrogen receptor modulators (SERMs) decrease bone resorption and increase bone density. They bind to estrogen receptors and may be either estrogen agonists or antagonists, depending on the drug or tissue involved. Calcitonin is approved for osteoporosis in women who are more than 5 years postmenopause. It increases bone density and reduces the risk of vertebral fractures. Calcitonin is available as a nasal spray or in injectable form. It is also indicated for Paget's disease and hypercalcemia. Hormone replacement therapy (HRT) is no longer used for osteoporosis. Until recently, HRT was a common treatment for osteoporosis; however, recent research shows increased risks of uterine cancer, thromboembolic disease, breast cancer, and other chronic disorders with use of hormone replacement therapy. (See Table 47.2 for a list of drugs used in the pharmacotherapy of osteoporosis.)

5. Osteomalacia is a MBD characterized by softening of bones due to demineralization. Worldwide, the most frequent cause of osteomalacia is a deficiency of vitamin D and calcium in the diet. This risk factor for the disease, however, is rare in the United States because many processed foods in this country are fortified with these vitamins. In the United States, osteomalacia is most prevalent in the elderly, in premature infants, and in individuals on strict vegetarian diets. The term *osteomalacia* is usually used for adults with this MBD; if it occurs in children, it is called rickets. Signs and symptoms of osteomalacia include hypocalcemia, muscle weakness, muscle spasms, and diffuse bone pain, especially in the hip area. Patients may also experience pain in the arms, legs, and spine. Classic signs of rickets in children include bowlegs and a pigeon breast. Children may also develop a slight fever and become restless at night. In extreme cases, surgical correction of disfigured limbs may be required.

6. **Pharmacotherapy of osteomalacia:** Drug therapy for children and adults consists of calcium supplements and vitamin D. Drugs used for these conditions are summarized in Table 47.1. Calcitriol reduces bone resorption and is useful in treating rickets. The effectiveness of calcitriol depends on an adequate amount of calcium; therefore, it is

© 2011 Pearson Education, Inc.

usually prescribed in combination with calcium supplements. It is available as oral tablets and solutions, and by the IV route.

7. Osteoarthritis is a degenerative, age-onset disease characterized by wearing away of cartilage at articular joint surfaces. Symptoms include muscle spasms, localized pain and stiffness, joint and bone enlargement. The etiology is poorly understood, though it is thought to be due to excessive wear of weight-bearing joints (hip, knee, and spine). (See Figure 47.4 for an illustration of a client with osteoarthritis.)

8. The goal in the pharmacotherapy of osteoarthritis is reduction of pain and inflammation. Medications used are topical medications such as capsaicin cream, nonsteroidal anti-inflammatory drugs (NSAIDs), aspirin, acetaminophen, COX-2 inhibitors, tramadol (Ultram), intra-articular glucocorticoids, and sodium hyaluronate (Hyalgan) injections into the joint.

9. Rheumatoid arthritis is a systemic autoimmune disorder, characterized by inflammation of multiple joints. Autoantibodies (rheumatoid factors) activate inflammatory response in joints. Other extra-articular systemic manifestations may develop, such as infections, pulmonary disease, pericarditis, blood abnormalities, and metabolic dysfunction. See Figure 47.5 for an illustration of a client with rheumatoid arthritis.

10. Pharmacotherapy for rheumatoid arthritis includes the same classes of drug used for osteoarthritis. Additional drugs are used for severe inflammation and immune aspects; they include glucocorticoids, disease-modifying antirheumatic drugs, and immunosuppressants. Several months may be needed before therapeutic results are achieved. (See Table 47.3 for a list of drugs used for rheumatoid arthritis.)

11. Gout is a form of acute arthritis caused by an accumulation of uric acid (urate) crystals in the joints and other body tissues, causing inflammation. Primary gout is caused by a hereditary defect in uric acid metabolism that causes uric acid to be produced faster than it can be excreted by the kidneys. *Secondary gout* is caused by diseases or drugs that increase the metabolic turnover of nucleic acids, or that interfere with uric acid excretion. Examples of drugs that may cause gout include thiazide diuretics, aspirin, cyclosporine, and alcohol, when ingested on a chronic basis. Conditions that can cause secondary gout include diabetic ketoacidosis, kidney failure, and diseases associated with a rapid cell turnover such as leukemia, hemolytic anemia, and polycythemia. Symptoms of acute attacks include red, swollen tissue, often in the big toes, ankles, fingers, wrists, knees, and elbows. Attacks are triggered by diet, injury, or other stress and often occur at night.

12. Goals of the pharmacotherapy of gout are termination of acute attacks and prevention of future attacks. Medications include NSAIDs, such as indomethacin (Indocin), for pain and inflammation. Uric acid–inhibiting drugs are used to block accumulation of uric acid in the blood and uric acid crystals in the joints. Prophylactic therapy of gout includes drugs that lower serum uric acid. Prophylactic therapy is used for patients who suffer frequent and acute gout attacks. Combination therapy using uric acid inhibitors such as colchicine and antigout medications like probenecid (Benemid) and allopurinol (Zyloprim) are the mainstay of gout prophylaxis. Colchicine reduces the accumulation of uric acid in the blood or uric acid crystals within the joints. Probenecid increases the excretion of uric acid by blocking its reabsorption in the kidney. Allopurinol blocks xanthine oxidase, thus inhibiting the formation of uric acid. When uric acid accumulation is blocked, symptoms associated with gout diminish. (Drugs for gout are listed in Table 47.4.)

13. Glucocorticoids may be used to treat exacerbations of acute gout, particularly when the symptoms are in a single joint, and the medication can be delivered intra-articularly.

LEARNING OUTCOME 5

Describe the nurse's role in the pharmacologic management of disorders related to bones and joints.

Concepts for Lecture

1. The role of the nurse in the pharmacologic management of disorders related to bones and joints involves careful monitoring of a client's condition and providing education as it relates to the prescribed drug treatment. Obtain baseline medical, surgical, and drug history; lifestyle and dietary habits, including use of herbal or alternative therapies; and a detailed description of symptomology and current therapies.

2. **The role of the nurse in bisphosphonate drug therapy:** Obtain a thorough history to determine risk factors, past medical history (especially a history of fractures), GI problems, and current medications and supplements. Clients with preexisting vitamin D deficiency or hypocalcemia should be placed on supplements and these conditions corrected prior to initiating bisphosphonate therapy. A complete physical examination should include complete blood count (CBC), pH, chemistry panel, renal- and liver-function studies, vital signs, and bone density studies such as a dual x-ray absorptiometry (DXA scan) to establish baseline data.

3. **The role of the nurse in calcium-supplement therapy:** Assess for signs and symptoms of hypercalcemia, such as drowsiness, lethargy, weakness, headache, anorexia, nausea, vomiting, thirst, and increased urination. Signs and symptoms to assess for hypocalcemia are facial twitching, muscle spasms, paresthesias, and seizures. Obtain baseline and periodic vital signs, labs, and ECG to determine the effectiveness of the medication. A history of fracture should be investigated. Calcium supplements are contraindicated in clients with a history of renal calculi, digoxin toxicity, dysrhythmias, or hypercalcemia.

4. **The role of the nurse in vitamin D therapy:** Obtain a thorough history to assess liver function, intake of fat-soluble vitamins, and current medications. Liver impairment and an accumulation of fat-soluble vitamins may cause toxicity. Assess sclera, skin pigment, and bowel movements. Monitor liver function tests, calcium, magnesium, and phosphate levels; and urinary calcium and phosphate levels during vitamin D therapy. Emphasize the importance of including extra dietary vitamin D in children and pregnant women.

5. **The role of the nurse in drug therapy with antigout medications** involves careful monitoring of a client's condition and providing education as it relates to the prescribed drug treatment. Obtain a thorough history, including current medications, vital signs, and a complete physical examination. The client should have the following lab studies: CBC, platelets, liver- and renal-function studies, uric acid levels, and urinalysis.

LEARNING OUTCOME 6

For each of the drug classes listed in Drugs at a Glance, know representative drugs and explain their mechanisms of action, primary actions, and important adverse effects.

Concepts for Lecture

1. **Calcium salts:** Prototype drug: calcium gluconate (Kalcinate). Mechanism of action: to return serum calcium levels to normal. Primary use: to correct hypocalcemia and for osteoporosis and Paget's disease. Adverse effects: hypercalcemia. Symptoms include drowsiness, lethargy, weakness,

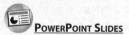

POWERPOINT SLIDES

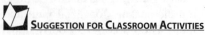

SUGGESTION FOR CLASSROOM ACTIVITIES

- Discuss the role of the nurse in the pharmacologic management of disorders related to bones and joints.

SUGGESTION FOR CLINICAL ACTIVITIES

- Assign students to care for patients receiving pharmacotherapy of disorders related to bones and joints.

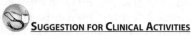

POWERPOINT SLIDES

Prototype Drug
- calcium salts
- calcitriol (Rocaltrol)
- alendronate (Fosamax)
- raloxifene (Evista)
- hydroxychloroquine sulfate (Plaquenil)
- colchicine

© 2011 Pearson Education, Inc.

headache, anorexia, nausea and vomiting, increased urination, and thirst. IV administration of calcium may cause hypotension, bradycardia, dysrhythmias, and cardiac arrest.

2. **Vitamin D therapy:** Prototype drug: calcitriol (Rocaltrol). Mechanism of action: as the active form of vitamin D. It promotes the intestinal absorption of calcium, reduces bone resorption, and elevates serum levels of calcium. Primary use: to treat impaired kidney function or hypoparathyroidism. It is also useful in treating rickets. Adverse effects: hypercalcemia, headache, weakness, dry mouth, thirst, increased urination, and muscle or bone pain.

3. **Bisphosphonates:** Prototype drug: etidronate disodium (Didronel). Mechanism of action: strengthens bones by slowing bone resorption. Primary use: for Paget's disease and to treat hypercalcemia due to malignancy. Adverse effects: diarrhea, nausea, vomiting, GI irritation, and a metallic- or altered-taste perception. Pathologic fractures may occur if the drug is taken longer than 3 months or in cases of chronic overdose. High IV doses can cause nephrotoxicity, though this is rare.

4. **Selective estrogen receptor modulators (SERMs):** Prototype drug: raloxifene (Evista). Mechanism of action: decreases bone resorption and increases bone mass and density by acting through the estrogen receptor. Primary use: for the prevention of osteoporosis in postmenopausal women. Adverse effects: hot flashes, migraine headache, flulike symptoms, endometrial disorder, breast pain, and vaginal bleeding. Raloxifene may cause fetal harm when administered to a pregnant woman.

5. **Disease-modifying antirheumatic drugs:** Prototype drug: hydroxychloroquine sulfate (Plaquenil). Mechanism of action: This drug relieves the severe inflammation characteristic of these disorders, although its mechanism of action is not known. Primary use: for rheumatoid arthritis and lupus erythematosus in clients who have not responded well to other anti-inflammatory drugs. Adverse effects: anorexia, GI disturbances, loss of hair, possible ocular effects, headache, and mood and mental changes.

6. **Uric acid inhibitor:** Prototype drugs: colchicine. Mechanism of action: inhibits the synthesis of microtubules, subcellular structures responsible for helping white blood cells infiltrate an area. Primary use: to reduce inflammation associated with acute gouty arthritis. Adverse effects: Nausea, vomiting, diarrhea, and GI upset are more likely to occur at the beginning of therapy. The drug may cause bone marrow toxicity, aplastic anemia, leucopenia, thrombocytopenia, or agranulocytosis. Colchicine may also directly interfere with the absorption of vitamin B_{12}.

Learning Outcome 7

Use the nursing process to care for patients receiving drug therapy for bone and joint disorders.

Concepts for Lecture

1. **Patients receiving pharmacotherapy for osteoporosis and other bone disorders—Assessment:** Obtain a complete health history including musculoskeletal, gastrointestinal, cardiovascular, neurologic, endocrine, hepatic, or renal disease. Obtain a drug history including allergies, signs of hypercalcemia or hypocalcemia, and possible drug interactions. Assess muscle strength, gait, and note any pain or discomfort on movement or at rest. Obtain bone density studies if ordered. Obtain a dietary history noting adequacy of essential vitamins, minerals, and nutrients obtained through food sources, particularly Ca,

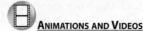

ANIMATIONS AND VIDEOS

- Mechanism in Action: Calcitriol (Galcijet, Racaltrol)

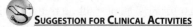

SUGGESTION FOR CLASSROOM ACTIVITIES

- Have each student make drug cards for each classification of drug used for disorders of bones and joints. The card should include actions, uses, routes of administration, dosages, and adverse effects.

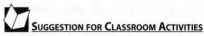

SUGGESTION FOR CLINICAL ACTIVITIES

- Divide students into small groups and have each group develop a teaching plan for a patient receiving pharmacologic management of disorders related to bones and joints.

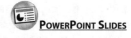

POWERPOINT SLIDES

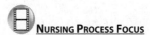

NURSING PROCESS FOCUS

- Clients receiving calcium supplements
- Clients receiving bisphosphonates
- Clients receiving colchicine

vitamin D, and Mg. Note amount of soda intake daily. Note sunscreen use and amount of sun exposure. Obtain baseline height, weight, and vital signs. Evaluate appropriate laboratory findings (e.g., CBC, electrolytes, calcium, phosphorus, and magnesium levels, hepatic and renal function studies).

2. **Patients receiving pharmacotherapy for osteoporosis and other bone disorders—Nursing diagnoses:** *Acute or Chronic Pain* (bone or joints), related to disease condition; *Deficient Knowledge* (drug therapy); *Risk for Injury, Risk for Falls* related to disease condition, adverse drug effects.

3. **Patients receiving pharmacotherapy for osteoporosis and other bone disorders—Planning:** The client will experience therapeutic effects (e.g., maintenance of adequate bone density, lessened fracture risk) and will be free from or experience minimal adverse effects. Verbalize an understanding of the drug's use, adverse effects, and required precautions. Demonstrate proper self-administration of the medication (e.g., dose, timing, when to notify provider).

4. **Patients receiving pharmacotherapy for osteoporosis and other bone disorders—Implementation:** Review the dietary history with the patient and discuss food source options for correcting any deficiencies, particularly calcium and vitamin D intake. Encourage the patient to adopt a healthy lifestyle of increased physical activity, adequate sun exposure, limited caffeine and soda intake, and limited or eliminated alcohol consumption. Monitor for GI irritation or abdominal pain. Monitor periodic lab work, especially Ca, Mg, phosphorus levels, and creatinine as needed. Assess for signs or symptoms of hypocalcemia or hypercalcemia. Increase fluid intake, avoiding caffeine or soda. Monitor compliance with recommended regimen. Instruct the patient and/or family in proper self-administration of drug.

5. **Patients receiving pharmacotherapy for osteoporosis and other bone disorders—Evaluation:** Experiences maintenance of adequate bone density, lessened fracture risk. Is free from or experiences minimal adverse effects. Verbalizes an understanding of the drug's use, adverse effects, and required precautions. Demonstrates proper self-administration of the medication (e.g., dose, timing, when to notify provider).

6. **Patients receiving anti-gout therapy—Assessment:** Obtain a complete health history including musculoskeletal, gastrointestinal, cardiovascular, neurologic, endocrine, hepatic, or renal disease. Obtain a drug history including allergies and possible drug interactions. Assess for inflammation, location, and note any pain or discomfort on movement or at rest. Obtain a dietary history, noting correlations between food intake, and increase in symptoms. Assess fluid intake. Obtain baseline weight and vital signs. Evaluate appropriate laboratory findings (e.g., uric acid level, CBC, hepatic and renal function studies, urinalysis). Assess for and promptly report adverse effects.

7. **Patients receiving anti-gout therapy—Nursing diagnoses:** *Acute Pain* related to acute stage of disease; *Activity Intolerance* related to joint pain; *Disturbed Body Image* related to joint inflammation and swelling; *Deficient Knowledge* (drug therapy); *Risk for Injury* related to acute inflammatory condition.

8. **Patients receiving anti-gout therapy—Planning:** The client will experience therapeutic effects (e.g., diminished inflammation, decreased or absent joint pain, increased ability to continue ADLs) and will be free from or experience minimal adverse effects. Verbalize an understanding of the drug's use, adverse effects and required precautions. Demonstrate proper self-administration of the medication (e.g., dose, timing, when to notify provider).

9. **Patients receiving anti-gout therapy—Implementation:** Review the dietary history, noting any correlation between diet and symptoms,

SUGGESTION FOR CLASSROOM ACTIVITIES

- Divide students into small groups, and have them prepare questions and answers for different categories of drugs used to treat disorders of bones and joints. Include questions on each drug's classification and mechanisms of action.

SUGGESTION FOR CLINICAL ACTIVITIES

- Direct students to implement a teaching plan for clients with disorders of bones and joints.

© 2011 Pearson Education, Inc.

especially after ingestion of purine-containing foods. Increase fluid intake to 2 to 4 liters per day. Monitor urine output and obtain periodic urinalysis. Monitor serum and urinary uric acid levels and symptoms associated with acute inflammatory period. Monitor daily weight and urinary output. Observe for skin rashes, fever, stomatitis, flulike symptoms, or general malaise. Instruct patient and/or family in proper self-administration of drug. Monitor lab results throughout therapy, and perform Coombs test for hemolytic anemia. Monitor for signs of toxicity. Monitor for signs of renal impairment, such as oliguria. Record intake and output. Ensure that medication is administered correctly. Monitor for pain and mobility.

10. **Patients receiving anti-gout therapy—Evaluation:** The client will experience diminished inflammation, decreased or absent joint pain, increased ability to continue ADLs) and be free from or experience minimal adverse effects. Verbalize an understanding of the drug's use, adverse effects, and required precautions. Demonstrate proper self-administration of the medication (e.g., dose, timing, when to notify provider).

GENERAL CHAPTER CONSIDERATIONS

1. Have students study and learn key terms listed at the beginning of the chapter.
2. Have students complete end-of-chapter exercises either in their book or on the MyNursingKit website.
3. Use the Classroom Response Questions provided in PowerPoint to assess students prior to lecture.

**MYNURSINGKIT
(www.mynursingkit.com)**

- Websites
- NCLEX® questions
- Critical Thinking Questions
- Case Studies
- Animations and Videos
- Drug Prototype Questions

**MYNURSINGLAB
(www.mynursinglab.com)**

- Knowledge Quick Check
- Pre/Posttests
- Customized study plans
- *Separate purchase*

STUDENT WORKBOOK AND RESOURCE GUIDE

- Chapter 47 activities
- *Separate purchase*

PEARSON NURSE'S DRUG GUIDE

- *Separate purchase*

PEARSON eTEXT

- Students can search, highlight, take notes, and more all in electronic format.
- *Separate purchase*

CLASSROOM RESPONSE QUESTION POWERPOINTS

TESTBANK

© 2011 Pearson Education, Inc.

CHAPTER 48
DRUGS FOR SKIN DISORDERS

LEARNING OUTCOME 1

Identify the structure and functions of the skin layers and associated structures.

Concepts for Lecture

1. The three layers of skin are the epidermis, dermis, and subcutaneous. The epidermis is the outermost layer and makes up 5% of the total skin thickness. There are five layers of epidermis. The stratum corneum is the outermost, strongest layer; it contains a large amount of keratin, which forms a barrier that repels bacteria and foreign matter. It is thickest in high-stress areas, such as the soles of the feet and the palms of the hands. The middle layers (innermost to outermost) include the stratum spinosum, stratum granulosum, and stratum lucidum. The stratum basale is the deepest layer and supplies new cells to the epidermis. Melanocytes are found in the deeper layers. They secrete the dark pigment melanin, which helps protect the skin from ultraviolet rays.
2. The dermis is the second layer of the skin and makes up 95% of the total skin thickness. It provides a foundation for hair and nails. Nerve endings, oil glands, sweat glands, and blood vessels are found in the dermis.
3. The subcutaneous or third layer of the skin is made of adipose tissue, which cushions, insulates, and provides a source of energy. It is not considered in the skin thickness but rather as a separate entity.

LEARNING OUTCOME 2

Explain the process by which superficial skin cells are replaced.

Concepts for Lecture

Skin cells are supplied by the stratum basale, which is the deepest epidermal layer. Old cells are damaged or lost by normal wear. New cells migrate up through the layers. As these cells are pushed to the surface, they are flattened and covered with a water-insoluble material, forming a protective seal. It takes 3 weeks for a new cell to reach the body surface. Pigment in the skin is determined by the amount of melanin, which also protects the skin from the ultraviolet in sunlight.

LEARNING OUTCOME 3

Describe drug therapies for skin infections, mite and lice infestations, acne vulgaris, rosacea, dermatitis, and psoriasis.

Concepts for Lecture

1. Skin disorders are difficult to classify. One simple method is to group them into the following general categories: infectious, inflammatory,

POWERPOINT SLIDES

SUGGESTION FOR CLASSROOM ACTIVITIES

- Provide pictures or models of the skin layers for students to view.

SUGGESTION FOR CLINICAL ACTIVITIES

- Direct students to do a complete skin assessment on their client this week in clinical.

POWERPOINT SLIDES

SUGGESTION FOR CLASSROOM ACTIVITIES

- Discuss how melanin protects the skin from ultraviolet rays and how sunblock can aid in that protection.

SUGGESTION FOR CLINICAL ACTIVITIES

- Assign students to a clinical in a dermatology clinic.

POWERPOINT SLIDES

© 2011 Pearson Education, Inc.

and neoplastic. (A summary of these disorders is given in Table 48.1.) Dermatologic signs and symptoms may be reflective of disease processes occurring elsewhere in the body. Skin abnormalities, including color, sizes, types, and character of surface lesions, and skin turgor and moisture may have potential systemic causes. (The relationship between the integumentary system and other body systems is depicted in Figure 48.1.)

2. Bacterial infections occur when there is a break in the skin's defenses. The two most common bacterial infections are staphylococcus and streptococcus. Many are mild and self-limiting or can be treated with topical antibiotics. Serious skin infections are those that are deep or systemic and require oral or parenteral antibiotics.

3. Fungal infections occur in warm, moist areas of skin. Tinea pedis (athlete's foot), tinea cruris (jock itch), tinea capitis (ringworm of the scalp), and tinea unguium (nails) are generally mild and treated with topical antifungals. Fungal infections of the skin and mucous membranes of immunocompromised clients are serious and require oral or parenteral antifungals.

4. Viral infections include childhood infections such as varicella (chickenpox), rubeola (measles), and rubella (German measles). Adult viral infections include herpes zoster (shingles) and herpes simplex (cold sores and genital lesions). Pharmacotherapy includes topical or oral antiviral therapy with acyclovir (Zovirax).

5. Common skin parasites include mites and lice. Mites (Sarcoptes scabiei) cause scabies. The female burrows into the skin and lays eggs, which causes intense itching. The common areas of infection are the fingers, extremities, trunk, axillary and gluteal folds, and pubic area. Scabies are spread by contact with upholstery and linens. (See Figure 48.2.) Lice (Pediculus) infest areas with hair. They lay eggs and leave debris called nits. Lice are transmitted by infected clothing or personal contact. (See Figure 48.3.) Scabicides kill mites, and pediculicides kill lice. The treatment of choice for lice and scabies is permethrin (Nix). Other treatment options are pyrethrins (RID) and malathion (Ovide). Lindane (Kwell, Scabene) is used only after other treatments fail because it has the potential to cause serious nervous system toxicity.

6. Sunburn is a common problem among the general public. It is associated with a light-skinned complexion and lack of sun protection. The dangers of skin exposure include eye injury, cataracts, and skin cancer. The best treatment for sunburn is prevention. When sunburn has already occurred, it is treated with soothing lotions, rest, prevention of dehydration, and topical anesthetic agents, such as benzocaine (Solarcaine), dibucaine (Nupercainal), lidocaine (Xylocaine), and tetracaine HCL (Pontocaine).

7. Acne vulgaris affects 80% of adolescents; it is also found in the over-30 population and is called mature acne or acne tardive. Factors associated with acne vulgaris include seborrhea, overproduction of sebum by the oil glands; abnormal formation of keratin that blocks oil glands; and androgens, which stimulate sebum production. Benzoyl peroxide (Benzalin, Triaz, others) is the most common topical OTC medication for acne. Other keratolytic agents used for severe acne include resorcinol, salicylic acid, and sulfur. Retinoids are a class of drug closely related to vitamin A and are used in the treatment of inflammatory skin conditions, dermatologic malignancies, and acne. Tretinoin (Retin-A) is an older drug that has an irritant action. Antibiotics are sometimes used in combination with acne medications. (See Table 48.2.) Oral contraceptives containing ethinyl estradiol and norgestimate may be used to help clear the skin of acne.

8. Rosacea is a progressive disorder with onset between 30 and 50 years of age. It is characterized by small papules without pus, flushed face

SUGGESTION FOR CLASSROOM ACTIVITIES

- Assign students to present a case study on one of the skin disorders presented in this chapter. Include the medications used to treat the disorder with the actions, indications, adverse effects, interactions, and mechanisms of action identified.

SUGGESTION FOR CLINICAL ACTIVITIES

- Assign students to care for patients receiving pharmacotherapy for skin disorders.

© 2011 Pearson Education, Inc.

around the nose and cheeks, and swelling of the soft tissues of the nose (rhinophyma). Rosacea is exacerbated by sunlight, stress, increased temperature, and agents that dilate facial blood vessels. Women are more often affected than men. (See Figure 48.4 for an illustration of rosacea.) Pharmacotherapy of acne and rosacea is very similar and includes benzoyl peroxide, a keratolytic, which dries and sheds the outer layer of the epidermis. Retinoids are used to reduce oil production and clogged pores. They should not be used if the client is pregnant. A common reaction to retinoids is sensitivity to sunlight. Other treatment options include antibiotics, estrogen, and antiprotozoals, which may also be prescribed for rosacea if hair follicle mites are present. (See Table 48.6 for a list of treatment options for acne and rosacea.)

9. Dermatitis is an inflammatory skin disorder characterized by pain, redness, and pruritus. Atopic dermatitis or eczema is chronic, with a genetic predisposition. Contact dermatitis is a hypersensitivity response. Seborrheic dermatitis is sometimes seen in newborns and in teenagers after puberty. Stasis dermatitis is a sign of poor venous circulation. The most effective treatment for dermatitis is topical glucocorticoids, which relieve local inflammation and itching. Adverse effects with long-term use include irritation, redness, thinning of the skin. Glucocorticoids are available in different doses and preparations, including creams, lotions, solutions, gels, and pads. (See Table 48.3 for a list of these medications.)

10. Psoriasis is a chronic skin disorder characterized by red patches of skin covered with flaky, silver-colored scales (plaques). The etiology may be a genetic immune reaction. Psoriasis causes an extremely fast skin-turnover rate; the plaques are shed rapidly, and underlying skin is inflamed and irritated. (See Figure 48.5 for an illustration of psoriasis.) The treatment goal is to reduce the erythema, plaques, and scales to improve appearance. There is no pharmacological cure. Topical therapies include topical glucocorticoids; topical immunomodulators (TIMs), which suppress the immune system; retinoid-like compounds; and tar treatment and anthralin, which inhibit DNA synthesis and arrest abnormal cell growth. Systemic therapies for psoriasis include methotrexate (Folex), acitretin (Soriatane), and etretinate (Tegison); these medications are taken orally to inhibit abnormal cell growth. Other drugs include immunosuppressive agents and biologic therapies. Nonpharmacological therapy includes phototherapy.

LEARNING OUTCOME 4

Describe the prevention and management of minor burns.

Concepts for Lecture

1. Burns are a unique type of stress that may affect all layers of the skin. Minor, first-degree burns affect only the outer layers of the epidermis, are characterized by redness, and are analogous to sunburn. Sunburn results from overexposure of the skin to UV light, and is associated with light skin complexions, prolonged exposure to the sun during the more hazardous hours of the day, and lack of protective clothing when outdoors. Chronic sun exposure can result in serious conditions, including eye injury, cataracts, and skin cancer. In addition to producing local skin damage, sun overexposure releases toxins that may produce systemic effects. The signs and symptoms of sunburn include erythema, intense pain, nausea, vomiting, chills, edema, and headache. These symptoms usually resolve within a matter of hours or days, depending on the

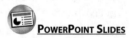 **POWERPOINT SLIDES**

SUGGESTION FOR CLASSROOM ACTIVITIES
- Invite a nurse from the burn unit to talk to students about burn injury.

SUGGESTION FOR CLINICAL ACTIVITIES
- Assign students to small groups and have them prepare a teaching plan that can be used to teach patients on prevention and treatment of minor burns. Have them present the teaching plan during postclinical conference.

© 2011 Pearson Education, Inc.

severity of the exposure. Once sunburn has occurred, medications can only alleviate the symptoms; they do not speed recovery time.

2. The best treatment for sunburn is prevention. Sunscreens are liquids or lotions applied for chemical or physical protection. Chemical sunscreens absorb the spectrum of UV light that is responsible for most sunburn. Chemical sunscreens include those that contain benzophenone for protection against UVA rays; those that work against UVB rays include cinnamates, p-aminobenzoic acid (PABA), and salicylates. Physical sunscreens such as zinc oxide, talc, and titanium dioxide reflect or scatter light to prevent the penetration of both UVA and UVB rays. Parsol is another sunscreen product that is being used more frequently as a key ingredient in lip balm. Treatment for sunburn consists of addressing symptoms with soothing lotions, rest, prevention of dehydration, and topical anesthetic agents, if needed. Treatment is usually done on an outpatient basis. Topical anesthetics for minor burns include benzocaine (Solarcaine), dibucaine (Nupercainal), lidocaine (Xylocaine), and tetracaine HCl (Pontocaine). Aloe vera is a popular natural therapy for minor skin irritations and burns. These same agents may also provide relief from minor pain due to insect bites and pruritus. In more severe cases, oral analgesics such as aspirin or ibuprofen may be indicated.

LEARNING OUTCOME 5

Describe the nurse's role in the pharmacologic management of skin disorders.

Concepts for Lecture

1. The role of the nurse in the pharmacological management of skin disorders involves careful monitoring of a client's condition and providing education as it relates to the prescribed drug treatment. Obtain baseline medical, surgical, and drug history; lifestyle and dietary habits, including use of herbal or alternative therapies; and a detailed description of symptomology and current therapies.

2. **Scabicide and pediculicide therapy:** Before assessing the client, be sure to don gloves. Assess the client's hair and skin for evidence of lice, nits, or scabies. Assess the axilla, neckline, hairline, groin, and beltline areas for evidence of lice, such as visualization of nits, erythema, and pruritus. Obtain a thorough history regarding onset of symptoms and possible exposure to others. Do not use scabicides or pediculicides, or use cautiously in pregnant or lactating women and young children. Use lindane cautiously in children ages 2 to 10 and only after other agents have been unsuccessful in treating the condition. Follow application instructions, and wear gloves when applying medication. Cleanse the lesions and surrounding areas with warm water and soap, and dry thoroughly prior to application of medication.

3. **Drug therapy for sunburn and minor skin irritation:** Assess the sunburn, including location, portion of body surface area, edema, erythema, and blistering. For severe cases, assess for fever, chills, weakness, and shock. If topical anesthetics or ointments are ordered, assess the skin for secondary infections, for which these medications are contraindicated. Topical benzocaine (Solarcaine) may cause a hypersensitivity reaction. For clients using the medication for the first time, a trial application on a small area of skin should be conducted to assess for an allergic reaction.

4. **Drug therapy for acne-related disorders:** Have the client undress so you can examine the extent of acne. Wear gloves when assessing the skin. Assess the anterior and posterior thorax because many acne lesions

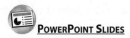

POWERPOINT SLIDES

SUGGESTION FOR CLASSROOM ACTIVITIES

• Discuss the role of the nurse in the pharmacologic treatment of clients with skin disorders.

SUGGESTION FOR CLINICAL ACTIVITIES

• Assign students to administer medication ordered for the treatment of skin disorders. Quiz students before medication administration as to the drug's classification, action, dosage, and adverse effects. Assess how students complete the six "rights" of medication administration.

may be found in these areas. Obtain a thorough history, including onset of acne, what treatments have been used and their effects, and whether or not the client is pregnant. Ask about allergies, past medical history, and current medications. Tretinoin (Avita, Retin-A, Trentin-X, and Isotretinoin [Accutane]) is contraindicated in individuals with a history of depression and suicidal ideation and during pregnancy. Individuals who are prescribed isotretinoin should sign a consent regarding the understanding of suicidal risks prior to treatment. Obtain a pregnancy test in all female clients of childbearing years.

Learning Outcome 6

For each of the classes listed in Drugs at a Glance, know representative drugs, and explain the mechanisms of drug action, primary actions, and important adverse effects.

Concepts for Lecture

1. **Scabicide, pediculicide:** Prototype drug: Permethrin (Acticin, Elimite, Nix). Mechanism of action: kills head and crab lice and mites and eradicates their ova. Primary use: marketed as a cream or lotion for mites and as a shampoo for head lice. A 1% lotion is approved for lice and a 5% lotion for mites. Adverse effects: Permethrin causes few systemic effects. Local reactions may occur and include pruritus, rash, transient tingling, burning, stinging, erythema, and edema of the affected area.
2. **Retinoids:** Prototype drug: Tretinoin (Avita, Retin-A, Trentin-X, others). Mechanism of action: a natural derivative of vitamin A that decreases comedone formation and increases extrusion of comedones from the skin. Also has the ability to improve photodamaged skin. Primary use: indicated for the early treatment and control of mild to moderate acne vulgaris. Adverse effects: Nearly all patients using topical tretinoin will experience redness, scaling, erythema, crusting and peeling of the skin. Very high oral doses can result in serious adverse effects, including bone pain, fever, headache, nausea, vomiting, rash, stomatitis, pruritus, sweating, and ocular disorders.

Learning Outcome 7

Use the nursing process to care for patients who are receiving drug therapy for skin disorders.

Concepts for Lecture

1. **Patients receiving therapy with scabicides and pediculicides—Assessment:** Obtain a complete history, including age, allergies, drug history, possible drug interactions, and seizure disorders. Obtain a social history of close contacts, including household members and sexual partners. Obtain baseline height, weight, and vital signs. Assess skin areas to be treated for signs of infestation (e.g., lice or nits in hair, reddened track areas between webs of fingers, around belt or elastic lines), irritation, excoriation, or drainage. Assess for adverse effects: localized tingling, pruritus, stinging, or burning.
2. **Patients receiving therapy with scabicides and pediculicides—Nursing diagnoses:** *Disturbed Body Image; Impaired Skin Integrity* related to pruritis and possible skin lesions; *Deficient Knowledge* (drug therapy); *Risk for Poisoning* related to incorrect use of the drug, adverse drug effects.

 PowerPoint Slides

Prototype Drug
- lindane (Kwell)
- benzocaine (Solarcaine)
- isotretinoin (13-cis-retinoic acid) (Accutane)

 Suggestion for Classroom Activities

- Have each student make drug cards for each classification of drug used to treat skin disorders. The card should include actions, uses, routes of administration, dosages, and adverse effects.

 Suggestion for Clinical Activities

- Divide students into small groups, and have each group develop a teaching plan for a patient receiving medications for skin disorders. Have the students implement these plans during clinical.

 PowerPoint Slides

 Nursing Process Focus

- Patients receiving therapy with scabicides and pediculicides
- Patients receiving anti-acne medications

 Suggestion for Classroom Activities

- Invite a nurse from a dermatology clinic to speak about treatments for the skin disorders covered in this chapter.

 Suggestion for Clinical Activities

- Direct students to implement a care plan for clients with skin disorders.

© 2011 Pearson Education, Inc.

3. **Patients receiving therapy with scabicides and pediculicides—Planning:** The client will experience therapeutic effects (e.g., infestation has cleared) and will be free from or experience minimal adverse effects. Verbalize an understanding of the drug's use, adverse effects, and required precautions. Demonstrate proper self-administration of the medication (e.g., dose, timing, when to notify provider).

4. **Patients receiving therapy with scabicides and pediculicides—Implementation:** Monitor appropriate medication administration for optimum results. Monitor affected area after treatment over the next 1 to 2 weeks to ensure infestation has been eliminated. Monitor family members, those in close care of patient, or sexual contacts for infestation. Bedding and personal objects should be cleansed before reuse. Monitor skin in areas that have been treated. Report any irritation, broken skin, erythema, rashes, or edema promptly. Instruct the patient or caregiver in proper self-administration of drug (e.g., use exactly as directed or per package directions).

5. **Patients receiving therapy with scabicides and pediculicides—Evaluation:** The client experiences therapeutic effects (e.g., infestation has cleared) and is free from or experiences minimal adverse effects. Verbalizes an understanding of the drug's use, adverse effects, and required precautions. Demonstrates proper self-administration of the medication (e.g., dose, timing, when to notify provider).

6. **Patients receiving anti-acne medications—Assessment:** Obtain a complete health history including dermatologic, hepatic or renal disease, psychiatric disorders, pregnancy or breast-feeding. Obtain a drug history including allergies and possible drug interactions. Evaluate appropriate laboratory findings (e.g., CBC, lipid profiles, hepatic or renal function labs). Obtain baseline vital signs. Assess for adverse effects: localized skin irritation, erythema, pruritus, dry or peeling skin; dry mouth, eyes, or nose may occur if on oral drug.

7. **Patients receiving anti-acne medications—Nursing diagnoses:** *Disturbed Body Image, Impaired Skin Integrity* related to skin condition or adverse drug effects; *Deficient Knowledge* (drug therapy); *Risk for Injury* related to adverse drug effects.

8. **Patients receiving anti-acne medications—Planning:** The client will experience therapeutic effects (e.g., acne lesions are clearing, appearance of wrinkles or skin damage is improving) and will be free from or experience minimal adverse effects. Verbalize an understanding of the drug's use, adverse effects, and required precautions. Demonstrate proper self-administration of the medication (e.g., dose, timing, when to notify provider).

9. **Patients receiving anti-acne medications—Implementation:** Monitor appropriate medication administration for optimum results. Monitor area under topical treatment for excessive dryness and irritation. Monitor patients on isotretinoin for emotional health or changes in mood. Monitor CBC, lipid levels, and hepatic function labs periodically for patients on oral medication. Monitor for vision changes. Monitor patient's exposure to sun and UV light. Monitor compliance with "iPledge" requirements for patients on isotretinoin. (iPledge is required of all patients on isotretinoin before receiving a prescription or refills of the drug.) Instruct the patient or caregiver in proper self-administration of drug (e.g., topical drug used appropriately, iPledge program is followed).

10. **Patients receiving anti-acne medications—Evaluation:** The client experiences therapeutic effects (e.g., acne lesions are clearing, appearance of wrinkles or skin damage is improving) and is free from or experiences minimal adverse effects. Verbalizes an understanding of the drug's use, adverse effects and required precautions. Demonstrates proper self-administration of the medication (e.g., dose, timing, when to notify provider).

© 2011 Pearson Education, Inc.

GENERAL CHAPTER CONSIDERATIONS

1. Have students study and learn key terms listed at the beginning of the chapter.
2. Have students complete end-of-chapter exercises either in their book or on the MyNursingKit website.
3. Use the Classroom Response Questions provided in PowerPoint to assess students prior to lecture.

 MyNursingKit
(www.mynursingkit.com)

- Websites
- NCLEX® questions
- Critical Thinking Questions
- Case Studies
- Animations and Videos
- Drug Prototype Questions

 MyNursingLab
(www.mynursinglab.com)

- Knowledge Quick Check
- Pre/Posttests
- Customized study plans
- *Separate purchase*

 Student Workbook and Resource Guide

- Chapter 48 activities
- *Separate purchase*

Pearson Nurse's Drug Guide

- *Separate purchase*

 Pearson eText

- Students can search, highlight, take notes, and more all in electronic format.
- *Separate purchase*

 Classroom Response Question PowerPoints

 Testbank

© 2011 Pearson Education, Inc.

CHAPTER 49
DRUGS FOR EYE AND EAR DISORDERS

LEARNING OUTCOME 1

Identify the basic anatomic structures of the eye.

Concepts for Lecture

The anterior cavity of the eye is filled with aqueous humor. It contains an anterior and posterior chamber. Aqueous humor is formed by the *ciliary body*, a muscular structure in the posterior chamber. Aqueous humor helps retain the shape of the eye and circulates to bring nutrients to the area and remove wastes. The trabecular network is connected to the canal of Schlemm, and aqueous humor drains from the anterior chamber into the canal of Schlemm and into the venous system, thus completing its circulation. Interference with either the inflow or outflow of aqueous humor, can lead to an increase in IOP.

 POWERPOINT SLIDES

Figure 49.1 Internal Structures of the Eye

 SUGGESTION FOR CLASSROOM ACTIVITIES

• Provide a picture or model of the eye for students to examine.

 SUGGESTION FOR CLINICAL ACTIVITIES

• Assign students to observe an ophthalmologic procedure in the surgical area.

LEARNING OUTCOME 2

Describe the major risk factors associated with glaucoma.

Concepts for Lecture

Glaucoma occurs when there is increased intraocular pressure, which leads to optic nerve damage and visual-field loss. It is the leading cause of preventable blindness. It is often a primary condition without an identifiable cause, occurring most frequently in those over 60 years of age and associated with genetic factors. Glaucoma can also occur secondary to eye trauma, diabetes, inflammation, hemorrhage, tumor, or cataracts. The risk factors for glaucoma include long-term use of glucocorticoids, antihypertensives, antihistamines, or antidepressants; hypertension; migraine headaches; severe nearsightedness or farsightedness; and normal aging.

 POWERPOINT SLIDES

 SUGGESTION FOR CLASSROOM ACTIVITIES

• Discuss risk factors for glaucoma and direct students to quiz each other on those factors.

 SUGGESTION FOR CLINICAL ACTIVITIES

• Invite an optometrist to speak to the students about glaucoma during postclinical conference.

LEARNING OUTCOME 3

Compare and contrast open-angle and closed-angle glaucoma.

Concepts for Lecture

1. Interference with either the inflow or outflow of aqueous humor, however, can lead to an increase in IOP. Glaucoma occurs when the IOP becomes so high (above 21 mmHg). There are two types of glaucoma, closed-angle and open-angle. Both types result from a buildup of aqueous humor, which can occur from either excessive production of aqueous humor or blockage of outflow. The difference is in how quickly it occurs and if there is a narrowing of the anterior angle. Glaucoma is diagnosed with tonometry, which measures intraocular pressure (IOP).

 POWERPOINT SLIDES

Figure 49.2 Forms of Primary Adult Glaucoma

 SUGGESTION FOR CLASSROOM ACTIVITIES

• Direct students to create concept maps of the development of both types of glaucoma.

 SUGGESTION FOR CLINICAL ACTIVITIES

• Assign students to an observation experience in an optometrist's office to watch testing of intraocular pressure.

2. Closed-angle glaucoma is also referred to as acute or narrow-angle glaucoma and accounts for 5% of all glaucoma. It is usually unilateral and is caused by stress, impact injury, or medications. The iris is pushed over the drainage area, causing the angle to narrow and close, which then causes a sudden increase in IOP. Symptoms include dull to severe eye pain, headache, bloodshot eyes, foggy vision with halos, and/or a bulging iris. Ocular pain may be so severe that it causes vomiting. Closed-angle glaucoma is a medical emergency requiring surgery.

3. Open-angle glaucoma is most common type and accounts for more than 90% of cases. It is usually bilateral, and increased intraocular pressure develops slowly over years. Open-angle is asymptomatic, and the iris does not cover the opening. It is treated with medications. (Forms of adult Primary glaucoma are illustrated in Figure 49.2.)

LEARNING OUTCOME 4

Explain the two primary mechanisms by which drugs reduce intraocular pressure.

Concepts for Lecture

Drugs for glaucoma work by one of two mechanisms: increasing the outflow of aqueous humor at the canal of Schlemm or decreasing the formation of aqueous humor at the ciliary body. Many agents for glaucoma act by affecting the autonomic nervous system. The goal of glaucoma pharmacotherapy is to prevent damage to the optic nerve by lowering intraocular pressure. Treatment begins when the IOP is between 21 and 30 mm/Hg or when signs of optic nerve damage or visual-field changes are present regardless of IOP. Combination therapy may be necessary to bring intraocular pressure under control. The drugs used for glaucoma decrease IOP by increasing the outflow of aqueous humor, or they decrease the formation of aqueous humor. Many antiglaucoma drugs affect the autonomic nervous system.

LEARNING OUTCOME 5

Describe the nurse's role in the pharmacologic management of eye and ear disorders.

Concepts for Lecture

1. The role of the nurse in the pharmacologic management of eye and ear disorders involves careful monitoring of a client's condition and providing education as it relates to the prescribed drug treatment. Obtain baseline medical, surgical, and drug history; lifestyle and dietary habits, including use of herbal or alternative therapies; and a detailed description of symptomology and current therapies.

2. **Drug therapy for glaucoma:** Determine if the client has a history of heart block, bradycardia, heart failure, or chronic obstructive pulmonary disease (COPD). Prior to starting drug therapy, establish a baseline blood pressure and pulse. When a beta blocker is used, teach the client how to check pulse and blood pressure before medication administration and review normal parameters. Determine any factors that could decrease compliance such as insufficient financial resources, lack of knowledge of the disease, lack of dexterity or skill in inserting eye drops, or difficulty in remembering the dosing schedule.

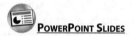

PowerPoint Slides

Suggestion for Classroom Activities

- Have students make concept maps showing the difference in the types of glaucoma, their treatment, causes, signs and symptoms, and how they are diagnosed.

Suggestion for Clinical Activities

- Direct students to administer eye drops to a client.

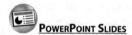

PowerPoint Slides

Suggestion for Classroom Activities

- Discuss the role of the nurse in the pharmacologic treatment of clients with eye and ear disorders.

Suggestion for Clinical Activities

- Invite a nurse who works in an ophthalmology office to speak to the class at postclinical conference about pharmacologic treatment of clients with eye disorders.

© 2011 Pearson Education, Inc.

It is crucial that the client is allowed to verbalize feelings; provide emotional support to the client and family.

3. **Drug therapy with otic preparations:** Assess the client's baseline hearing and auditory status, symptoms, and any current medical conditions. Obtain information regarding hypersensitivity to hydrocortisone, neomycin sulfate, or polymyxin B. The use of these medications is contraindicated in the presence of a perforated eardrum. Chloramphenicol ear drops are contraindicated in hypersensitivity and eardrum perforation. Side effects include burning, redness, rash, swelling, and other signs of topical irritation. When instilling otic preparations, cleanse the ear thoroughly and remove the cerumen through irrigation. Otic drugs should be warmed to body temperature (but not higher) before instillation.

LEARNING OUTCOME 6

Identify drugs for treating glaucoma and explain their basic actions and adverse effects.

Concepts for Lecture

1. Pharmacotherapy of glaucoma includes pros taglandins, which dilate the trabecular meshwork and increase aqueous humor outflow. Beta-adrenergic blockers decrease the production of aqueous humor; adverse effects include bronchoconstriction, dysrhythmias, and hypotension. Alpha$_2$-adrenergic agonists decrease production of aqueous humor.

2. Drugs for glaucoma—Prostaglandins. Prototype drug: latanoprost (Xalatan). Mechanism of action: believed to reduce IOP by increasing the outflow of aqueous humor. Primary use: for treatment of open-angle glaucoma. Adverse effects: conjunctival edema, tearing, dryness, burning, pain, irritation, itching, a sensation of a foreign body in the eye, photophobia, and visual disturbances. The eyelashes on the treated eye may grow thicker and/or darker. Changes may occur in the pigmentation of the iris of the treated eye and in the periocular skin.

3. Drugs for glaucoma—Beta-adrenergic blocker. Prototype drug: timolol (Betimol, Istalol, Timoptic). Mechanism of action: reduces the formation of aqueous humor. Primary use: to reduce elevated intraocular pressure in chronic open-angle glaucoma. Adverse effects: local burning and stinging upon instillation.

4. Other medications used in the pharmacotherapy of glaucoma include carbonic anhydrase inhibitors, which decrease the production of aqueous humor; nonselective sympathomimetics (mydriatics), which dilate the pupil to increase the outflow and may also cause increased IOP and increased BP and HR (rarely used for glaucoma); cholinergic agonists (miotics), which constrict the pupil to allow more room for outflow; and osmotic diuretics, which reduce the formation of aqueous humor.

LEARNING OUTCOME 7

Identify drugs that dilate or constrict pupils, relax ciliary muscles, constrict ocular blood vessels, or moisten eye membranes.

Concepts for Lecture

1. Drugs used in eye examinations include mydri atics, which dilate the pupil to allow better visualization. Adversely, they cause photophobia, can increase IOP, and can cause CNS effects. Another drug type used is

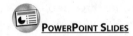
POWERPOINT SLIDES

Table 49.1 Selected Drugs for Glaucoma

Prototype Drug
- latanoprost (Xalatan)
- timolol (Betimol, Istalol, Timoptic)

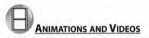
ANIMATIONS AND VIDEOS
- Mechanism in Action: Pilocarpine (Adsorbocarpine)

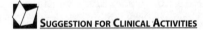
SUGGESTION FOR CLASSROOM ACTIVITIES
- Divide students into small groups, and have them prepare questions and answers for different categories of drugs used to treat glaucoma. Include questions on each drug's classification and mechanisms of action.

SUGGESTION FOR CLINICAL ACTIVITIES
- Assign students to care for patients receiving pharmacotherapy for glaucoma.

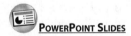
POWERPOINT SLIDES

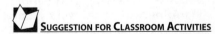
SUGGESTION FOR CLASSROOM ACTIVITIES
- Direct students to make a drug cards for mydriatics, cycloplegics, and eye lubricants.

cycloplegics, which cause both dilation and relaxation of the ciliary muscle. Adversely, they cause severe blurred vision, loss of near vision, and angle-closure glaucoma attacks.
2. Drugs for irritation and dryness include vasoconstrictors, cycloplegics, mydriatics, and lubricant drugs. They are used to lubricate the eye's surface or penetrate a specific area of the eye.

LEARNING OUTCOME 8

Identify drugs for treating ear conditions.

Concepts for Lecture

1. The ear has two major sensory functions, hearing and equilibrium and balance. There are three important structural areas—the outer ear, the middle ear, and the inner ear. (See Figure 49.3 for structures of the ear.)
2. **Otitis** is inflammation of the ear. External otitis is associated with water (swimmer's ear). Otitis media is associated with upper respiratory infections, allergies, and auditory tube irritation.
3. **Mastoiditis** is an inner ear infection of the mastoid sinus. It can result in hearing loss if untreated.
4. Pharmacotherapy for ear disorders includes antibiotics to treat infections, topical medication (eardrops) for the external ear, and systemic antibiotics for middle and inner ear infections and also for extensive outer ear infections. Other otic medications are glucocorticoids, which are used when inflammation is present, and cerumen (earwax) softeners to remove accumulated earwax buildup.

LEARNING OUTCOME 9

Use the nursing process to care for patients who are receiving drug therapy for eye and ear disorders.

Concepts for Lecture

1. **Patients receiving opthalmic solutions for glaucoma—Assessment:** Obtain a complete health history, including allergies, drug history, and possible drug interactions. Obtain a complete physical examination, focusing on visual acuity and visual-field assessments. Assess for the presence or history of ocular pain. Assess for history of recent eye trauma or infection. Obtain baseline vital signs. Assess for adverse effects. Assess for desired therapeutic effects dependent on reason drug is given (e.g., intraocular pressure remains below 20 mmHg or at target value, no changes in visual acuity or fields).
2. **Patients receiving opthalmic solutions for glaucoma—Nursing diagnoses:** *Disturbed Sensory Perception* (visual); *Anxiety* related to concerns of loss of vision, eye pain; *Pain* (disease condition, treatment adverse effects); *Deficient Knowledge* (drug therapy); *Risk for Injury* related to visual acuity deficits; *Deficient Self-care* related to impaired vision.
3. **Patients receiving opthalmic solutions for glaucoma—Planning:** The client will experience therapeutic effects (e.g., eye pressure has normalized, visual acuity and visual fields remain stable) and will be free from or experience minimal adverse effects. Verbalize an understanding of the drug's use, adverse effects, and required precautions. Demonstrate proper self-administration of the medication (e.g., dose, timing, when to notify provider).

 SUGGESTION FOR CLINICAL ACTIVITIES
- Assign students to care for clients receiving mydriatics, cycloplegics, and eye lubricants.

 POWERPOINT SLIDES

Figure 49.3 Structures of the External Ear, Middle Ear, and Inner Ear
Table 49.3 Otic Preparations

 SUGGESTION FOR CLASSROOM ACTIVITIES
- Divide students into small groups, and have each group develop a teaching plan for a client receiving medication for an ear disorder.

 SUGGESTION FOR CLINICAL ACTIVITIES
- Assign students to a client who is receiving an eardrop. Observe the student administering this medication.

 POWERPOINT SLIDES

 NURSING PROCESS FOCUS
- Clients Receiving Ophthalmic Solutions for Glaucoma

 SUGGESTION FOR CLASSROOM ACTIVITIES
- Direct students to create a nursing-care plan for a client with glaucoma.

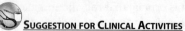 **SUGGESTIONS FOR CLINICAL ACTIVITIES**
- Direct students to create a nursing-care plan for a client with glaucoma.
- Direct students to implement a teaching plan for a client with an eye or ear disorder.

© 2011 Pearson Education, Inc.

4. **Patients receiving opthalmic solutions for glaucoma—Implementation:** Monitor visual acuity, vision fields, and intraocular eye pressure. Monitor appropriate administration of drug to avoid extra-ocular effects. Monitor intraocular pressure periodically. Monitor for increasing eye redness, pain, light sensitivity, or changes in visual acuity. Remove contact lenses before administering ophthalmic solutions. Monitor vital signs periodically for signs of systemic absorption of topical preparations. Provide for eye comfort such as adequately lighted room. Instruct the patient or caregiver in proper self-administration of drug (e.g., appropriate instillation of eye drops).

5. **Patients receiving opthalmic solutions for glaucoma—Evaluation:** The client experiences normalized eye pressure, stable visual acuity, and visual fields and is free from or experiences minimal adverse effects. Verbalizes an understanding of the drug's use, adverse effects and required precautions. Demonstrates proper self-administration of the medication (e.g., dose, timing, when to notify provider).

GENERAL CHAPTER CONSIDERATIONS

1. Have students study and learn key terms listed at the beginning of the chapter.
2. Have students complete end-of-chapter exercises either in their book or on the MyNursingKit website.
3. Use the Classroom Response Questions provided in PowerPoint to assess students prior to lecture.

MYNURSINGKIT
(www.mynursingkit.com)

- Websites
- NCLEX® questions
- Critical Thinking Questions
- Case Studies
- Animations and Videos
- Drug Prototype Questions

MYNURSINGLAB
(www.mynursinglab.com)

- Knowledge Quick Check
- Pre/Posttests
- Customized study plans
- *Separate purchase*

STUDENT WORKBOOK AND RESOURCE GUIDE

- Chapter 49 activities
- *Separate purchase*

PEARSON NURSE'S DRUG GUIDE

- *Separate purchase*

PEARSON ETEXT

- Students can search, highlight, take notes, and more all in electronic format.
- *Separate purchase*

CLASSROOM RESPONSE QUESTION
POWERPOINTS

TESTBANK